Diagnosis and Treatment of Kidney Diseases

Diagnosis and Treatment of Kidney Diseases

Edited by Jordan Bryan

hayle medical

New York

Hayle Medical,
750 Third Avenue, 9th Floor,
New York, NY 10017, USA

Visit us on the World Wide Web at:
www.haylemedical.com

ISBN: 978-1-64647-546-9

Cataloging-in-Publication Data

Diagnosis and treatment of kidney diseases / edited by Jordan Bryan.
p. cm.
Includes bibliographical references and index.
ISBN 978-1-64647-546-9
1. Kidneys--Diseases. 2. Kidneys--Diseases--Diagnosis.
3. Kidneys--Diseases--Treatment. I. Bryan, Jordan.
RC902 .K53 2023
616.61--dc23

Table of Contents

Preface

This book aims to highlight the current researches and provides a platform to further the scope of innovations in this area. This book is a product of the combined efforts of many researchers and scientists, after going through thorough studies and analysis from different parts of the world. The objective of this book is to provide the readers with the latest information of the field.

Kidneys are the two bean-shaped organs and each kidney is approximately the size of a fist. They filter unnecessary water and waste from the blood and produce urine. Kidney disease refers to the impairment of kidneys where the kidneys are damaged to an extent where they are incapable of filtering blood efficiently. The cells of the kidneys can be damaged due to ischemic, immunological and toxic complaints, which cause organ dysfunction and failure in certain cases. Acute kidney injury is a prevalent occurrence that is linked to negative renal and patient outcomes. The human kidneys have a limited capacity for regeneration. The immune system plays a significant role in the regeneration capacity of the kidneys, as it first promotes inflammation and then promotes tissues healing. This book explores all the important aspects of kidney diseases in the present day scenario. It provides the readers with a thorough understanding of the diagnosis and treatment of these diseases. With state-of-the-art inputs by acclaimed experts of nephrology, this book targets students and professionals.

I would like to express my sincere thanks to the authors for their dedicated efforts in the completion of this book. I acknowledge the efforts of the publisher for providing constant support. Lastly, I would like to thank my family for their support in all academic endeavors.

Editor

1

Lysophosphatidic Acid Signaling in Diabetic Nephropathy

Jong Han Lee [1,2], Donghee Kim [2], Yoon Sin Oh [3] and Hee-Sook Jun [1,2,4,*]

1 College of Pharmacy, Gachon University, Incheon 21936, Korea; jhleecw@gachon.ac.kr
2 Lee Gil Ya Cancer and Diabetes Institute, Gachon University, Incheon 21999, Korea; dh2388@gachon.ac.kr
3 Department of Food and Nutrition, Eulji University, Seongnam 13135, Korea; ysoh@eulji.ac.kr
4 Gachon University Gil Medical Center, Gachon Medical and Convergence Institute, Incheon 21565, Korea
* Correspondence: hsjun@gachon.ac.kr

Abstract: Lysophosphatidic acid (LPA) is a bioactive phospholipid present in most tissues and body fluids. LPA acts through specific LPA receptors (LPAR1 to LPAR6) coupled with G protein. LPA binds to receptors and activates multiple cellular signaling pathways, subsequently exerting various biological functions, such as cell proliferation, migration, and apoptosis. LPA also induces cell damage through complex overlapping pathways, including the generation of reactive oxygen species, inflammatory cytokines, and fibrosis. Several reports indicate that the LPA–LPAR axis plays an important role in various diseases, including kidney disease, lung fibrosis, and cancer. Diabetic nephropathy (DN) is one of the most common diabetic complications and the main risk factor for chronic kidney diseases, which mostly progress to end-stage renal disease. There is also growing evidence indicating that the LPA–LPAR axis also plays an important role in inducing pathological alterations of cell structure and function in the kidneys. In this review, we will discuss key mediators or signaling pathways activated by LPA and summarize recent research findings associated with DN.

Keywords: diabetic nephropathy; lysophosphatidic acid; lysophosphatidic acid receptor; chronic kidney injury

---

1. Introduction

Diabetic nephropathy (DN) is a microvascular complication of diabetes and develops in approximately 20–40% patients with diabetes, including type 1 and type 2 diabetes patients [1,2]. It has become the main risk factor for the development of chronic kidney diseases, such that most DN patients progress to end-stage renal disease (ESRD) and require renal replacement in the end [2]. Thus, DN not only increases the health cost for individuals and the society at large but is also a risk factor for morbidity and mortality. Intensive glycemic control is a well-established strategy for the prevention of DN. Despite the efforts for the management of hyperglycemia and hypertension using current therapies, such as angiotensin converting enzyme (ACE) inhibitors and angiotensin II receptor blockers (ARBs) [3,4], the risk of DN progression has still not been reduced. Currently available drugs only delay the progress of the disease, rather than curing it. Therefore, a novel and effective therapeutic approach is urgently needed for patients with DN.

Phospholipids are generally known to be structural components of plasma membranes, but growing evidence indicates that membrane phospholipids also play crucial roles as signaling molecules and exert a wide range of physiological responses. Lysophosphatidic acid (LPA) is a small, naturally occurring glycerophospholipid, which is composed of a glycerol backbone with an ester-linked acyl chain and a phosphate group. It is also produced by the action of various lysophospholipases, including autotaxin (ATX), and phospholipases A1 or A2 (PLA1 and PLA2). LPA acts through specific LPA receptors (LPAR1 to LPAR6) coupled with G protein and is associated with a wide range of cell responses, such as proliferation and migration [5,6], and pathologies of a number of diseases, including fibrosis, cancer, neuronal disorders, and bone metabolism [5,7–10]. Hyperglycemia, advanced glycation end product (AGE), and pro-inflammatory cytokines are considered the three main initial mediators of DN development [11,12]. However, some recent studies also showed that the LPA–LPA receptor axis may play an important role in the pathogenesis of diabetic kidney disease.

In this review article, we review the key mediators and signaling pathways activated by LPA and summarize newly reported signaling pathways modulated by different LPA receptor antagonists in different DN models.

2. Biosynthesis and Degradation of LPA

LPA is the smallest bioactive lysophospholipid (MW 430–480 Da) derived from membrane phospholipids [13] and acts as an extracellular signaling molecule via its receptors, regulating various cellular processes, including cell proliferation, survival, migration, differentiation, remodeling, and cytokine/chemokine secretion [13]. LPA is known to be water soluble and is present in most tissues and biological fluids, such as plasma, saliva, tears, follicular fluid, and cerebrospinal fluid [5,14]. LPA is produced by several enzymes, either in the intracellular or extracellular compartment, as shown in Figure 1. In the intracellular compartment, LPA is naturally synthesized through the action of glycerol-3-phosphate acyltransferase (GPAT) during the process of triglyceride and phospholipid anabolism, which is found mainly in the mitochondria and endoplasmic reticulum of various cell types [15,16]. LPA is also synthesized by the action of intra/extra-cellular PLA1 or PLA2 from phosphatidic acid (PA). Ubiquitously expressed PLA1 and PLA2 in the body hydrolyze the bond between the fatty acid chain and the glycerol backbone at *sn1* (saturated) or *sn2* (unsaturated) positions of PA [17,18]. Membrane phospholipids are major sources for LPA production. Metabolically, they are first converted into lysophospholipids, such as lysophosphatidylethanolamine (LPE), lysophosphatidylcholine (LPC), lysophosphatidylserine (LPS), and then, subsequently cleaved by ATX, also known as ectonucleotidepyrophosphatases/ phosphodiesterases-2. This pathway is considered a determinant for the LPA level in plasma [19,20].

LPA is converted by several classes of enzymes, including lipid phosphate phosphatases (LPPs), LPA acyltransferase, and phospholipases [21–23], as shown in Figure 1. LPPs (LPP1, LPP2, and LPP3) exist extracellularly and intracellularly in the endoplasmic reticulum and Golgi, and dephosphorylate LPA and degrade it into monoacylglycerol (MAG). LPA can also be converted to PA by the action of the acylglycerophosphate acyltransferase (AGPAT) enzyme, also known as LPA acyltransferase [24]. The third alternative pathway for LPA degradation is mediated by the action of lysophospholipases, via formation of glycerol-3-phosphate [25].

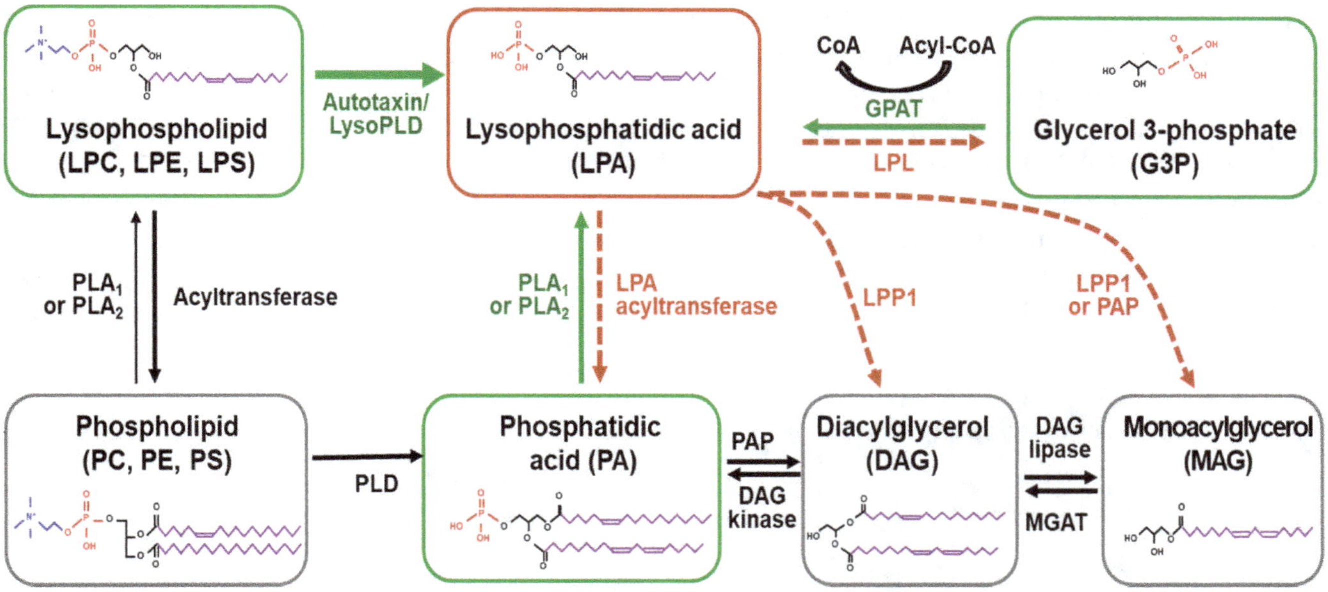

Figure 1. The enzymatic pathways of lysophosphatidic acid (LPA) synthesis and degradation. LPA can be synthesized from different precursors, including lysophospholipids, phosphatidic acid, and glycerol 3-phosphate. The enzymes and pathways involved in LPA production are indicated using green text and a green solid line, respectively. LPA is converted into either monoacylglycerol or phosphatidic acid. The enzymes and pathways involved in LPA conversion are indicated using red text and a red dotted line, respectively. Lysophosphatidylcholine (LPC), lysophosphatidylethanolamine (LPE), lysophosphatidylserine (LPS), lysophospholipase D (Lyso PLD), lysophospholipase (LPL), glycerol 3-phosphate acyltransferase (GPAT), phospholipase C (PLC), phospholipase A1 or A2 (PLA1 and PLA2), diacylglycerol (DAG), monoacylglycerol (MAG), MAG acyltransferase (MGAT), lipid phosphate phosphatase 1 or 2 (LPP1 and LPP2), phosphatidate phosphatase (PAP), phosphatidylcholine (PC), phosphatidylethanolamine (PE), phosphatidylserine (PS), and phospholipase D (PLD).

3. LPA Receptors and Intracellular Signaling Pathways

LPA induces various cellular effects by binding to specific G protein-coupled LPA receptors (LPARs) and activates downstream intracellular signaling pathways, resulting in various physiological and pathophysiological responses [5]. Till now, six LPARs have been identified and classified into A rhodopsin-like G protein-coupled receptors [26]. They can be further grouped into two groups, according to their distinct protein homology, such as LPAR1 to LPAR3 belonging to the endothelial differentiation gene (*Edg*) family, and LPAR4 to LPAR6 belonging to the *P2Y* purinergic gene cluster [6,8]. These receptors have the ability to interact with at least one or more heterotrimeric G subunits, such as Gαi/o, Gαq/11, Gα12/13, and Gs [6]. LPAR1/Edg2 and LPAR2/Edg4 receptors couple with Gαi/o, Gαq/11, and Gα12/13. Once bound together, the complexes transduce extracellular signals into intracellular pathways through molecules, such as the Ras homologous (Rho) protein family of GTPases, phospholipase C (PLC), diacylglycerol (DAG), mitogen-activated protein kinase (MAPK), and phosphatidylinositol 3-kinase (PI3K)-protein kinase B (Akt). Activation of these receptors mostly ends up promoting cell proliferation, survival, and migration [27,28]. LPAR3/Edg7 couples with Gαi/o and Gαq/11, and participates in LPA-induced Ca^{2+} mobilization, PLC, adenylyl-cyclase inhibition, and MAPK activation [28]. LPAR4/GPR23/P2Y9 and LPAR5/GPR92 induce stress fiber formation and neurite retraction through Gα12/13 and downstream Rho/Rho-associated protein kinase (ROCK) pathway [29,30]. LPAR4 is known as the only LPA receptor that can increase intracellular cAMP accumulation by coupling to Gs [29]. LPAR5 interacts with Gαq/11 and increases intracellular Ca^{2+} levels [31]. LPA6/P2Y5 receptor binds to either Gαi/o or Gα12/13, and induces Rho-dependent alteration of cellular morphology [32,33]. In addition, other G protein-coupled receptors, including GPR35 [34] and P2Y10 [35], were also identified as LPARs, which induced Ca^{2+} responses by LPA stimulation.

LPA can also bind to and activate non-GPCR targets, the receptor for advanced glycation end products (RAGE) [36], and the cation channel transient receptor potential vanilloid 1 (TRPV1) [37]. RAGE participates in LPA-induced nicotinamide adenine dinucleotide phosphate (NADPH) oxidase (Nox), reactive oxygen species (ROS) induction, and activation of NFκB, serum response factor (SRF), PI3K, and Akt [38]. TRPV1 increases intracellular Ca^{2+} levels following LPA stimulation [37]. Another non-GPCR, peroxisome proliferator-activated receptor gamma (PPARγ), is the intracellular receptor for LPA, and is critically important for mediating the effects of LPA on vascular remodeling [39]. Among them, the expression of LPAR1-4 has been detected in renal tissue [40]. Although many LPA receptors and their signaling pathways have been identified, as shown in Figure 2, the functional role of each receptor is poorly understood. Further studies will be required.

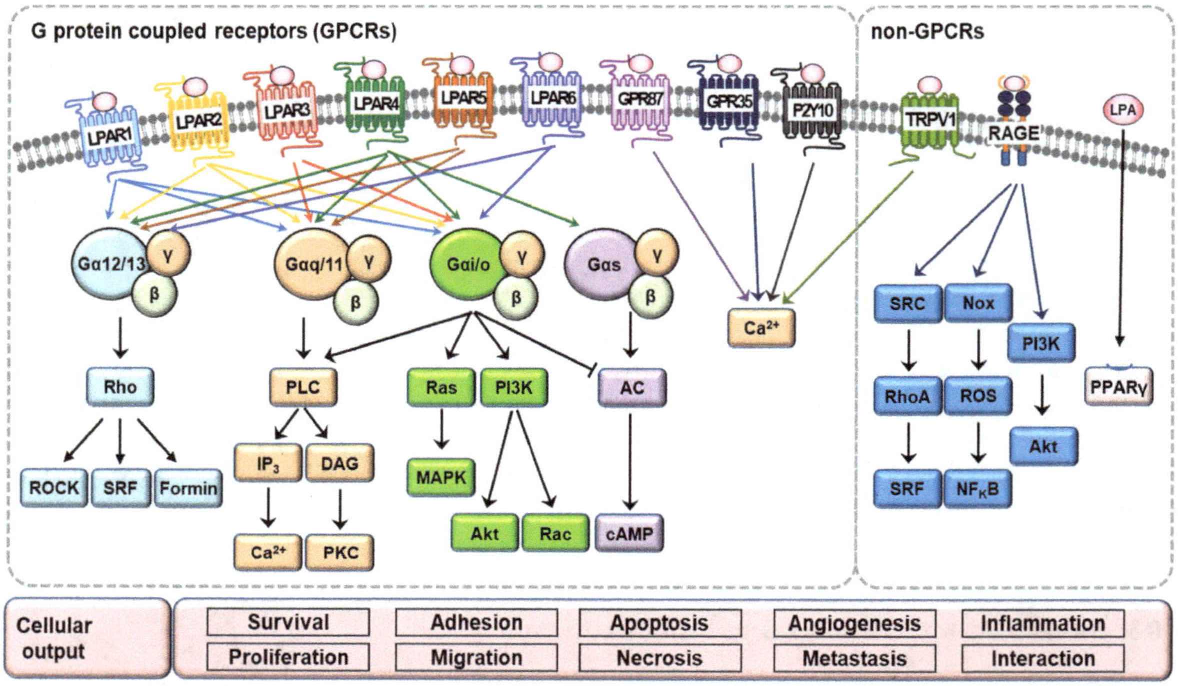

Figure 2. LPA signaling pathways. LPA can induce multiple cellular effects via binding to specific GPCRs, including LPAR1–LPAR6, as well as binding to non-GPCRs, such as transient receptor potential vanilloid 1 (TRPV1), receptor for advanced glycation end products (RAGE), and intracellular peroxisome proliferator-activated receptor gamma (PPARγ). After binding to receptors, LPA activates downstream intracellular signaling pathways, thereby resulting in various physiological and pathophysiological responses, as described in detail in the text.

4. Pathogenesis of DN

4.1. Definition of Chronic Kidney Disease

Kidney disease is a heterogeneous group of disorders affecting kidney structure and function, which can be further classified into two distinct syndromes, acute and chronic kidney disease (CKD) [6]. Acute kidney injury is characterized by rapid diminution of kidney function, resulting in excretion of creatinine [41]. It occurs over several hours or days but not more than three months, whereas chronic kidney injury is in cases of more than three months. Acute kidney injury often leads to the development of chronic kidney failure [41]. Conversely, chronic kidney disease increases the risk of incidence of acute kidney injury [42,43]. Whatever the initial injury, the final pathogenesis of CKD involves renal fibrosis, characterized by excessive extracellular matrix (ECM) accumulation in glomerular and tubular interstitial cells [44,45]. Renal fibrosis changes tissue architecture and function, which leads to kidney dysfunction and failure.

4.2. *Glomerulosclerosis*

Glomerulosclerosis is hardening of glomeruli in the kidney and is frequently referred to as focal segmental glomerulosclerosis or nodular glomerulosclerosis [46]. The initial pathogenic events start in glomerular endothelium, including the activation and dysfunction of endothelial cells, hemodynamic alterations, as well as loss of glomerular basement membrane (GBM) electrical charge. These alterations subsequently trigger an inflammatory response in the glomerular apparatus, which further affects mesangial cells and induces proliferation and dysfunction of mesangial cells [43,47]. Excessive ECM production is the underlying mechanism for mesangial expansion. Podocytes are the cells located inside the Bowman's capsule of the kidney, which anatomically wrap around capillaries of the glomerulus [48]. The damage in podocytes decreases their number and increases foot process effacement and denudation of GBM. The accumulated damage increases cell death by apoptosis or necrosis, and replacement of glomerular cells by ECM, which, in turn, increases hardening of glomeruli and eventually leads to glomerulosclerosis [16,44].

4.3. *Tubular Interstitial Fibrosis*

Although the initial glomerular damage and glomerulosclerosis are the major factors for the development of CKDs, the fibrosis in the tubulo-interstitial compartment is also a major contributor [43,49]. Initial glomerular damage increases the leakage of abnormally filtered proteins, including albumin, complement, and cytokines. These proteins and immune effectors or molecules activate tubular cells and initiate an inflammatory response. Simultaneously, different types of inflammatory cells (macrophages, monocytes, lymphocytes, mast cells, and dendritic cells) are recruited from circulation by increasing the expression of chemokines (monocyte chemoattractant protein 1, CCL2/MCP1; regulated upon activation, normal T cell expressed, and secreted, CCL5/RANTES), and adhesion molecules (E and P selectins, intercellular adhesion molecule-1, ICAM-1; vascular cell adhesion molecule-1, VCAM-1) [50]. In particular, the recruited monocytes transdifferentiate into macrophages in the kidney interstitium. Myofibroblasts are responsible for producing fibrillar matrix in the renal interstitium [51]. Under normal conditions, a lower population of myofibroblasts is maintained. However, they are activated, and their number is increased through various ways (proliferation, epithelial mesenchymal transition (EMT), and recruitment of circulating fibrocytes derived from bone marrow cells) in a pathological environment. In addition, accumulation of ECM proteins within the kidney interstitium is the consequence of imbalance between synthesis and degradation of ECM. Thus, the expression of plasminogen activator inhibitor-1 (PAI-1, a specific inhibitor of urokinase-type and tissue-type plasminogen activator (uPA and tPA)) and tissue inhibitor of metalloproteinase 1 (tissue inhibitor matrix metalloproteinase-1, TIMP-1; a specific inhibitor of MMPs) are increased during fibrosis, resulting in the inhibition of ECM degradation [52–54]. Beyond the abovementioned pathological events, hemodynamic alterations also reduce post-glomerular blood flow to peritubular capillaries, which, in turn, leads to hypoxic conditions and damage to tubular epithelium [55].

5. Cellular Signaling Pathways Involved in Pathogenesis of DN

In the diabetic milieu, such as hyperglycemia and dyslipidemia, metabolic alteration increases the production of ROS mainly through the Polyol and/or Nox pathway [56,57]. In addition, an increased intracellular glucose level increases AGE production and ROS by activating the AGEs receptor (RAGE) axis [58]. These abnormal metabolic and physiological consequences directly induce both vascular endothelial cell dysfunction and hemodynamic alterations, including activation of the renin–angiotensin system. Subsequently, this impact triggers a number of cellular signaling cascades, including the protein kinase c (PKC), mitogen-activated protein kinases (MAPKs; p38 and c-Jun N-terminal kinases (JNK)), Janus kinase/signal transducer and activator of transcription protein (JAK/STAT), and transforming growth factor (TGF)-β/Smad, thereby inducing a cellular response via activation of key transcription factors, such as NF-κB [56,57]. In particular, several vasoactive factors (angiotensin II, thromboxane, and endothelin-1) enhance their fibrotic action in diabetic renal diseases via secondary induction of TGF-β expression [56,59].

The Smad signaling pathway has also been reported to be associated with the renal hypertrophy and accumulation of ECM molecules through TGF-β signaling in DN [56,60,61]. Accumulation of AGEs within the glomerular apparatus, mesangial matrix, and tubular cells also directly causes serious alteration of diabetic kidney structure by reacting with plasma proteins and extra vascular proteins. As a consequence, AGEs lead to the transcriptional upregulation of TGF-β1, IL-6, and NF-κB, possibly via activation of PKC and/or oxidative stress [59,62]. PKCs are important players for the onset and progression of DN via hyperglycemia-induced upregulation of vascular endothelial growth factor (VEGF) expression in the mesangial cells [63]. In response to such molecules or signals, chemokines, growth factors, and profibrotic factors are ultimately upregulated in renal cells, such as tubular epithelial cells, podocytes, and mesangial cells, which contribute to cellular injury, progressive fibrosis, and loss of glomerular filtration rate, thereby increasing proteinuria during the development and progression of DN [56,57].

Recently, new molecules or potential signaling pathways have been added to the established pathways, which has made the pathogenesis of DN more complex. However, new observations simultaneously increase the possibility of identifying new targets for the treatment of DN. Interleukin (IL)-33-mediated suppression of the tumorigenicity 2 receptor (ST2) axis is one such pathway, which is very attractive due to its association with inflammatory response. IL-33 was first identified as a member of the IL-1 family in 2005 [64]. IL-33 acts through ST2 [65], which plays an important role in the immunity against pathogens, type 2 inflammation, tissue homeostasis, and repair [66,67]. Soluble ST2 level elevates in the serum of CKD and is associated with the severity of the disease [68], possibly suggesting its role in the development of CKD. However, these studies are very limited.

Sodium–glucose cotransporter (SGLT)-2 may be a potential contributor to CKD. Under normal physiological conditions, urine does not contain glucose, owing to its effective reabsorption by two transporters, SGLT-1 and SGLT-2 [69]. The SGLT-2 transporter is located on the luminal side of the first segment of the proximal tubule in the kidney. It is a high-capacity, low-affinity transporter, but is responsible for the reabsorption of approximately 90% of all filtered glucose [70]. SGLT-2 inhibitor induces glycosuria and natriuresis by blocking reabsorption of glucose and sodium in the proximal tubule [71]. As a consequence, afferent arteriolar vasoconstriction is induced, thereby reducing intraglomerular pressure, decreasing hyperfiltration, and improving renal function [72].

Current evidence also suggests that autophagy is critical in kidney physiology and homeostasis. In the diabetic milieu, increased oxidative stress, inflammation, and mitochondrial dysfunction modulate the autophagy activation and inhibition as well as lead to cellular recycling dysfunction [73]. Reduction of autophagy induces loss of podocytes, damage in proximal tubular cells, and glomerulosclerosis [74, 75]. High glucose treatment has activated autophagy in podocytes and protected the podocytes from hyperglycemia-related apoptosis [76]. Similarly, autophagy related 5 (Atg5)-knockout diabetic mice (deficiency of autophagy activation) showed more severe proteinuria and impaired renal function [77,78]. Autophagy also protects mesangial cells from apoptosis induced by TGF-β1 via transforming growth factor β-activated kinase (TAK)1 and PI3K–AKT-dependent pathways [79]. Several studies have consistently indicated that DN is associated with decreased autophagy and increased apoptosis [80–82].

6. Chronic Kidney Injury and LPA–LPAR Axis

CKD has been becoming a major public health problem globally. It involves a progressive loss of kidney function over a period of months or years, which frequently leads to end-stage renal failure [1]. The main risk factors of CKD include high blood pressure, diabetes, cardiac disease, and a family history of kidney failure with genetic problems [83]. The potential role of LPA in the pathogenesis of kidney disease was suggested for the first time following the discovery of a positive correlation between circulation LPA levels and renal dysfunction in patients with kidney disorder at the end of the 1990s [84]. Later on, Grove KJ et al. also reported that the LPA level was elevated in glomeruli of eNOS

(–/–) *db/db* mice, a robust model of DN [85]. Furthermore, LPA induced renal tubulointerstitial fibrosis, a classical hallmark of CKD, in a mouse model of unilateral ureteral obstruction [86]. More recently, LPA was identified as a biomarker of CKD in metabolic screening assay, using plasma samples from CKD patients with diverse etiologies and two different CKD rodent models [87]. Consistent with results of other studies, the LPA and LPC forms (16:0, 18:0, 18:1, and 18:2) were also detected in urine of DN patients [88]. On the contrary, several studies showed similar or reduced LPA levels in the plasma, but an increased urinary LPA level in CKD patients and animal models, suggesting that the local expression levels of LPA and LPARs are more important for the development of CKD [88–90]. LPA regulates various biological responses by binding to G-protein–coupled receptors (LPAR1–LPAR6) [5].

Recently, we and another group reported that the LPAR1 and/or LPAR3 were upregulated in different DN mouse models [91–93]. Treatment with a dual LPAR1/3 antagonist (Ki16425 or BMS002) or AM095 (a novel antagonist of LPAR1) reduced renal injury in the *db/db* mice (leptin receptor-deficient mouse with human type 2 diabetic phenotype) and streptozotocin (STZ)-induced diabetic mice (pancreatic beta cell-destroyed mouse with human type 1 diabetic phenotype) [91–93]. The expression of ATX and LPA production increases and activates the LPAR1-mediated signaling pathway in mesangial cells' exposure to high-glucose media and in the kidney cortex of diabetic *db/db* mice [91]. LPA–LPAR1 activation increases the phosphorylation of glycogen synthase kinase (GSK)3β at serine 9 residue (Ser9) and induces translocation of sterol regulatory element-binding protein (SREBP) 1 into the nucleus [91]. Subsequently, it induces TGF-β expression, which contributes to the development of glomerular injury in *db/db* mice. However, treatment of ki16425 reduces proteinuria, glomerular tuft area and volume, and mesangial matrix expansion by regulating the LPA–GSK3β–SREBP1 axis [91]. In line with our observation, LPAR1 deletion in unilateral ureteral obstruction-induced mice prevents renal fibrosis by suppressing the expression of connective tissue growth factor in proximal tubular epithelial cells [86]. Additionally, Diao et al. reported that LPAR3 deletion affects the spatiotemporal expression of collagen types I, III, IV, and VI in peri-implantation of the mouse uterus [94]. All of these studies suggest that the LPA–LPAR axis regulates renal fibrosis differently for different kidney cell types or different tissues, and that at least two receptors, LPAR1 and LPAR3, might be important contributors to renal fibrosis.

Similarly, Zhang et al. showed improvements in renal function, using a different dual LPAR1/3 antagonist, BMS002, in the endothelial nitric oxide synthase-deficient (eNOS (–/–)) *db/db* mouse [92]. The expressions of ATX, LPAR1, and LPAR3 proteins in these mice significantly increased in the glomerular podocytes and tubular epithelial cells in the renal cortex [92]. Blockading the LPAR1/3 activity ameliorated glomerular injury and reverses kidney dysfunction by reducing podocyte loss and increased the phosphorylation of Akt2 (known to be essential for maintaining podocyte viability and function) [95], which prevented reduction in the glomerular filtration rate and reduced proteinuria without affecting blood pressure [92]. However, the underlying molecular mechanism in their study was not fully addressed and further studies will be needed.

Furthermore, our studies showed that increased LPA levels in STZ-induced diabetic mice increases Toll-like receptor (TLR) 4 expression and directly activates the NF-κB, the master transcription factor responsible for inflammatory cytokine expression. Simultaneously, activated TLR4 also produces ROS through the nicotinamide adenine dinucleotide phosphate (NADPH) oxidase system [93]. All these intracellular changes synergistically activate NF-κB and/or JNK by increasing phosphorylation of p65 and JNK [93]. Ultimately, it leads to renal fibrosis via upregulation of pro-inflammatory cytokines and fibrotic factors, including TGF-β1, TIMP-1, and fibronectin. In contrast, AM095 treatment attenuates DN by downregulation of these signaling pathways in vivo. In mesangial cells, LPA treatment activates these signaling pathways similar to that in mice; however, this degree of activation was reduced by AM095 treatment [93]. We also observed some beneficial effects of AM095 treatment on glycemic control. However, the underlying mechanism should be addressed in future studies.

Mesangial cell proliferation and accumulation in the pathogenesis of DN is a major risk factor contributing to glomerulosclerosis. LPA treatment increased the proliferation of mouse mesangial cells (SV40 MES13), concomitant with the increased expression levels of cyclin D1 and CDK4 and decreased expression of $p27^{Kip1}$. The expression of Krüppel-like factor 5 (KLF5) was upregulated by activating MAPK and elevating the expression of early growth response 1 (Egr1) in the kidney cortex of *db/db* mice and LPA-treated SV40 MES13 cells. Moreover, LPA significantly increased the activity of Rac1 GTPase in SV40 MES13 cells, and the dominant–negative form of Rac1 blunted the phosphorylation of p38, the upregulation of Egr1, and the LPA-mediated induction of KLF5, indicating that the downstream pathway of Rac1 was involved in LPA-induced mesangial cell proliferation [96]. Taken together, these observations suggested that the Rac1/MAPK/KLF5 signaling pathway is one of the underlying mechanisms contributing to glomerular hyper proliferation during the progression of DN. Recently, Guo et al. showed that LPA activates β-catenin, a downstream mediator of Wnt signaling, in colon cancer cells and KLF5 plays a critical role in β-catenin activation [97]. Several studies directly indicated that the Wnt/β-catenin signaling pathway was implicated in renal fibrosis and apoptosis in CKD models [98,99]. Thus, the regulation of these pathways may provide a potential therapeutic target for the treatment of DN.

Some studies have also suggested that LPA may bind to the receptor for RAGE, a member of the immunoglobulin superfamily [36,100]. Under in vitro conditions, this interaction is essential for LPA-induced ovarian tumor implantation and metastasis, as well as for LPA-mediated proliferation and migration of vascular smooth muscle cells [36]. In addition, LPA failed to activate vascular Akt signaling in mice that were administered soluble RAGE or genetic deletion of RAGE [36]. These observations indicated that RAGE-mediated signal transduction may play an important role in diabetic microvascular complication, including DN. Zaslaysky et al. also revealed that three major LPARs (LPAR1-3) form homo- or hetero-dimers within the LPAR subgroup and hetero-dimers with sphingosine 1 phosphate receptor (S1PR), pH-sensing G protein-coupled receptor (GPR4), and ovarian cancer G-protein coupled receptor-1 (OGR1/GPR68) [101], thereby activating the downstream signaling pathways linked to inflammation and fibrosis. S1PR signaling activation promotes renal fibrosis in the diabetic condition [102–104]. In the terminal ileum of inflammatory bowel diseases, the expression of OGR1/GPR68 positively increases the expression of pro-fibrotic genes and collagen deposition, suggesting the potential involvement of these receptors, signaling for the pathogenesis of DN [105]. However, there is no direct evidence connecting DN pathogenesis with dimer formation between LPARs and these receptors. Another potential LPA receptor is the TRPV1 ion channel [37]. However, there have been no reports demonstrating its role in DN.

7. Conclusions and Future Research Directions

DN is the main risk factor for chronic kidney diseases, which mostly progress to the development of ESRD in the end. The best treatment regimen for DN is kidney replacement; however, it is highly restricted, due to various reasons, such as rare donors and rejection of the transplanted organ. Several medications are currently available for DN, but they are not sufficient for the recovery from kidney injury and restoration of kidney function in DN patients. Alternative drugs are thus required. Accumulated evidence indicates that the LPA–LPAR axis plays an important role in inducing pathological alterations of cell structure and function in the kidneys. Current studies showed that LPAR antagonism using pharmacological inhibitors significantly decreases the abnormality of kidney structure, such as GBM thickness, and increases of renal function, such as reducing proteinuria in different types of diabetic mouse models by regulating several signaling pathways, as shown in Figure 3.

The currently available data suggest that LPA signaling may regulate fibrosis, proliferation, and the inflammatory response in mesangial cells and podocytes or induce apoptosis via the following signaling pathways: 1) PI3K-AKT-GSK3β-TGF-β axis for fibrosis; 2) Rac1GTPase-MAPK-KLF5-CDK4/Cyclin D1 axis for proliferation; 3) TLR4-NADPH oxidase-ROS–NF-κB/MAPK or TLR4-NF-κB/MAPK axis for inflammatory response; 4) PI3K-AKT-GSK3α axis for apoptosis; 5) LPA-RAGE axis for glomerular injury; and 6) Wnt/β-catenin axis for fibrosis and apoptosis. For further details, please see above. LPAR: LPA receptor, RAGE: AGE receptor, Rac1: Ras-related C3 botulinum toxin substrate 1, NADPH:

Nicotinamide adenine dinucleotide phosphate oxidase, TLR4: Toll-like receptor 4, NF-κB: Nuclear factor-κB, KLF5: Krüppel-like factor 5.

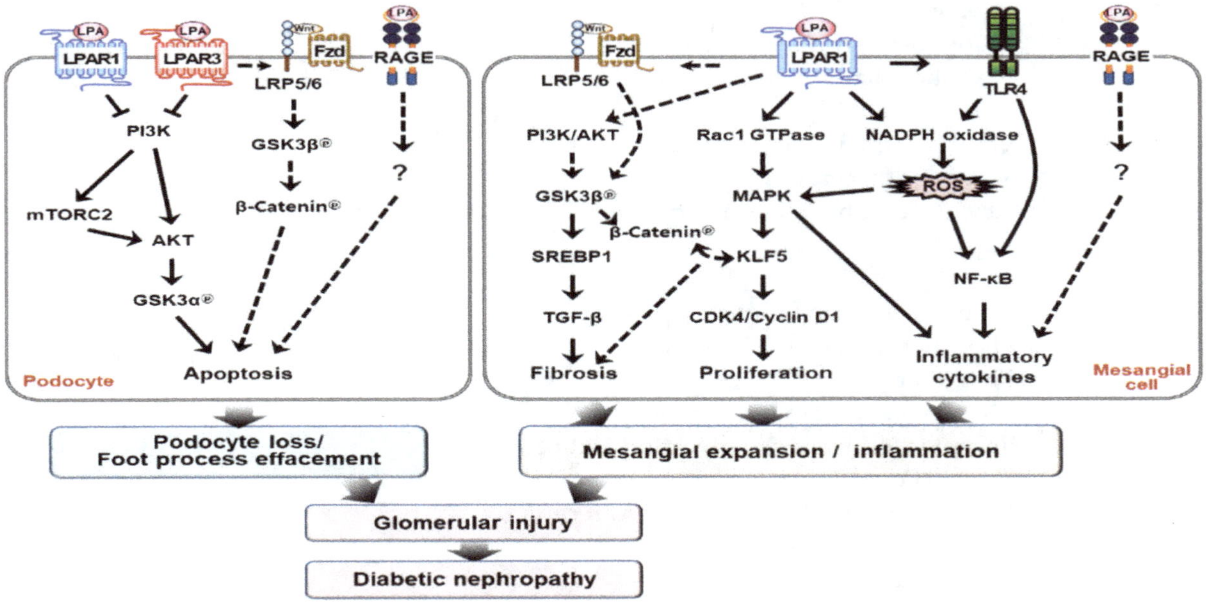

Figure 3. Schematic representation of LPA signaling in diabetic nephropathy models.

However, there are still many unanswered questions. Further studies should be performed in the following directions: Since the kidney consists of heterogeneous cells (such as podocytes, mesangial microvascular endothelial cells, and renal proximal tubule epithelial cells) and the LPAR expression level may be different in different cell types, further studies should first determine the LPAR expression level under different physiological and pathophysiological conditions. In addition, the studies should investigate the effects of LPAR antagonism on each type of kidney cell, using not only pharmacological inhibitors, but also genetically engineered in vivo models. Moreover, there are many different forms of LPA, which exhibit different affinities for each LPAR type. Each LPAR also exhibits various interaction affinities with one or more G protein subunits, thereby promoting different biological effects. These aspects should be further elucidated. Furthermore, the LPA–LPAR-mediated signaling pathway is also modulated by a cross-talk with other signaling pathways, such as epidermal growth factor (EGF) or vasoactive (angiotensin II) receptor-mediated signals [106], which will be defined in future studies. Since LPA regulates local blood flow, systemic blood pressure, and platelet function, and these factors directly play a critical role in renal function [40,107], future studies need to investigate the effect of LPA on the physiological and pathophysiological conditions in the renal vasculature and the tubular system. In addition, there are no studies demonstrating the relationship between the LPA–LPAR axis and the IL-33-ST2 axis and SGLT2 and autophagy. These new avenues should also be investigated in the future. Further understanding of the precise mechanisms underlying LPA action under physiological and pathophysiological conditions may facilitate the development of new therapeutic targets for DN.

Author Contributions: J.H.L. and H.-S.J. collected information and wrote the manuscript; J.H.L, D.K, Y.S.O, and H.-S.J. edited and revised the manuscript; J.H.L. and H.-S.J. approved the final version of the manuscript.

Abbreviations

DN	Diabetic nephropathy
ESRD	End-stage renal disease
ACE	Angiotensin converting enzyme
ARBs	Angiotensin II receptor blockers
LPA	Lysophosphatidic acid
ATX	Autotaxin

AGE	Advanced glycation end (product)
GPAT	Glycerol-3-phosphate acyltransferase
PLA1 and PLA2	Phospholipases A1 or A2
PA	Phosphatidic acid
LPE	Lysophosphatidylethanolamine
LPC	Lysophosphatidylcholine
LPS	Lysophosphatidylserine
LPPs	Lipid phosphate phosphatases
MAG	Monoacylglycerol
AGPAT	Acylglycerophosphate acyltransferase
PLC	Phospholipase C
DAG	Diacylglycerol
MAPK	Mitogen-activated protein kinase
PI3K	Phosphatidylinositol 3 kinase
PKB	Protein kinase B
ROCK	Rho-associated protein kinase
RAGE	Receptor for advanced glycation end products
Nox	NADPH oxidase
PPARγ	Peroxisome proliferator-activated receptor γ
CKD	Chronic kidney disease
ECM	Extracellular matrix
GBM	Glomerular basement membrane
EMT	Epithelial mesenchymal transition
CCL2/MCP1	Monocyte chemoattractant protein 1
CCL5/RANTES	Regulated upon activation, normal T cell expressed, and secreted
ICAM-1	Intercellular adhesion molecule-1
VCAM-1	Vascular cell adhesion molecule-1
PAI-1	Plasminogen activator inhibitor-1
uPA and tPA	Urokinase-type and tissue-type plasminogen activator
TIMP-1	Tissue inhibitor matrix metalloproteinase-1
JNK	c-Jun N-terminal kinases
VEGF	Vascular endothelial growth factor
SGLT-2	Sodium–glucose cotransporter-2
GSK3β	Glycogen synthase kinase 3β
SREBP 1	Sterol regulatory element-binding protein1
TGF-β	Transforming growth factor-β
TLR 4	Toll-like receptor 4
NF-κB	Nuclear factor-κB
KLF5	Krüppel-like factor 5
Egr1	Early growth response 1
S1PR	Sphingosine 1 phosphate receptor
GPR4	pH-sensing G protein-coupled receptor
OGR1/GPR68	Ovarian cancer G-protein coupled receptor-1

References

1. Gheith, O.; Farouk, N.; Nampoory, N.; Halim, M.A.; Al-Otaibi, T. Diabetic kidney disease: World wide difference of prevalence and risk factors. *J. Nephropharmacol.* **2016**, *5*, 49–56. [CrossRef] [PubMed]
2. Alicic, R.Z.; Rooney, M.T.; Tuttle, K.R. Diabetic kidney disease: Challenges, progress, and possibilities. *Clin. J. Am. Soc. Nephrol.* **2017**, *12*, 2032–2045. [CrossRef] [PubMed]
3. Dounousi, E.; Duni, A.; Leivaditis, K.; Vaios, V.; Eleftheriadis, T.; Liakopoulos, V. Improvements in the management of diabetic nephropathy. *Rev. Diabet. Stud.* **2015**, *12*, 119–133. [CrossRef] [PubMed]
4. Bash, L.D.; Selvin, E.; Steffes, M.; Coresh, J.; Astor, B.C. Poor glycemic control in diabetes and the risk of incident chronic kidney disease even in the absence of albuminuria and retinopathy: Atherosclerosis risk in communities (ARIC) study. *Arch. Intern. Med.* **2008**, *168*, 2440–2447. [CrossRef] [PubMed]

5. Yung, Y.C.; Stoddard, N.C.; Chun, J. LPA receptor signaling: Pharmacology, physiology, and pathophysiology. *J. Lipid Res.* **2014**, *55*, 1192–1214. [CrossRef] [PubMed]
6. Park, F.; Miller, D.D. Role of lysophosphatidic acid and its receptors in the kidney. *Physiol. Genom.* **2017**, *49*, 659–666. [CrossRef] [PubMed]
7. Aikawa, S.; Hashimoto, T.; Kano, K.; Aoki, J. Lysophosphatidic acid as a lipid mediator with multiple biological actions. *J. Biochem.* **2015**, *157*, 81–89. [CrossRef] [PubMed]
8. Choi, J.W.; Herr, D.R.; Noguchi, K.; Yung, Y.C.; Lee, C.W.; Mutoh, T.; Lin, M.E.; Teo, S.T.; Park, K.E.; Mosley, A.N.; et al. LPA receptors: Subtypes and biological actions. *Annu. Rev. Pharmacol. Toxicol.* **2010**, *50*, 157–186. [CrossRef]
9. Budd, D.C.; Qian, Y. Development of lysophosphatidic acid pathway modulators as therapies for fibrosis. *Future Med. Chem.* **2013**, *5*, 1935–1952. [CrossRef] [PubMed]
10. Chu, X.; Wei, X.; Lu, S.; He, P. Autotaxin-lpa receptor axis in the pathogenesis of lung diseases. *Int. J. Clin. Exp. Med.* **2015**, *8*, 17117–17122. [PubMed]
11. Rhee, S.Y.; Kim, Y.S. The role of advanced glycation end products in diabetic vascular complications. *Diabetes Metab. J.* **2018**, *42*, 188–195. [CrossRef] [PubMed]
12. Rabbani, N.; Thornalley, P.J. Advanced glycation end products in the pathogenesis of chronic kidney disease. *Kidney Int.* **2018**, *93*, 803–813. [CrossRef] [PubMed]
13. Valdes-Rives, S.A.; Gonzalez-Arenas, A. Autotaxin-lysophosphatidic acid: From inflammation to cancer development. *Mediat. Inflamm.* **2017**, *2017*, 9173090. [CrossRef]
14. Aoki, J. Mechanisms of lysophosphatidic acid production. *Semin. Cell Dev. Biol.* **2004**, *15*, 477–489. [CrossRef] [PubMed]
15. Prentki, M.; Madiraju, S.R. Glycerolipid metabolism and signaling in health and disease. *Endocr. Rev.* **2008**, *29*, 647–676. [CrossRef] [PubMed]
16. Mirzoyan, K. The Role of lpa in Kidney Pathologies. Ph.D. Thesis, Université Toulouse 3 Paul Sabatier, Toulouse, France, 2018.
17. Nakajima, K.; Sonoda, H.; Mizoguchi, T.; Aoki, J.; Arai, H.; Nagahama, M.; Tagaya, M.; Tani, K. A novel phospholipase a1 with sequence homology to a mammalian sec23p-interacting protein, p125. *J. Biol. Chem.* **2002**, *277*, 11329–11335. [CrossRef] [PubMed]
18. Richmond, G.S.; Smith, T.K. The role and characterization of phospholipase a1 in mediating lysophosphatidylcholine synthesis in trypanosoma brucei. *Biochem. J.* **2007**, *405*, 319–329. [CrossRef] [PubMed]
19. Aoki, J.; Inoue, A.; Okudaira, S. Two pathways for lysophosphatidic acid production. *Biochim. Biophys. Acta* **2008**, *1781*, 513–518. [CrossRef]
20. Nakanaga, K.; Hama, K.; Aoki, J. Autotaxin—An LPA producing enzyme with diverse functions. *J. Biochem.* **2010**, *148*, 13–24. [CrossRef]
21. Brindley, D.N.; Pilquil, C. Lipid phosphate phosphatases and signaling. *J. Lipid Res.* **2009**, *50* (Suppl. 1), S225–S230. [CrossRef]
22. Saba, J.D. Lysophospholipids in development: Miles apart and edging in. *J. Cell. Biochem.* **2004**, *92*, 967–992. [CrossRef] [PubMed]
23. Kok, B.P.; Venkatraman, G.; Capatos, D.; Brindley, D.N. Unlike two peas in a pod: Lipid phosphate phosphatases and phosphatidate phosphatases. *Chem. Rev.* **2012**, *112*, 5121–5146. [CrossRef] [PubMed]
24. Aguado, B.; Campbell, R.D. Characterization of a human lysophosphatidic acid acyltransferase that is encoded by a gene located in the class iii region of the human major histocompatibility complex. *J. Biol. Chem.* **1998**, *273*, 4096–4105. [CrossRef] [PubMed]
25. Wang, A.; Dennis, E.A. Mammalian lysophospholipases. *Biochim. Biophys. Acta* **1999**, *1439*, 1–16. [CrossRef]
26. Pasternack, S.M.; von Kugelgen, I.; Al Aboud, K.; Lee, Y.A.; Ruschendorf, F.; Voss, K.; Hillmer, A.M.; Molderings, G.J.; Franz, T.; Ramirez, A.; et al. G protein-coupled receptor P2Y5 and its ligand LPA are involved in maintenance of human hair growth. *Nat. Genet.* **2008**, *40*, 329–334. [CrossRef] [PubMed]
27. Fukushima, N.; Kimura, Y.; Chun, J. A single receptor encoded by VZG-1/LPA1/EDG-2 couples to g proteins and mediates multiple cellular responses to lysophosphatidic acid. *Proc. Natl. Acad. Sci. USA* **1998**, *95*, 6151–6156. [CrossRef] [PubMed]
28. Ishii, I.; Contos, J.J.; Fukushima, N.; Chun, J. Functional comparisons of the lysophosphatidic acid receptors, lp(a1)/vzg-1/edg-2, lp(a2)/edg-4, and lp(a3)/edg-7 in neuronal cell lines using a retrovirus expression system. *Mol. Pharmacol.* **2000**, *58*, 895–902. [CrossRef]

29. Lee, C.W.; Rivera, R.; Dubin, A.E.; Chun, J. LPA(4)/GPR23 is a lysophosphatidic acid (LPA) receptor utilizing g(s)-, g(q)/g(i)-mediated calcium signaling and G(12/13)-mediated rho activation. *J. Biol. Chem.* **2007**, *282*, 4310–4317. [CrossRef]
30. Noguchi, K.; Ishii, S.; Shimizu, T. Identification of P2Y9/GPR23 as a novel g protein-coupled receptor for lysophosphatidic acid, structurally distant from the edg family. *J. Biol. Chem.* **2003**, *278*, 25600–25606. [CrossRef]
31. Lee, C.W.; Rivera, R.; Gardell, S.; Dubin, A.E.; Chun, J. GPR92 as a new G12/13- and GQ-coupled lysophosphatidic acid receptor that increases camp, lpa5. *J. Biol. Chem.* **2006**, *281*, 23589–23597. [CrossRef]
32. Yanagida, K.; Masago, K.; Nakanishi, H.; Kihara, Y.; Hamano, F.; Tajima, Y.; Taguchi, R.; Shimizu, T.; Ishii, S. Identification and characterization of a novel lysophosphatidic acid receptor, P2Y5/LPA6. *J. Biol. Chem.* **2009**, *284*, 17731–17741. [CrossRef] [PubMed]
33. Riaz, A.; Huang, Y.; Johansson, S. G-protein-coupled lysophosphatidic acid receptors and their regulation of akt signaling. *Int. J. Mol. Sci.* **2016**, *17*, 215. [CrossRef] [PubMed]
34. Oka, S.; Ota, R.; Shima, M.; Yamashita, A.; Sugiura, T. GPR35 is a novel lysophosphatidic acid receptor. *Biochem. Biophys. Res. Commun.* **2010**, *395*, 232–237. [CrossRef] [PubMed]
35. Murakami, M.; Shiraishi, A.; Tabata, K.; Fujita, N. Identification of the orphan gpcr, p2y(10) receptor as the sphingosine-1-phosphate and lysophosphatidic acid receptor. *Biochem. Biophys. Res. Commun.* **2008**, *371*, 707–712. [CrossRef] [PubMed]
36. Rai, V.; Toure, F.; Chitayat, S.; Pei, R.; Song, F.; Li, Q.; Zhang, J.; Rosario, R.; Ramasamy, R.; Chazin, W.J.; et al. Lysophosphatidic acid targets vascular and oncogenic pathways via rage signaling. *J. Exp. Med.* **2012**, *209*, 2339–2350. [CrossRef] [PubMed]
37. Nieto-Posadas, A.; Picazo-Juarez, G.; Llorente, I.; Jara-Oseguera, A.; Morales-Lazaro, S.; Escalante-Alcalde, D.; Islas, L.D.; Rosenbaum, T. Lysophosphatidic acid directly activates TRPV1 through a c-terminal binding site. *Nat. Chem. Biol.* **2011**, *8*, 78–85. [CrossRef] [PubMed]
38. Bowman, M.A.; Schmidt, A.M. The next generation of rage modulators: Implications for soluble rage therapies in vascular inflammation. *J. Mol. Med.* **2013**, *91*, 1329–1331. [CrossRef] [PubMed]
39. McIntyre, T.M.; Pontsler, A.V.; Silva, A.R.; St Hilaire, A.; Xu, Y.; Hinshaw, J.C.; Zimmerman, G.A.; Hama, K.; Aoki, J.; Arai, H.; et al. Identification of an intracellular receptor for lysophosphatidic acid (LPA): Lpa is a transcellular ppargamma agonist. *Proc. Natl. Acad. Sci. USA* **2003**, *100*, 131–136. [CrossRef]
40. Pradere, J.P.; Gonzalez, J.; Klein, J.; Valet, P.; Gres, S.; Salant, D.; Bascands, J.L.; Saulnier-Blache, J.S.; Schanstra, J.P. Lysophosphatidic acid and renal fibrosis. *Biochim. Biophys. Acta* **2008**, *1781*, 582–587. [CrossRef]
41. Makris, K.; Spanou, L. Acute kidney injury: Definition, pathophysiology and clinical phenotypes. *Clin. Biochem. Rev.* **2016**, *37*, 85–98.
42. Levey, A.S.; Levin, A.; Kellum, J.A. Definition and classification of kidney diseases. *Am. J. Kidney Dis.* **2013**, *61*, 686–688. [CrossRef] [PubMed]
43. Hewitson, T.D.; Holt, S.G.; Smith, E.R. Progression of tubulointerstitial fibrosis and the chronic kidney disease phenotype—Role of risk factors and epigenetics. *Front. Pharmacol.* **2017**, *8*, 520. [CrossRef] [PubMed]
44. Ke, B.; Fan, C.; Yang, L.; Fang, X. Matrix metalloproteinases-7 and kidney fibrosis. *Front. Physiol.* **2017**, *8*, 21. [CrossRef] [PubMed]
45. Xiao, Z.; Chen, C.; Meng, T.; Zhang, W.; Zhou, Q. Resveratrol attenuates renal injury and fibrosis by inhibiting transforming growth factor-β pathway on matrix metalloproteinase 7. *Exp. Biol. Med.* **2016**, *241*, 140–146. [CrossRef] [PubMed]
46. Rosenberg, A.Z.; Kopp, J.B. Focal segmental glomerulosclerosis. *Clin. J. Am. Soc. Nephrol.* **2017**, *12*, 502–517. [CrossRef]
47. Humphreys, B.D. Mechanisms of renal fibrosis. *Annu. Rev. Physiol.* **2018**, *80*, 309–326. [CrossRef]
48. Reiser, J.; Altintas, M.M. Podocytes. *F1000 Res.* **2016**, *5*. [CrossRef]
49. Iwano, M.; Neilson, E.G. Mechanisms of tubulointerstitial fibrosis. *Curr. Opin. Nephrol. Hypertens.* **2004**, *13*, 279–284. [CrossRef]
50. Lee, S.B.; Kalluri, R. Mechanistic connection between inflammation and fibrosis. *Kidney Int. Suppl.* **2010**, S22–S26. [CrossRef]
51. Grgic, I.; Duffield, J.S.; Humphreys, B.D. The origin of interstitial myofibroblasts in chronic kidney disease. *Pediatr. Nephrol.* **2012**, *27*, 183–193. [CrossRef]

52. Ye, Y.; Vattai, A.; Zhang, X.; Zhu, J.; Thaler, C.J.; Mahner, S.; Jeschke, U.; von Schonfeldt, V. Role of plasminogen activator inhibitor type 1 in pathologies of female reproductive diseases. *Int. J. Mol. Sci.* **2017**, *18*, 1651. [CrossRef] [PubMed]
53. Hu, C.; Sun, L.; Xiao, L.; Han, Y.; Fu, X.; Xiong, X.; Xu, X.; Liu, Y.; Yang, S.; Liu, F.; et al. Insights into the mechanisms involved in the expression and regulation of extracellular matrix proteins in diabetic nephropathy. *Curr. Med. Chem.* **2015**, *22*, 2858–2870. [CrossRef] [PubMed]
54. Hodgkins, K.S.; Schnaper, H.W. Tubulointerstitial injury and the progression of chronic kidney disease. *Pediatr. Nephrol.* **2012**, *27*, 901–909. [CrossRef] [PubMed]
55. Singh, D.K.; Winocour, P.; Farrington, K. Mechanisms of disease: The hypoxic tubular hypothesis of diabetic nephropathy. *Nat. Clin. Pract. Nephrol.* **2008**, *4*, 216–226. [CrossRef] [PubMed]
56. Bhattacharjee, N.; Barma, S.; Konwar, N.; Dewanjee, S.; Manna, P. Mechanistic insight of diabetic nephropathy and its pharmacotherapeutic targets: An update. *Eur. J. Pharmacol.* **2016**, *791*, 8–24. [CrossRef] [PubMed]
57. Kawanami, D.; Matoba, K.; Utsunomiya, K. Signaling pathways in diabetic nephropathy. *Histol. Histopathol.* **2016**, *31*, 1059–1067. [PubMed]
58. Kanwar, Y.S.; Wada, J.; Sun, L.; Xie, P.; Wallner, E.I.; Chen, S.; Chugh, S.; Danesh, F.R. Diabetic nephropathy: Mechanisms of renal disease progression. *Exp. Biol. Med.* **2008**, *233*, 4–11. [CrossRef]
59. Nowotny, K.; Jung, T.; Hohn, A.; Weber, D.; Grune, T. Advanced glycation end products and oxidative stress in type 2 diabetes mellitus. *Biomolecules* **2015**, *5*, 194–222. [CrossRef]
60. Sureshbabu, A.; Muhsin, S.A.; Choi, M.E. TGF-β signaling in the kidney: Profibrotic and protective effects. *Am. J. Physiol. Ren. Physiol.* **2016**, *310*, F596–F606. [CrossRef]
61. Chang, A.S.; Hathaway, C.K.; Smithies, O.; Kakoki, M. Transforming growth factor-β1 and diabetic nephropathy. *Am. J. Physiol. Ren. Physiol.* **2016**, *310*, F689–F696. [CrossRef]
62. Volpe, C.M.O.; Villar-Delfino, P.H.; Dos Anjos, P.M.F.; Nogueira-Machado, J.A. Cellular death, reactive oxygen species (ROS) and diabetic complications. *Cell Death Dis.* **2018**, *9*, 119. [CrossRef] [PubMed]
63. Tufro, A.; Veron, D. Vegf and podocytes in diabetic nephropathy. *Semin. Nephrol.* **2012**, *32*, 385–393. [CrossRef] [PubMed]
64. Schmitz, J.; Owyang, A.; Oldham, E.; Song, Y.; Murphy, E.; McClanahan, T.K.; Zurawski, G.; Moshrefi, M.; Qin, J.; Li, X.; et al. IL-33, an interleukin-1-like cytokine that signals via the IL-1 receptor-related protein ST2 and induces t helper type 2-associated cytokines. *Immunity* **2005**, *23*, 479–490. [CrossRef] [PubMed]
65. Gao, Q.; Li, Y.; Li, M. The potential role of IL-33/ST2 signaling in fibrotic diseases. *J. Leukoc. Biol.* **2015**, *98*, 15–22. [CrossRef] [PubMed]
66. Tonacci, A.; Quattrocchi, P.; Gangemi, S. IL33/ST2 axis in diabetic kidney disease: A literature review. *Medicina* **2019**, *55*, 50. [CrossRef] [PubMed]
67. Cao, Q.; Wang, Y.; Niu, Z.; Wang, C.; Wang, R.; Zhang, Z.; Chen, T.; Wang, X.M.; Li, Q.; Lee, V.W.S.; et al. Potentiating tissue-resident type 2 innate lymphoid cells by IL-33 to prevent renal ischemia-reperfusion injury. *J. Am. Soc. Nephrol.* **2018**, *29*, 961–976. [CrossRef]
68. Bao, Y.S.; Na, S.P.; Zhang, P.; Jia, X.B.; Liu, R.C.; Yu, C.Y.; Mu, S.H.; Xie, R.J. Characterization of interleukin-33 and soluble ST2 in serum and their association with disease severity in patients with chronic kidney disease. *J. Clin. Immunol.* **2012**, *32*, 587–594. [CrossRef]
69. Wilding, J.P. The role of the kidneys in glucose homeostasis in type 2 diabetes: Clinical implications and therapeutic significance through sodium glucose co-transporter 2 inhibitors. *Metab. Clin. Exp.* **2014**, *63*, 1228–1237. [CrossRef]
70. Vallon, V.; Thomson, S.C. Targeting renal glucose reabsorption to treat hyperglycaemia: The pleiotropic effects of SGLT2 inhibition. *Diabetologia* **2017**, *60*, 215–225. [CrossRef]
71. Sano, M.; Takei, M.; Shiraishi, Y.; Suzuki, Y. Increased hematocrit during sodium-glucose cotransporter 2 inhibitor therapy indicates recovery of tubulointerstitial function in diabetic kidneys. *J. Clin. Med. Res.* **2016**, *8*, 844–847. [CrossRef]
72. Dekkers, C.C.J.; Gansevoort, R.T.; Heerspink, H.J.L. New diabetes therapies and diabetic kidney disease progression: The role of SGLT-2 inhibitors. *Curr. Diabetes Rep.* **2018**, *18*, 27. [CrossRef] [PubMed]
73. Susztak, K.; Raff, A.C.; Schiffer, M.; Bottinger, E.P. Glucose-induced reactive oxygen species cause apoptosis of podocytes and podocyte depletion at the onset of diabetic nephropathy. *Diabetes* **2006**, *55*, 225–233. [CrossRef] [PubMed]
74. Lin, T.A.; Wu, V.C.; Wang, C.Y. Autophagy in chronic kidney diseases. *Cells* **2019**, *8*, 61. [CrossRef] [PubMed]
75. Tagawa, A.; Yasuda, M.; Kume, S.; Yamahara, K.; Nakazawa, J.; Chin-Kanasaki, M.; Araki, H.; Araki, S.;

Koya, D.; Asanuma, K.; et al. Impaired podocyte autophagy exacerbates proteinuria in diabetic nephropathy. *Diabetes* **2016**, *65*, 755–767. [CrossRef]

76. Lenoir, O.; Jasiek, M.; Henique, C.; Guyonnet, L.; Hartleben, B.; Bork, T.; Chipont, A.; Flosseau, K.; Bensaada, I.; Schmitt, A.; et al. Endothelial cell and podocyte autophagy synergistically protect from diabetes-induced glomerulosclerosis. *Autophagy* **2015**, *11*, 1130–1145. [CrossRef] [PubMed]
77. Liu, N.; Xu, L.; Shi, Y.; Zhuang, S. Podocyte autophagy: A potential therapeutic target to prevent the progression of diabetic nephropathy. *J. Diabetes Res.* **2017**, *2017*, 3560238. [CrossRef] [PubMed]
78. Ma, T.; Zhu, J.; Chen, X.; Zha, D.; Singhal, P.C.; Ding, G. High glucose induces autophagy in podocytes. *Exp. Cell Res.* **2013**, *319*, 779–789. [CrossRef]
79. Ding, Y.; Kim, J.K.; Kim, S.I.; Na, H.J.; Jun, S.Y.; Lee, S.J.; Choi, M.E. TGF-β1 protects against mesangial cell apoptosis via induction of autophagy. *J. Biol. Chem.* **2010**, *285*, 37909–37919. [CrossRef]
80. Yasuda-Yamahara, M.; Kume, S.; Tagawa, A.; Maegawa, H.; Uzu, T. Emerging role of podocyte autophagy in the progression of diabetic nephropathy. *Autophagy* **2015**, *11*, 2385–2386. [CrossRef]
81. Ding, Y.; Choi, M.E. Autophagy in diabetic nephropathy. *J. Endocrinol.* **2015**, *224*, R15–R30. [CrossRef]
82. Yamahara, K.; Kume, S.; Koya, D.; Tanaka, Y.; Morita, Y.; Chin-Kanasaki, M.; Araki, H.; Isshiki, K.; Araki, S.; Haneda, M.; et al. Obesity-mediated autophagy insufficiency exacerbates proteinuria-induced tubulointerstitial lesions. *J. Am. Soc. Nephrol.* **2013**, *24*, 1769–1781. [CrossRef] [PubMed]
83. Macisaac, R.J.; Ekinci, E.I.; Jerums, G. Markers of and risk factors for the development and progression of diabetic kidney disease. *Am. J. Kidney Dis.* **2014**, *63*, S39–S62. [CrossRef] [PubMed]
84. Sasagawa, T.; Suzuki, K.; Shiota, T.; Kondo, T.; Okita, M. The significance of plasma lysophospholipids in patients with renal failure on hemodialysis. *J. Nutr. Sci. Vitaminol.* **1998**, *44*, 809–818. [CrossRef] [PubMed]
85. Grove, K.J.; Voziyan, P.A.; Spraggins, J.M.; Wang, S.; Paueksakon, P.; Harris, R.C.; Hudson, B.G.; Caprioli, R.M. Diabetic nephropathy induces alterations in the glomerular and tubule lipid profiles. *J. Lipid Res.* **2014**, *55*, 1375–1385. [CrossRef] [PubMed]
86. Sakai, N.; Chun, J.; Duffield, J.S.; Lagares, D.; Wada, T.; Luster, A.D.; Tager, A.M. Lysophosphatidic acid signaling through its receptor initiates profibrotic epithelial cell fibroblast communication mediated by epithelial cell derived connective tissue growth factor. *Kidney Int.* **2017**, *91*, 628–641. [CrossRef] [PubMed]
87. Zhang, Z.H.; Chen, H.; Vaziri, N.D.; Mao, J.R.; Zhang, L.; Bai, X.; Zhao, Y.Y. Metabolomic signatures of chronic kidney disease of diverse etiologies in the rats and humans. *J. Proteome Res.* **2016**, *15*, 3802–3812. [CrossRef] [PubMed]
88. Saulnier-Blache, J.S.; Feigerlova, E.; Halimi, J.M.; Gourdy, P.; Roussel, R.; Guerci, B.; Dupuy, A.; Bertrand-Michel, J.; Bascands, J.L.; Hadjadj, S.; et al. Urinary lysophopholipids are increased in diabetic patients with nephropathy. *J. Diabetes Its Complicat.* **2017**, *31*, 1103–1108. [CrossRef]
89. Michalczyk, A.; Dolegowska, B.; Heryc, R.; Chlubek, D.; Safranow, K. Associations between plasma lysophospholipids concentrations, chronic kidney disease and the type of renal replacement therapy. *Lipids Health Dis.* **2019**, *18*, 85. [CrossRef]
90. Mirzoyan, K.; Baiotto, A.; Dupuy, A.; Marsal, D.; Denis, C.; Vinel, C.; Sicard, P.; Bertrand-Michel, J.; Bascands, J.L.; Schanstra, J.P.; et al. Increased urinary lysophosphatidic acid in mouse with subtotal nephrectomy: Potential involvement in chronic kidney disease. *J. Phys. Biochem.* **2016**, *72*, 803–812. [CrossRef]
91. Li, H.Y.; Oh, Y.S.; Choi, J.W.; Jung, J.Y.; Jun, H.S. Blocking lysophosphatidic acid receptor 1 signaling inhibits diabetic nephropathy in db/db mice. *Kidney Int.* **2017**, *91*, 1362–1373. [CrossRef]
92. Zhang, M.Z.; Wang, X.; Yang, H.; Fogo, A.B.; Murphy, B.J.; Kaltenbach, R.; Cheng, P.; Zinker, B.; Harris, R.C. Lysophosphatidic acid receptor antagonism protects against diabetic nephropathy in a type 2 diabetic model. *J. Am. Soc. Nephrol.* **2017**, *28*, 3300–3311. [CrossRef] [PubMed]
93. Lee, J.H.; Sarker, M.K.; Choi, H.; Shin, D.; Kim, D.; Jun, H.S. Lysophosphatidic acid receptor 1 inhibitor, am095, attenuates diabetic nephropathy in mice by downregulation of TLR4/NF-κB signaling and NADPH oxidase. *Biochim. Biophys. Acta. Mol. Basis Dis.* **2019**, *1865*, 1332–1340. [CrossRef] [PubMed]
94. Diao, H.; Aplin, J.D.; Xiao, S.; Chun, J.; Li, Z.; Chen, S.; Ye, X. Altered spatiotemporal expression of collagen types i, iii, iv, and vi in LPAR3-deficient peri-implantation mouse uterus. *Biol. Reprod.* **2011**, *84*, 255–265. [CrossRef] [PubMed]
95. Canaud, G.; Bienaime, F.; Viau, A.; Treins, C.; Baron, W.; Nguyen, C.; Burtin, M.; Berissi, S.; Giannakakis, K.; Muda, A.O.; et al. Akt2 is essential to maintain podocyte viability and function during chronic kidney disease. *Nat. Med.* **2013**, *19*, 1288–1296. [CrossRef] [PubMed]

96. Kim, D.; Li, H.Y.; Lee, J.H.; Oh, Y.S.; Jun, H.S. Lysophosphatidic acid increases mesangial cell proliferation in models of diabetic nephropathy via RAC1/MAPK/KLF5 signaling. *Exp. Mol. Med.* **2019**, *51*, 18. [CrossRef] [PubMed]
97. Guo, L.; He, P.; No, Y.R.; Yun, C.C. Kruppel-like factor 5 incorporates into the β-catenin/TCF complex in response to LPA in colon cancer cells. *Cell. Signal.* **2015**, *27*, 961–968. [CrossRef] [PubMed]
98. Lin, X.; Zha, Y.; Zeng, X.Z.; Dong, R.; Wang, Q.H.; Wang, D.T. Role of the wnt/β-catenin signaling pathway in inducing apoptosis and renal fibrosis in 5/6-nephrectomized rats. *Mol. Med. Rep.* **2017**, *15*, 3575–3582. [CrossRef] [PubMed]
99. Tan, R.J.; Zhou, D.; Zhou, L.; Liu, Y. Wnt/β-catenin signaling and kidney fibrosis. *Kidney Int. Suppl.* **2014**, *4*, 84–90. [CrossRef]
100. Manigrasso, M.B.; Juranek, J.; Ramasamy, R.; Schmidt, A.M. Unlocking the biology of rage in diabetic microvascular complications. *Trends Endocrinol. Metab.* **2014**, *25*, 15–22. [CrossRef]
101. Zaslavsky, A.; Singh, L.S.; Tan, H.; Ding, H.; Liang, Z.; Xu, Y. Homo- and hetero-dimerization of LPA/S1P receptors, OGR1 and GPR4. *Biochimi. Biophys. Acta* **2006**, *1761*, 1200–1212. [CrossRef]
102. Yaghobian, D.; Don, A.S.; Yaghobian, S.; Chen, X.; Pollock, C.A.; Saad, S. Increased sphingosine 1-phosphate mediates inflammation and fibrosis in tubular injury in diabetic nephropathy. *Clin. Exp. Pharmacol. Physiol.* **2016**, *43*, 56–66. [CrossRef] [PubMed]
103. Ishizawa, S.; Takahashi-Fujigasaki, J.; Kanazawa, Y.; Matoba, K.; Kawanami, D.; Yokota, T.; Iwamoto, T.; Tajima, N.; Manome, Y.; Utsunomiya, K. Sphingosine-1-phosphate induces differentiation of cultured renal tubular epithelial cells under rho kinase activation via the S1P2 receptor. *Clin. Exp. Nephrol.* **2014**, *18*, 844–852. [CrossRef] [PubMed]
104. Huang, K.; Liu, W.; Lan, T.; Xie, X.; Peng, J.; Huang, J.; Wang, S.; Shen, X.; Liu, P.; Huang, H. Berberine reduces fibronectin expression by suppressing the S1P-S1P2 receptor pathway in experimental diabetic nephropathy models. *PLoS ONE* **2012**, *7*, e43874. [CrossRef]
105. Hutter, S.; van Haaften, W.T.; Hunerwadel, A.; Baebler, K.; Herfarth, N.; Raselli, T.; Mamie, C.; Misselwitz, B.; Rogler, G.; Weder, B.; et al. Intestinal activation of ph-sensing receptor OGR1 [GPR68] contributes to fibrogenesis. *J. Crohn Colitis* **2018**, *12*, 1348–1358. [CrossRef] [PubMed]
106. Colin-Santana, C.C.; Avendano-Vazquez, S.E.; Alcantara-Hernandez, R.; Garcia-Sainz, J.A. Egf and angiotensin ii modulate lysophosphatidic acid LPA(1) receptor function and phosphorylation state. *Biochim. Biophys. Acta* **2011**, *1810*, 1170–1177. [CrossRef] [PubMed]
107. Xu, K.; Ma, L.; Li, Y.; Wang, F.; Zheng, G.Y.; Sun, Z.; Jiang, F.; Chen, Y.; Liu, H.; Dang, A.; et al. Genetic and functional evidence supports lpar1 as a susceptibility gene for hypertension. *Hypertension* **2015**, *66*, 641–646. [CrossRef]

No Cytotoxic and Inflammatory Effects of Empagliflozin and Dapagliflozin on Primary Renal Proximal Tubular Epithelial Cells under Diabetic Conditions In Vitro

Patrick C. Baer [1,*], Benjamin Koch [1], Janina Freitag [1], Ralf Schubert [2] and Helmut Geiger [1]

1 Division of Nephrology, Department of Internal Medicine III, University Hospital, Goethe-University, 60596 Frankfurt/M., Germany; b.koch@med.uni-frankfurt.de (B.K.); janinafreitag@gmx.net (J.F.); h.geiger@em.uni-frankfurt.de (H.G.)

2 Division of Allergology, Pneumology and Cystic Fibrosis, Department for Children and Adolescents, University Hospital, Goethe-University, 60596 Frankfurt/M., Germany; ralf.schubert@kgu.de

* Correspondence: patrick.baer@kgu.de or p.baer@em.uni-frankfurt.de

Abstract: Gliflozins are inhibitors of the renal proximal tubular sodium-glucose co-transporter-2 (SGLT-2), that inhibit reabsorption of urinary glucose and they are able to reduce hyperglycemia in patients with type 2 diabetes. A renoprotective function of gliflozins has been proven in diabetic nephropathy, but harmful side effects on the kidney have also been described. In the current project, primary highly purified human renal proximal tubular epithelial cells (PTCs) have been shown to express functional SGLT-2, and were used as an in vitro model to study possible cellular damage induced by two therapeutically used gliflozins: empagliflozin and dapagliflozin. Cell viability, proliferation, and cytotoxicity assays revealed that neither empagliflozin nor dapagliflozin induce effects in PTCs cultured in a hyperglycemic environment, or in co-medication with ramipril or hydro-chloro-thiazide. Oxidative stress was significantly lowered by dapagliflozin but not by empagliflozin. No effect of either inhibitor could be detected on mRNA and protein expression of the pro-inflammatory cytokine interleukin-6 and the renal injury markers KIM-1 and NGAL. In conclusion, empa- and dapagliflozin in therapeutic concentrations were shown to induce no direct cell injury in cultured primary renal PTCs in hyperglycemic conditions.

Keywords: renal tubular cells; epithelial cells; proximal tubule; cytotoxicity; injury; inflammation; empagliflozin; dapagliflozin; kidney

---

1. Introduction

Over 90% of the filtered glucose in the kidney is reabsorbed by the sodium-glucose co-transporter 2 (SGLT-2) expressed in the apical brush border membrane of tubular epithelial cells [1,2]. Inhibition of SGLT-2 blocks the reabsorption of glomerularly filtered glucose (and sodium) in the ensuing proximal S1/S2 segment, a mechanism that has been exploited to reduce hyperglycemia in patients with type 2 diabetes mellitus [1]. Based on the selective inhibition of SGLT-2, gliflozins increase urinary glucose excretion by reducing the reabsorption into the bloodstream. Gliflozins are a class of antidiabetic drugs used to lower glucose in type 2 diabetes mellitus [3,4]. The mechanism of action is independent of endogenous insulin and shows a very low risk of hypoglycemia. In the last few years, the renoprotective function of gliflozins has been described in diabetic nephropathy, which affects approximately 40% of patients with diabetes and is a leading cause of chronic kidney disease worldwide. SGLT2 inhibition has been described as reducing inflammation and attenuating the progression of diabetic nephropathy [4].

As the first active substance, the European Medicines Agency granted marketing authorization for dapagliflozin in 2012. Empagliflozin and ertugliflozin have also been approved; in the meantime, canagliflozin has been taken off the market in Germany. Other substances are in advanced clinical trials or are approved in the United States. The pleiotropic effects of SGLT2 inhibitors have the potential to generate benefits beyond the inhibition of glucose reuptake, and there is increasing evidence that gliflozins may reduce the risk of progression of renal impairment in diabetic patients [5]. It has been shown that in patients with type 2 diabetes and kidney disease, the risk of kidney failure and cardiovascular events was lower in the canagliflozin group than in the placebo group [6]. A post-hoc analysis from recent published trial revealed the risk of AKI may be lower under SGLT2 inhibition [7]. In another study of patients with diabetes, initiation of SGLT2 inhibitor therapy has been shown to be associated with a slower rate of kidney function decline and lower risk of major kidney events compared with initiation of other glucose-lowering drugs [8]. Although current evidence supports their safety, additional efforts are needed to elucidate the long-term impact of these compounds on chronic kidney disease, mineral metabolism, and bone health. Indeed, the limited study follow-up precludes a definitive answer on the impact of gliflozins (e.g., on electrolyte and mineral metabolism changes), especially in high-risk subgroups of patients [9]. The findings of ongoing and future clinical trials will help shed further light on the role of gliflozins in the long-term protection of renal function.

Nevertheless, despite overall good clinical tolerability [10], harmful effects also can occur during daily gliflozin intake. Reported adverse events are especially acute kidney injury (AKI) [11,12], acute tubular necrosis [13], genital infections, and bone fractures [3]. Although current evidence supports their safety, additional efforts are needed to elucidate the long-term impact of these compounds on chronic kidney disease, mineral metabolism, and bone health. Indeed, the limited follow-up studies and the heterogeneity of the case-mix of different randomized controlled trials preclude a definitive answer on the impact of these compounds on long-term outcomes such as the risk of bone fracture.

The US Food and Drug Administration (FDA) issued a warning in June 2016 covering the increased risk of AKI following the use of gliflozins [14]. A total of 101 cases were reported between March 2013 and October 2015, but a much higher number is expected worldwide. The FDA warning was based on data suggesting a link between the development of AKI and two approved gliflozins [3]. In this alert, patients with diabetes and heart failure, chronic renal insufficiency, and/or decreased circulating blood volume were included in the risk group. The risk is potentiated by the additional intake of ACE inhibitors, diuretics, and/or nonsteroidal anti-inflammatory drugs, warned the FDA. In November 2019, the German Drug Commission concluded that treatment with gliflozins should be stopped if patients are hospitalized due to major surgery or acute serious illness [15]. However, despite these relevant safety issues, the points are still under investigation and no firm conclusion can be currently drawn.

Possible pathophysiologic mechanisms of AKI induced by SGLT-2 inhibitors have been highlighted recently [16]. Osmotic diuresis can lead to volume depletion, while uricosuria as a consequence of increased glucose–uric acid exchange in the proximal tubule, has the potential of direct tubular damage through crystal formation. High glucose concentrations in renal tubules may lead to altered fructose metabolism in proximal tubular cells and, thus, to local cytotoxicity and tubular injury from increased oxidative stress and the release of inflammatory molecules [16]. Summing up all current data, it can be concluded that a very detailed study of why some patients on gliflozin therapy develop acute renal failure, but not others, and details about the underlying cellular pathomechanisms in the kidney are needed urgently. To date, there is only speculation about the exact pathomechanisms of the renal side effect of gliflozins. No clear investigations have been published to elucidate these mechanisms.

In this project, highly purified and cultured human renal proximal tubular epithelial cells (PTCs) were used as an in vitro model to study the cellular damage of gliflozins. This is the first study using primary highly differentiated PTCs to investigate possible effects of two gliflozins: empa- and dapagliflozin. As PTCs are the direct site of action for SGLT2 inhibitors, a simulation of different environmental variables, such as high glucose, or combinations with other drugs were used to investigate the influence on the renal tubule system in the in vitro model and possibly to simulate the conditions in the human nephron.

2. Results

2.1. Characterization of SGLT-2 Expression and Function in PTCs

Immunofluorescence staining clearly showed the expression of SGLT-2 in the apical membrane of cells of the proximal tubule in situ (Figure 1A) and PTCS in vitro (Figure 1C). The staining of human renal sections showed that SGLT-2 is exclusively expressed in the apical brush border membrane of tubular epithelial cells.

Cultured PTCs displayed an epithelial morphology with a highly compact cell monolayer (Figure 1B). The expression of SGLT2 mRNA and protein in cultured PTCs was also proven by standard PCR analysis (Figure 1D) and western blotting (Figure 1E). The RNA and protein isolated from human kidneys (renal extracts) were used as positive controls in both verifications (Figure 1D,E).

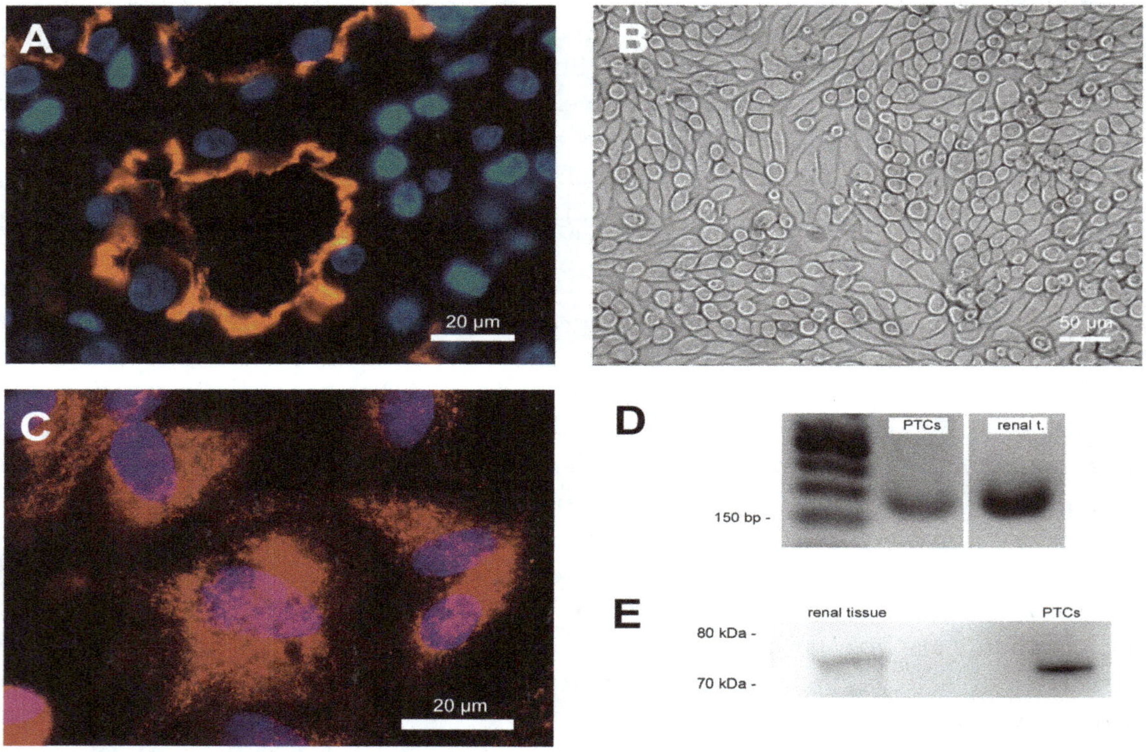

Figure 1. Cell characterization. (**A**) Immunofluorescence staining of human renal paraffin-embedded tissue sections showing sodium-glucose co-transporter 2 (SGLT-2) expression on the apical cell membrane in the proximal tubular nephron. Nuclei were counterstained with 4,6-diamino-2-phenylindole (DAPI; blue). (**B**) Characteristic phase contrast microscopy of confluent PTCs cultured in standard cell culture. (**C**) Immunofluorescence staining of SGLT-2 expression in cultured PTCs. Nuclei were counterstained with DAPI (blue). (**D**) Proof of SGLT-2 mRNA expression in cultured PTCs and RNA from human renal tissue extracts using PCR. (**E**) Proof of SGLT-2 protein expression in cultured PTCs and protein from human renal tissue extracts using western blotting.

As a functional assay, the glucose uptake was evaluated using the fluorescent glucose analog NBDG-2. Loading of NBDG-2 into PTCs was shown by the measurement of unloaded cells as a negative control. The SGLT2-mediated NBDG-2 influx from the cell culture medium into the cells was sensitive to inhibition by the SGLT inhibitors in a dose-dependent manner (Figure 2). Incubation of PTC with 10 nM empa- or dapagliflozin had no inhibitory effect on the glucose uptake of PTCs. The

NBDG-2 assay confirms the activity of the sodium-glucose co-transporter in cultured PTCs and the inhibitory effect of the gliflozins.

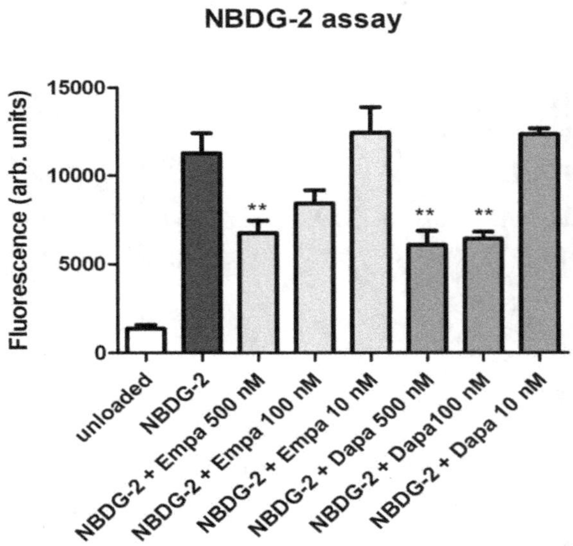

Figure 2. Functional assay. NBDG-2, a fluorescent glucose analog, was used to monitor glucose uptake in cultured PTCs. NBDG-2 was added either alone or with decreasing concentrations of gliflozins (500, 100, 10 nM) for 60 min at 37 °C. Cells incubated in buffer without NBDG-2 were used as background controls (unloaded). Fluorescence was measured using a fluorescence reader with excitation and emission wavelengths of 485 and 538 nm (arbitrary units, mean ± standard deviation (SD), $n = 4$, ** $p<0.01$ versus NBDG-2).

2.2. Cell Viability, Proliferation, and Cytotoxicity Assays

We used two viability assays using calcein-acetoxymthyl (calcein-AM) and XTT to investigate the effects of empa- and dapagliflozin on PTCs viability. Calcein-AM is a cell-permeant non-fluorescent dye, which is exclusively in viable cells converted into calcein, a dye with intense green fluorescence. The XTT assay is a colorimetric assay used to estimate the metabolic activity of viable cells.

Both assays demonstrated that empa- and dapagliflozin induce no cytotoxic effects on cultured PTCs. Depending on the experiment, media were additionally supplemented by a combination of empa- or dapagliflozin with ramipril or hydro-chloro-thiazide (HCT). Nevertheless, no statistically significant difference could be detected compared to the control (high glucose medium: HG) either with the calcein assay (Figure 3A) or the XTT assay (Figure 3B). In addition, we used different internal negative controls within the two assays. In the calcein assay, we used a mixture of cytokines which significantly reduced the viability of PTCs over the incubation period (43.5 ± 8.4% versus HG (=100%)) (Figure 3A). For the XTT, we used a low glucose medium 199 (LG) as a control. Incubation in LG resulted in a reduced metabolic activity, due to reduced cell proliferation (72.2 ± 5.5% versus HG (=100%)) (Figure 3B).

In addition, both a proliferation and a cytotoxicity assay were used to detect further effects of empa- and dapagliflozin on PTCs. The fluorometric assay with 4,6-diamino-2-phenylindole (DAPI), measuring the DNA content as an indirect determination of cell number and proliferation, verified that both gliflozins had no influence on cell proliferation. Furthermore, the combinations with ramipril or HCT also showed no effects on cell proliferation, whereas the negative control (LG) reduced proliferation of PTCs significantly (77.8 ± 2.5% versus HG (=100%)) (Figure 4A). Cytotoxic effects, measured by quantification of lactate dehydrogenase (LDH) in the supernatant of PTCs after incubation in gliflozin-containing media or co-medications, were also not detectable (Figure 4B). Only the incubation with the cytomix induced a significant increase in LDH activity in the supernatant (148.3 ± 16.7% versus HG (=100%)) (Figure 4B).

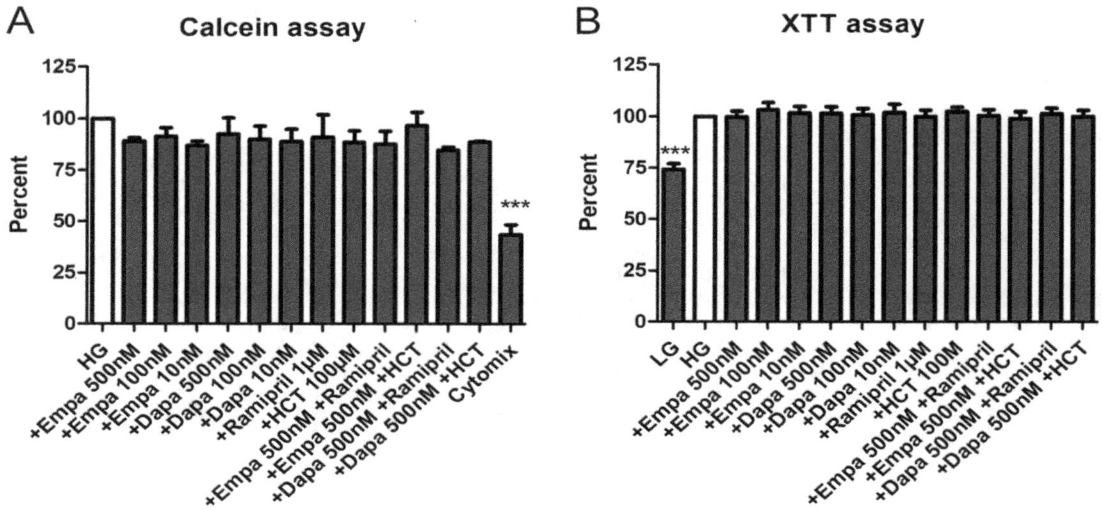

Figure 3. Cell viability assays. The PTCs cultured in 96-well plates were incubated for 6 d in media containing empa- or dapagliflozin and co-medications. No significant effects of the different pretreatments on the cell viability were detected. (**A**) Calcein assay. After loading with calcein-AM for 1h, fluorescence was measured immediately using a fluorescence reader (ex 485 nm, em 538 nm, arbitrary units, calculated as percent in relation to the control (high glucose medium: HG), mean ± SD, $n = 5$). Cells incubated with a mixture of cytokines (Cytomix) were used as a negative control (*** $p < 0.001$). (**B**) XTT assay. The XTT assay was performed and optical density (OD) was measured in a microplate reader at 490 vs. 650 nm (arbitrary units, calculated as percent in relation to the control (HG), mean ± SD, $n = 4$). Cells cultured in low glucose medium 199 (LG) were used as a negative control (*** $p < 0.001$).

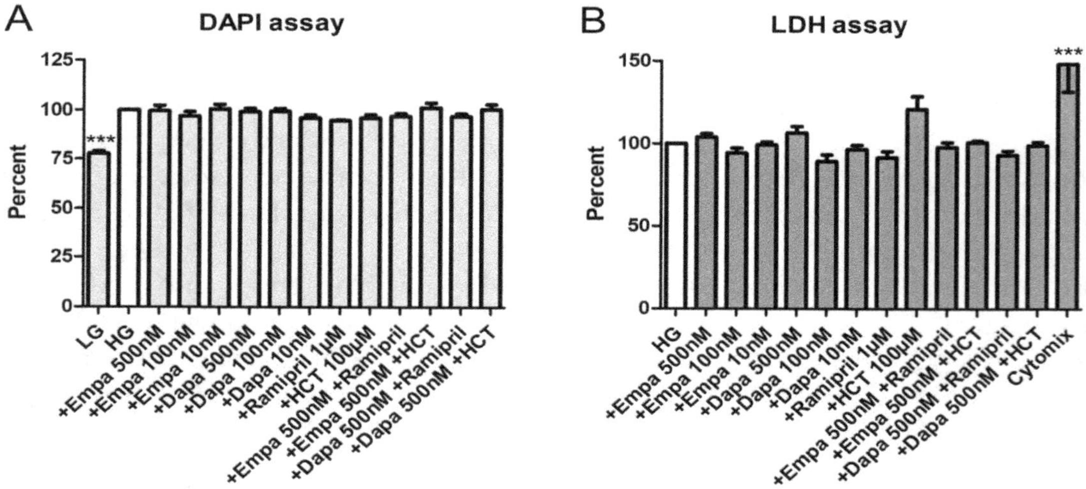

Figure 4. Cell proliferation and cytotoxicity assays. (**A**) DAPI assay. The assay was used to measure the DNA content as an indirect determination of cell number and proliferation [17]. Fluorescence was measured using a fluorescence reader (ex 355 nm, em 460 nm, arbitrary units, calculated as percent in relation to the control (HG), mean ± SD, $n = 4$). Cells cultured in LG were used as a negative control. (**B**) Lactate dehydrogenase (LDH) assay. The measurement of LDH activity released from the cytosol of damaged cells into the supernatant was used for the quantification of cell death and cell lysis. Absorbance was measured in a microplate reader (490 vs. 650 nm, arbitrary units, calculated as percent in relation to the control (HG), mean ± SD, $n = 4$–6). A mixture of pro-inflammatory cytokines was used as a positive control (*** $p < 0.001$).

2.3. *Measurement of Oxidative Stress and Tubular Injury Markers*

Formation of intracellular oxidative stress was proven using fluorescence measurements of intracellular 2′,7′-dichlorofluorescein (DCF). Incubation of PTCs in HG increased oxidative stress levels in a significant manner. Addition of empagliflozin (500 nM) to HG could not reduce the oxidative stress level (Figure 5). By contrast, oxidative stress generation evoked by high glucose exposure was significantly suppressed by the treatment with dapagliflozin (500 nM). We further checked the effect of H_2O_2 (250 μM) after loading for establishment of the DCF measurements, resulting in a maximum signal (positive control, data not shown). Unloaded cells were used as negative controls and compared with cells after DCF loading (data not shown).

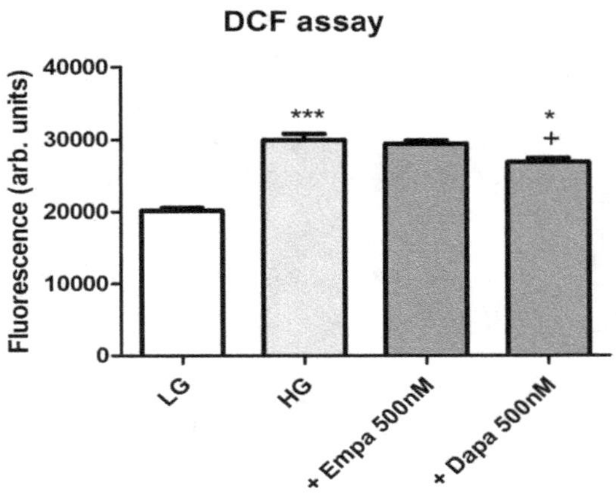

Figure 5. Formation of oxidative stress under diabetic culture conditions. Confluent PTCs in 96-well plates were cultured in LG, HG or with gliflozins (500 nM) for 6 d. Then, 2′,7′-dichlorodihydrofluorescein diacetate (20 μM in Hank's buffered saline solution) was added for 30 min at 37 °C. Fluorescence of intracellular DCF was measured using a fluorescence reader with excitation and emission wavelengths of 485 and 538 nm (arbitrary units, mean ± SD, $n = 6$, *** $p < 0.001$ vs. LG, + $p < 0.05$ vs. HG, * $p < 0.05$ vs. Empa 500 nM).

We further studied the role of SGLT2 inhibition in the induction and release of pro-inflammatory and injury markers. Firstly, we checked the mRNA levels of the pro-inflammatory cytokine interleukin-6 (IL-6) and two renal tubular injury markers (kidney injury molecule-1 (KIM-1), and neutrophil gelatinase-associated lipocalin (NGAL)) after 24 h incubation in HG with gliflozins. As shown in Figure 6, neither empagliflozin nor dapagliflozin influenced the mRNA expression of all three readouts. Comparison between LG and HG showed an induction of IL-6 and NGAL mRNA after incubation for 24 h, but not of KIM-1 (data not shown). Stimulation with a mixture of cytokines was used as a positive control. The cytomix induced a significant induction of IL-6 and NGAL mRNA but not KIM-1 mRNA expression (Figure 6).

We then checked the release of all three molecules in the supernatant of PTCs (Figure 7). At the protein level, IL-6 is constitutively released by PTCs cultured in HG (11.9 ± 1.7 ng/mL; mean ± SD, $n = 6$). When the cells were incubated with gliflozins, no significant effect on the release of IL-6 protein was detected. Incubation in the presence of the cytomix increased the release of IL-6 protein significantly (417 ± 117 %, calculated as percent in relation to the control (HG), $n = 6$). In addition, we also found no effect of empa- or dapagliflozin on the release of KIM-1 and NGAL. The cytomix induced the release of NGAL protein in a significant manner (269 ± 57 %, $n = 4$), whereas release of KIM-1 was not increased. At the protein level, KIM-1 and NGAL are also constitutively released by PTCs cultured in HG (11.6 ± 2.1 ng/mL and 115.7 ± 26.2 ng/mL, respectively; mean ± SD, $n = 4$).

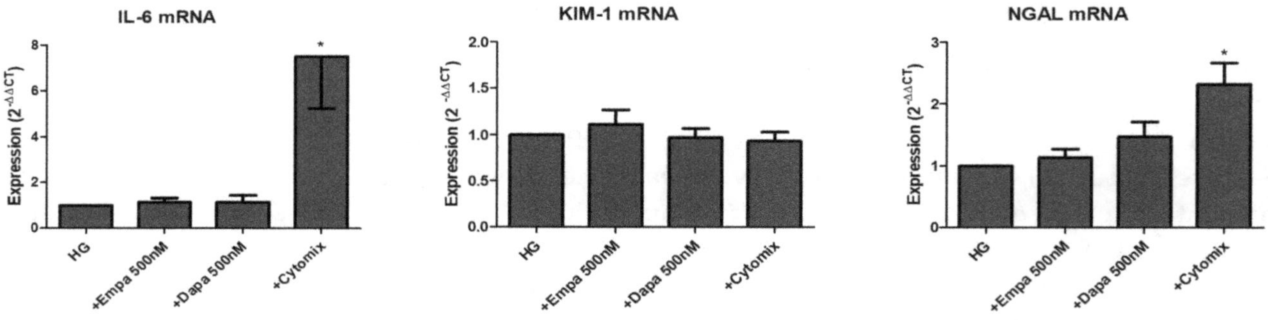

Figure 6. Effect of empagliflozin and dapagliflozin on mRNA expression of selected factors. Cells were grown in small culture flasks until confluence, serum depleted for 2 h and stimulated in HG for 24 h. The expression levels in each experiment were normalized to a housekeeping gene (β-actin) and are expressed relative to the control using the ΔΔCT method. A mixture of pro-inflammatory cytokines (cytomix) was used as a control, whereas only IL-6 mRNA was significantly increased after incubation with the cytomix (* $p < 0.05$ versus HG; IL-6 and NGAL $n = 6$; KIM-1 $n = 7$).

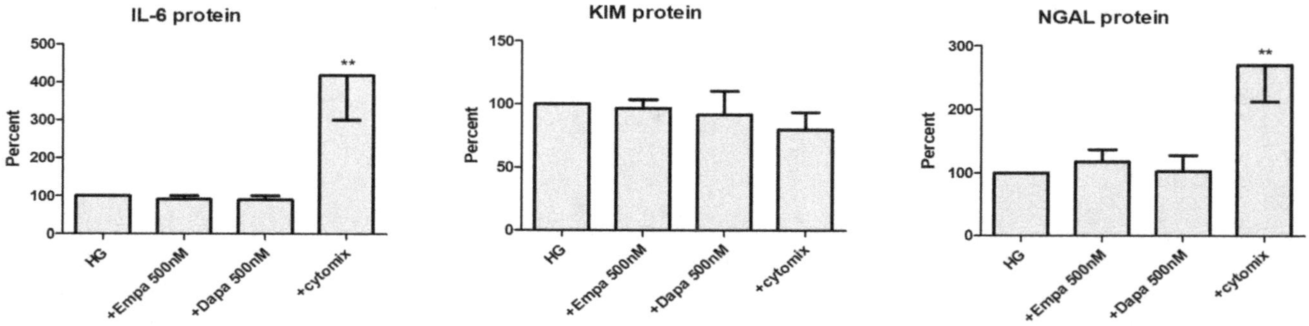

Figure 7. Effect of empagliflozin and dapagliflozin on the release of pro-inflammatory and injury proteins. Cells were grown in a 24-well plate until confluence, serum depleted for 2 h and stimulated in HG for 48 h. Supernatants were then harvested and quantified using commercially available immunoassays (optical density 450/620 nm, calculated as percent in relation to the control (HG), mean ± SD). A mixture of pro-inflammatory cytokines (cytomix) was used as a positive control. (** $p < 0.01$ versus HG, IL-6 $n = 6$, KIM-1 and NGAL $n = 4$).

3. Discussion

Gliflozins are the latest class of hypoglycemic agents for the treatment of diabetes mellitus type 2 and have a unique mechanism of lowering glucose by the inhibition of renal proximal tubular sodium-glucose co-transporter-2. SGLT-2 inhibitors have been shown to increase urinary glucose excretion and decrease serum glucose and HbA1c. In addition, compared to other topical antidiabetic medications, gliflozin intake can also reduce body weight. The drug group is further attributed to an improvement in hypertension, a reduction in cardiovascular mortality risk, and multiple effects on the kidney. Nevertheless, despite good overall clinical tolerability, several harmful effects have been published related to daily intake. Caution is still advised regarding possible adverse events described such as AKI and acute tubular necrosis [3,13]. Under certain circumstances—possibly dehydration of the patient, low blood pressure, or certain co-medications—gliflozin may damage the organ. Currently, however, there is only speculation about the exact pathomechanisms of the renal side effects [16]. No clear investigations have been published to elucidate these mechanisms. The influence of osmotic pressure and the development of excess uric acid on the function of tubular epithelial cells in the nephron might be involved in this context [18]. Increased osmotic pressure (hyperosmolarity) in the tubular system may activate the polyol pathway in epithelial cells [19], leading to osmotic damage via the accumulation of sorbitol and the formation of oxidative stress with cellular damage, inflammation, and pathological tissue change [20,21]. The main site of action of SGLT-2 inhibition raises the question whether inhibition of the transporter induces direct cytotoxic or inflammatory effects on renal proximal tubular epithelial cells.

In the current study, we focus on the effects of two currently available gliflozins on renal proximal tubular epithelial cells. For the first time, we examined the cytotoxic and inflammatory effects of empa- and dapagliflozin on primary and highly differentiated PTCs under diabetic conditions in vitro. High levels of circulating glucose and inflammation are the main causes of tissue damage in diabetes mellitus by inducing cell injury and high levels of oxidative stress in the kidney [22]. In this case, it should also be mentioned that diabetes itself is a systemic pro-inflammatory condition, involving not only the kidney, but also the cardiovascular system and bone [23,24].

Several in vitro studies using immortalized human tubular epithelial cells (e.g., HK2 cell line) [25–28], murine tubular epithelial cells [29] or non-renal cells [30,31] investigated either the effects of empa- or of dapagliflozin. Some of them have shown that SGLT2 inhibition reduced the release of inflammatory or fibrotic factors induced by high glucose levels [25–27], others found effects on oxidative stress responses [26,30,31]. Our current study looked at whether high glucose induced changes were influenced by either of the two gliflozins. Whereas we found no effect on cell viability, proliferation, and cytotoxicity, a significant reduction in the oxidative stress was found after incubation with dapagliflozin. Chen and co-workers also demonstrated decreased reactive oxidative species after incubation with dapagliflozin in a fructose-induced diabetic milieu [31]. Others investigated the subcellular mechanisms underlying the protective effects of empagliflozin from high glucose-mediated injuries on HK-2 cells [26]. As oxidative stress plays pathologic roles in diabetic kidneys [32] and empagliflozin may reduce this effect [33], the authors analyzed the effects of empagliflozin and described the protection of HK-2 cells from high glucose-mediated injuries through a mitochondrial mechanism.

In addition, a series of in vitro cytotoxicological investigations were conducted to evaluate a mode of action for gliflozin-associated effects. In addition to the in vitro studies, the effects of gliflozins on the kidney were also assessed in several in vivo studies and in clinical trials (currently reviewed by Ninčević and co-workers [34]), which should not be discussed here. Cytotoxicity and inflammation mediated by high glucose is directly responsible for pathological changes in diabetic nephropathy [35]. The in vitro data presented by Smith and co-workers demonstrated no genotoxic, cytotoxic, or mitogenic role for empagliflozin. However, the data indicate that an oxidative metabolite of empagliflozin is cytotoxic to renal tubular cells, but is not genotoxic [29]. Others described a canagliflozin-induced cytotoxicity at particularly low concentrations in proliferating immortalized tubular epithelial cells in vitro [36]. We also checked the influence of often used co-medications, such as ramipril or HCT, on the cytotoxicity and viability of PTCs. Co-incubation of gliflozins with either ramipril, clinically used to lower hypertension via inhibition of the renal angiotensin-converting enzyme, or HCT, clinically used as diuretic medication, did not induce significant effects on PTCs. We did not check the co-medications by PCR and enzyme-linked immunosorbent assay (EIA) due the negative results of the cytotoxicity and viability assays (and also to the low availability of primary isolated PTCs). Measurement of the inflammatory marker (IL-6) and two injury markers (KIM-1 and NGAL) showed that the gliflozins did not influence their expression in vitro. In contrast to our study, other have shown that SGLT-2 inhibition with empagliflozin reduces high glucose-induced IL-6 release in HK-2 cells [27]. Dekkers and co-workers further described in a post-hoc analysis of a clinical trial that dapagliflozin decreased urinary KIM-1 and IL-6 excretion, suggesting that dapagliflozin may beneficially affect renal inflammation and reduces tubular cell injury [37].

In summary, our current study describes the expression and function of SGLT-2 on primary, highly differentiated PTCs and investigated the effects of SGLT-2 inhibition using two gliflozins: empa- and dapagliflozin. Cell viability, proliferation and cytotoxicity assays revealed that neither empagliflozin nor dapagliflozin induces effects in PTCs cultured in diabetic medium, or co-medication with ramipril or HCT. Oxidative stress was significantly lowered by dapagliflozin but not empagliflozin. No effect of either inhibitor could be detected on the mRNA and protein expression of inflammatory or injury markers. In conclusion, empa- and dapagliflozin in therapeutic concentrations (C_{max} 500 nM) induce no direct cell injury in cultured primary renal proximal tubular cells. Nevertheless, further future studies are needed to investigate potential specific factors leading to tubular injury. First, the effects of incubation in high concentrations of fructose and in hyperosmotic media, both in the presence of gliflozins and high glucose media, should be investigated. High fructose, in vivo generated due to consumption of high fructose dietary products, may also affect tubular epithelial cells [38]. Dietary fructose has been shown to cause tubular injury in vitro and in vivo [21,39]. In addition, an increment in osmotic pressure, generated in vivo by dehydration, may cause activation of the polyol pathway also leading in the accumulation of fructose [16,20]. On the other hand, high concentrations of uric acid could be another factor involved [18], whereas it has been shown that canagliflozin therapy decreased serum uric acid in patients with type 2 diabetes [40]. Finally, the in vitro effects of supratherapeutic gliflozin concentrations that may mimic the accumulation of the drug in conditions of renal failure in vivo should also be investigated in future studies.

4. Materials and Methods

4.1. Isolation and Culture of Primary Human Renal Proximal Tubular Epithelial Cells

Human renal tissue was obtained from patients undergoing tumor nephrectomies. The donors gave written informed consent. The study was approved by the ethics committee of the clinic of the Goethe University, Frankfurt (05 Dec 2014, UGO 03/10, Amendment). The ethical standards defined by the World Medical Association Declaration of Helsinki were complied with.

Primary human renal proximal tubular epithelial cells (PTC) were separated as described previously [41]. In brief, cells were isolated after tumor nephrectomies from renal tissue not involved in renal cell carcinoma. The tissue was disintegrated using crossed blades, digested with collagenase/dispase, and passed through a 106 μm mesh. Remaining cohered cells were then incubated with collagenase IV, DNase, and $MgCl_2$ and further purified by a Percoll density gradient centrifugation. The cells were then isolated by a mAb against aminopeptidase M (CD13) and the Mini-MACS system (Miltenyi, Bergisch Gladbach, Germany) to enrich highly purified PTC. Primary isolated PTC were strongly positive for aminopeptidase M (98.6 %). Ultrastructural analysis revealed highly preserved brush border microvilli, a well-developed endocytosis apparatus, and numerous mitochondria [41,42]. Isolated cells were seeded in 6-well plates. Medium 199 (M4530, Sigma-Aldrich, Taufkirchen, Germany) with a physiologic glucose concentration (100 mg/dl) was supplemented with 10% fetal bovine serum (FBS; Biochrom, Berlin, Germany), used as standard culture medium and replaced every three to four days. Confluent cells were passaged by trypsinization. Cells between passages 2 and 5 were used for the experiments.

4.2. Characterization of SGLT-2 Expression

Regarding histological staining, a small portion of human renal tissue normally used for PTC isolation was fixed with 10% formalin at room temperature for 4–6 h. Subsequently, paraffin-embedded tissue sections (4 μm) were dewaxed and rehydrated in xylol, 100, 96, and 70 % ethanol, boiled in TRIS-buffer (10 mM Tris Base, 1 mM EDTA, 0.05 % Tween 20, pH 9.0) for 20 min for antigen retrieval and washed with phosphate-buffered saline (PBS). Samples were blocked with normal goat serum at 37 °C for 30 min and incubated with anti-SGLT-2 (Santa Cruz Biotechnology, Heidelberg, Germany, no. sc-393350, 1:50) overnight at 4 °C. After washing with PBS, a Cy3-conjugated goat-anti-mouse IgG (Jackson Immuno Research, Cambridgeshire, UK, no. 115-165-062; 1:300) was applied for 1 h at 37 °C. Sections were subsequently, mounted in mounting medium and examined using Zeiss fluorescence microscope equipment.

Regarding fluorescence microscopy, PTC cultured on chamber slides was rinsed three times with PBS, and fixed with paraformaldehyde (4%) for 10 min. The fixed cells were washed twice. Unspecific binding sites were blocked by PBS containing 5% normal goat serum for 20 min. Primary antibody anti-SGLT-2 (Santa Cruz Biotechnology, no. sc-393350; 1:50) was applied without washing and incubated for 30 min at 37 °C with gentle shaking. After washing with PBS, cells were incubated with a Cy3-conjugated goat-anti-mouse IgG (1:300) for 30 min at 37 °C. Controls of autofluorescence or non-specific fluorescence were performed on fixed cells processed without the primary antibody. Monolayers were mounted in mounting medium and examined using Zeiss fluorescence microscope equipment.

Proof of SGLT-2 mRNA expression in cultured PTCs was done by PCR analysis (described in Section 4.7). The expression of SGLT-2 protein on PTC was examined using western blotting, as described previously [43]. In brief, the cells were lysed using 10 mM Tris pH 7.4, 0.1% sodium dodecyl sulphate (SDS), 0.1% Tween20, 0.5 % TritonX100, 150 mM NaCl, 10 mM EDTA, 1 M urea, 10 mM NEM, 4 mM benzamidine, and 1 mM PMSF and collected by scraping. After centrifugation, the pellet was suspended in Laemmli's buffer and heated at 95 °C for 5 min prior to electrophoresis on a 10 % SDS polyacrylamide gel. The protein content was determined by a standard assay and an equal volume of protein was loaded into each lane. The separated proteins were transferred electrophoretically to Immobilon transfer membrane (Millipore). Membranes were blocked for 2 h. Immunoblotting was performed by incubating with antibodies against SGLT-2 (resulting in a 73 kDa band; Santa Cruz Biotechnology, no. sc-393350; 1:200), followed by a secondary antibody (horseradish peroxidase-conjugated anti-mouse IgG; DAKO P0447, 1:1000). Protein bands were made visible using the Peqlab Fusion FX system (VWR, Darmstadt, Germany).

4.3. *Stimulations*

Cells were grown in 24- or 96-well culture plates, or small culture flasks (25cm^2) in standard cell culture medium (described in Section 4.1) until confluence. PTCs in selected experiments were grown to subconfluence and used for the assays (as indicated). The cells were then washed and kept in serum-free medium 199 for 2 h and stimulated as indicated in the particular assay. In most assays, LG with 10 % FBS (glucose content 100 mg/dl (5.5 mM)) was used as a negative control. Stimulations were done in HG with 10% FBS (glucose content 450 mg/dl (25 mM)) which induced a diabetic milieu in the cultures. In case of protein measurements in the supernatants (EIA, Section 4.8), stimulations were done in high glucose medium 199 without 10% FBS. For stimulations, empagliflozin (Adipogen, San Diego, CA, USA; no. AG-CR1-3619) was dissolved in dimethylsulfoxide and diluted in medium (500, 100, 10 nM). Dapaglifozin (Cayman Chemical, Ann Arbor, MI, USA; no. 11574) was dissolved in dimethyl sulfoxid and diluted in medium (500, 100, 10 nM). Maximal concentration of both gliflozins (500 nM) is matched to the published maximal therapeutic concentration observed (C_{max}) [44,45]. The interactions of gliflozin with ramipril (Cayman Chemicals, no. 15558; stock solution 1mM in dimethyl sulfoxide) or HCT (Sigma-Aldrich, Taufkirchen, Germany, no. H-4759; stock solution 100mM in dH_2O) were investigated in selected experiments (viability, cytotoxicity, and proliferation assays).

4.4. *Functional Assay*

We used 2-Deoxy-2-[(7-nitro-2,1,3-benzoxadiazol-7-yl)amino]-D-glucose (NBDG-2; Hoelzel Diagnostika, Köln, Germany, no. M6327), a fluorescent glucose analogon for usage in fluorescence measurements [46], to monitor glucose uptake in cultured PTCs. Confluent PTCs in 96-well plates were washed with pre-warmed HBSS. The HBSS containing NBDG-2 (100 µg/mL) either alone or with decreasing concentrations of gliflozins (500, 100, 10 nM) was added for 60 min at 37 °C (in quadruplicate for each biological replicate). Cells incubated in buffer without NBDG-2 were used as background controls. The cells were then washed with HBSS and fluorescence was measured directly using a fluorescence reader (BMG Fluostar, Ortenberg, Germany) with excitation and emission wavelengths of 485 nm and 538 nm, respectively. Data are expressed as arbitrary fluorescence units.

4.5. *Cell Viability, Proliferation, and Cytotoxicity Assays*

The cell viability of PTC was determined by two viability assays, a photometric assay using 2,3-Bis-(2-Methoxy-4-Nitro-5-Sulfophenyl)-2*H*-Tetrazolium-5-Carboxanilide (XTT) and a fluorescence-based assay using calcein-AM (Biolegend, San Diego, CA, USA) to investigate any possible cytotoxic effects, as described previously [43]. In brief, confluent PTCs in 96-well plates were incubated for 6 d in media containing empa- or dapagliflozin and co-medications (in quintuplicate for each biological replicate). The XTT reagent was then added to the wells, as described by the manufacturer (AppliChem, Darmstadt, Germany), and incubated at 37 °C for 4 h. Absorbance was measured in an Apollo LB911 microplate reader (Berthold, Bad Wildbad, Germany) at 492 nm vs. 650 nm. For the fluorescence assay, cells were washed and calcein-AM (1 μM) was added incubated at 37 °C for 30 min. Fluorescence was then measured immediately using a fluorescence reader (BMG Fluostar, Ortenberg, Germany) with excitation and emission wavelengths of 485 nm and 515 nm, respectively. Cells incubated in buffer without calcein-AM were used as background controls. Data are calculated as a percent in relation to the control (HG). Cells cultured in LG were used as a negative control.

Epithelial cell proliferation was determined by a fluorometric assay using DAPI, measuring the DNA content as an indirect determination of cell number and proliferation [17]. In brief, subconfluent PTCs in 96-well plates were incubated for 6 d in media containing empa- or dapagliflozin and co-medications (in quintuplicate for each biological replicate). Then, cells were permeabilized using 0.02% SDS, 150 mM NaCl, and 15 mM sodium citrate. Finally, DAPI (2 μg/mL) was added to each well. Fluorescence was measured in a fluorescence reader (FluoStar, BMG Labtech, Offenburg, Germany) with excitation and emission wavelengths of 355 nm and 460 nm, respectively. Data are calculated as a percent in relation to the control (HG). Cells cultured in LG were used as a negative control.

The measurement of LDH activity released from the cytosol of damaged cells into the supernatant was used for the quantification of cell death and cell lysis to determine cytotoxic effects. Supernatants were harvested after incubation in gliflozin-containing media for 6 d and processed as described by the manufacturer (Sigma-Aldrich, Taufkirchen, Germany, no. 11644793001). Absorbance was measured in a microplate reader at 490 nm vs. 650 nm. Data are calculated as a percent in relation to the control (HG). Cells cultured in medium 199 containing a mixture of cytokines (Cytomix: γ-interferon, 200 U/mL; IL-1β, 25 U/mL; and tumor necrosis factor-α, 10 ng/mL) were used as a positive control.

4.6. *Measurement of Oxidative Stress*

The cell-permeant 2′,7′-dichlorodihydrofluorescein diacetate (H_2DCFDA) was used to detect reactive oxygen species in PTCs. Upon cleavage of the acetate groups by intracellular esterases and oxidation, nonfluorescent H_2DCFDA is converted to highly fluorescent DCF. Confluent PTCs in 96-well plates were cultured in LG, HG or with gliflozins (500 nM) for 6 d. The cells were then washed with pre-warmed HBSS and H_2DCFDA (20 μM in HBSS) was added for 30 min at 37 °C (in quintuplicate for each biological replicate). Cells incubated in buffer without DCF were used as background controls. The cells were then washed with HBSS and fluorescence was measured immediately using a fluorescence reader (BMG Fluostar, Ortenberg, Germany) with excitation and emission wavelengths of 485 nm and 538 nm, respectively. Data are expressed as arbitrary fluorescence units.

4.7. *PCR*

The RNA extraction was performed using single-step RNA isolation from cultured PTC by a standard protocol. After the RNA extraction, cDNAs were synthesized for 30 min at 37 °C using 1 μg RNA, 50 μM random hexamers, 1 mM deoxynucleotide-triphosphate-mix, 50 units of reverse transcriptase (Fermentas, St. Leon-Rot, Germany) in 10× PCR buffer, 1 mM β-mercaptoethanol and 5 mM $MgCl_2$. A Hot FIREPol EvaGreen Mix Plus was used (Solis Biodyne, Tartu, Estonia) for the master mix; the primer mix and RNAse-free water were added. Quantitative PCR was carried out in 96-well plates using the following conditions: 12 min at 95 °C for enzyme activation, 15 s at 95 °C for denaturation, 20 s at 63 °C for annealing, and 30 s at 72 °C for elongation (40 cycles). Finally, a melting curve analysis was conducted. Products were checked by agarose gel electrophoresis in selected experiments. The PCR fragment quantification was realized using the ABI Prism ® 7900HT Fast Real-Time PCR System with a Sequence Detection System SDS 2.4.1 (Thermo Fisher Scientific,

Waltham, MA, USA). Relative quantification was estimated by the ΔΔCT method [47] with β-actin as a housekeeper. The level of target gene expression was calculated using $2^{-\Delta\Delta Ct}$. The PCR products in selected experiments were separated by agarose electrophoresis (2 %) and observed under ultraviolet illumination. Primer pairs were synthesized by Invitrogen (Karlsruhe, Germany) and are listed in Table 1.

Table 1. Primer used for PCR analyses

Gene	Primer Forward	Primer Reverse	Product Length (bp)	NCBI Reference Sequence
SGLT-2	TGG GCT GGA ACA TCT ATG CC	GTG GAA GGC GTA ACC CAT GA	155	NM_003041.3
IL-6	AAA GAT GGC TGA AAA AGA TGG ATG C	ACA GCT CTG GCT TGT TCC TCA CTA C	150	NM_000600.4
KIM-1	CAG TGG CGT ATA TTG TTG CCG	CAG TCG TGA CGG TTG GAA CA	134	NM_001173393.2
NGAL	GAC CCG CAA AAG ATG TAT GCC	CTC ACC ACT CGG ACG AGG TA	197	NM_005564.4
β-Actin	ACT GGA ACG GTG AAG GGT GAC	AGA GAA GTG GGG TGG CTT TT	169	NM_001101

4.8. *Immunoassays*

After stimulation for 48 h (described in Section 4.3), supernatants were harvested, centrifuged at 300× *g* for 5 min and used for the quantification of IL-6, KIM-1 or NGAL, or stored at −20 °C for later measurement. Interleukin-6 was quantified using a commercially available EIA kit (Immunotools, Friesoythe, Germany; no. 31670069). KIM-1 was quantified using a commercially available EIA DuoSet (R&DSystems, Wiesbaden, Germany; no. DY1750). NGAL was quantified using a commercially available EIA DuoSet (R&DSystems, Wiesbaden, Germany; no. DY1757). All assays were processed as described by the manufacturer. In brief, the wells of 96-well microtiter plates were coated with the capture antibody overnight at room temperature. Nonspecific binding sites were blocked with blocking buffer for 1 h. The plates were then washed with PBS/0.05 % Tween and the standard (IL-6 assay: 8–500 pg/mL; KIM-1: 15.5–1000 pg/mL; NGAL: 78.1–5000 pg/mL), and the samples were added for 2 h at room temperature. All samples were diluted in assay buffer (IL-6: 1:25; KIM-1: 1:20; NGAL 1:20) and run in duplicate. The plates were washed and incubated with biotinylated detection antibody for 2 h at room temperature, washed again and incubated with horseradish-peroxidase-streptavidin for 30 min. After washing, TMB was added for 5–20 min and the substrate reaction was stopped and measured (450 vs. 620 nm). The data are calculated as ng/mL in the supernatant and presented as percent versus the related control.

4.9. *Statistical Analysis*

The data are expressed as mean ± SD. Analysis of variance with Dunnett's Multiple Comparison Test or Student's *t*-test were used for statistical analysis. Analyses were performed using Prism 5.0 (GraphPad Software, San Diego, CA, USA). p values < 0.05 were considered significant.

Author Contributions: Investigation, P.C.B. and J.F.; Conceptualization, P.C.B., B.K., R.S., and H.G.; Formal analysis, P.C.B., B.K., and J.F.; Writing, review, and editing, P.C.B., B.K., R.S., and H.G. All authors have read and agreed to the published version of the manuscript.

Acknowledgments: We thank Rita Schmitt-Prokopp and Michael Lein, SANA, Klinik für Urologie und Kinderurologie, Offenbach, Germany, for providing us with human renal tissue. We also thank Felix Chun, Klinik für Urologie, Goethe Universität, Frankfurt, Germany, for providing us with human renal tissue.

Abbreviations

AKI	Acute kidney injury
Dapa	Dapagliflozin
DAPI	4,6-diamino-2-phenylindole
DCF	2′,7′-dichlorofluorescein
EIA	Enzyme immune assay
Empa	Empagliflozin
FBS	Fetal bovine serum
HCT	Hydro-chloro-thiazide
HG	High glucose medium 199 (450 mg/dl)
IL-6	Interleukin-6
KIM-1	Kidney injury molecule-1
LDH	Lactate dehydrogenase
LG	Low glucose medium 199 (100 mg/dl)
NBDG-2	2-Deoxy-2-[(7-nitro-2,1,3-benzoxadiazol-7-yl)amino]-D-glucose
NGAL	Neutrophil gelatinase-associated lipocalin (Lipocalin-2)
PCR	Polymerase chain reaction
PTC	Primary human renal proximal tubular epithelial cells
SGLT	Sodium-glucose co-transporter
XTT	2,3-Bis-(2-Methoxy-4-Nitro-5-Sulfophenyl)-2*H*-Tetrazolium-5-Carboxanilide

References

1. Gerich, J.E. Role of the kidney in normal glucose homeostasis and in the hyperglycaemia of diabetes mellitus: Therapeutic implications. *Diabet. Med.* **2010**, *27*, 136–142. [CrossRef] [PubMed]
2. Vallon, V. The proximal tubule in the pathophysiology of the diabetic kidney. *Am. J. Physiol. Regul. Integr. Comp. Physiol.* **2011**, *300*, R1009–R1022. [CrossRef] [PubMed]
3. Faillie, J.-L. Pharmacological aspects of the safety of gliflozins. *Pharmacol. Res.* **2017**, *118*, 71–81. [CrossRef] [PubMed]
4. De Nicola, L.; Gabbai, F.B.; Liberti, M.E.; Sagliocca, A.; Conte, G.; Minutolo, R. Sodium/glucose cotransporter 2 inhibitors and prevention of diabetic nephropathy: Targeting the renal tubule in diabetes. *Am. J. Kidney Dis.* **2014**, *64*, 16–24. [CrossRef]
5. Bae, J.H.; Park, E.-G.; Kim, S.; Kim, S.G.; Hahn, S.; Kim, N.H. Effects of Sodium-Glucose Cotransporter 2 Inhibitors on Renal Outcomes in Patients with Type 2 Diabetes: A Systematic Review and Meta-Analysis of Randomized Controlled Trials. *Sci. Rep.* **2019**, *9*, 13009. [CrossRef]
6. Perkovic, V.; Jardine, M.J.; Neal, B.; Bompoint, S.; Heerspink, H.J.L.; Charytan, D.M.; Edwards, R.; Agarwal, R.; Bakris, G.; Bull, S.; et al. Canagliflozin and Renal Outcomes in Type 2 Diabetes and Nephropathy. *N. Engl. J. Med.* **2019**, *380*, 2295–2306. [CrossRef]
7. Mayer, G.J.; Wanner, C.; Weir, M.R.; Inzucchi, S.E.; Koitka-Weber, A.; Hantel, S.; von Eynatten, M.; Zinman, B.; Cherney, D.Z.I. Analysis from the EMPA-REG OUTCOME® trial indicates empagliflozin may assist in preventing the progression of chronic kidney disease in patients with type 2 diabetes irrespective of medications that alter intrarenal hemodynamics. *Kidney Int.* **2019**, *96*, 489–504. [CrossRef]
8. Heerspink, H.J.L.; Karasik, A.; Thuresson, M.; Melzer-Cohen, C.; Chodick, G.; Khunti, K.; Wilding, J.P.H.; Garcia Rodriguez, L.A.; Cea-Soriano, L.; Kohsaka, S.; et al. Kidney outcomes associated with use of SGLT2 inhibitors in real-world clinical practice (CVD-REAL 3): A multinational observational cohort study. *Lancet Diabetes Endocrinol.* **2020**, *8*, 27–35. [CrossRef]
9. Cianciolo, G.; de Pascalis, A.; Capelli, I.; Gasperoni, L.; Di Lullo, L.; Bellasi, A.; La Manna, G. Mineral and Electrolyte Disorders with SGLT2i Therapy. *JBMR Plus* **2019**, *3*, e10242. [CrossRef]
10. Di Lullo, L.; Mangano, M.; Ronco, C.; Barbera, V.; de Pascalis, A.; Bellasi, A.; Russo, D.; Di Iorio, B.; Cozzolino, M. The treatment of type 2 diabetes mellitus in patients with chronic kidney disease: What to expect from new oral hypoglycemic agents. *Diabetes Metab. Syndr.* **2017**, *11*, S295–S305. [CrossRef]

11. Perlman, A.; Heyman, S.N.; Matok, I.; Stokar, J.; Muszkat, M.; Szalat, A. Acute renal failure with sodium-glucose-cotransporter-2 inhibitors: Analysis of the FDA adverse event report system database. *Nutr. Metab. Cardiovasc. Dis.* **2017**, *27*, 1108–1113. [CrossRef] [PubMed]
12. Hassani-Ardakania, K.; Lipman, M.L.; Laporta, D.; Yu, O.H.Y. A Case of Severe Acute Kidney Injury Exacerbated by Canagliflozin in a Patient with Type 2 Diabetes. *Case Rep. Endocrinol.* **2019**. [CrossRef] [PubMed]
13. Pleros, C.; Stamataki, E.; Papadaki, A.; Damianakis, N.; Poulidaki, R.; Gakiopoulou, C.; Tzanakis, I. Dapagliflozin as a cause of acute tubular necrosis with heavy consequences: A case report. *CEN Case Rep.* **2018**, *7*, 17–20. [CrossRef] [PubMed]
14. FDA. *FDA Drug Safety Communication: FDA Strengthens Kidney Warnings for Diabetes Medicines Canagliflozin (Invokana, Invokamet) and Dapagliflozin (Farxiga, Xigduo XR) (06-14-2016)*; US Food and Drug Administration: Silver Spring, MD, USA, 2016.
15. Arzneimittelkommission der deutschen Ärzteschaft. *Drug Safety Mail No. 2019-064*; Bundesärztekammer: Berlin, Germany, 2019.
16. Hahn, K.; Ejaz, A.A.; Kanbay, M.; Lanaspa, M.A.; Johnson, R.J. Acute kidney injury from SGLT2 inhibitors: Potential mechanisms. *Nat. Rev. Nephrol.* **2016**, *12*, 711–712. [CrossRef] [PubMed]
17. Blaheta, R.A.; Franz, M.; Auth, M.K.; Wenisch, H.J.; Markus, B.H. A rapid non-radioactive fluorescence assay for the measurement of both cell number and proliferation. *J. Immunol. Methods* **1991**, *142*, 199–206. [CrossRef]
18. Hahn, K.; Kanbay, M.; Lanaspa, M.A.; Johnson, R.J.; Ejaz, A.A. Serum uric acid and acute kidney injury: A mini review. *J. Adv. Res.* **2017**, *8*, 529–536. [CrossRef]
19. Soltani, Z.; Rasheed, K.; Kapusta, D.R.; Reisin, E. Potential role of uric acid in metabolic syndrome, hypertension, kidney injury, and cardiovascular diseases: Is it time for reappraisal? *Curr. Hypertens. Rep.* **2013**, *15*, 175–181. [CrossRef]
20. Handler, J.S.; Kwon, H.M. Kidney cell survival in high tonicity. *Comp. Biochem. Physiol. A Physiol.* **1997**, *117*, 301–306. [CrossRef]
21. Cirillo, P.; Gersch, M.S.; Mu, W.; Scherer, P.M.; Kim, K.M.; Gesualdo, L.; Henderson, G.N.; Johnson, R.J.; Sautin, Y.Y. Ketohexokinase-dependent metabolism of fructose induces proinflammatory mediators in proximal tubular cells. *J. Am. Soc. Nephrol.* **2009**, *20*, 545–553. [CrossRef]
22. Mittal, M.; Siddiqui, M.R.; Tran, K.; Reddy, S.P.; Malik, A.B. Reactive oxygen species in inflammation and tissue injury. *Antioxid. Redox Signal.* **2014**, *20*, 1126–1167. [CrossRef]
23. Tousoulis, D.; Economou, E.K.; Oikonomou, E.; Papageorgiou, N.; Siasos, G.; Latsios, G.; Kokkou, E.; Mourouzis, K.; Papaioannou, S.; Deftereos, S.; et al. The Role and Predictive Value of Cytokines in Atherosclerosis and Coronary Artery Disease. *Curr. Med. Chem.* **2015**, *22*, 2636–2650. [CrossRef] [PubMed]
24. Mazzaferro, S.; Cianciolo, G.; De Pascalis, A.; Guglielmo, C.; Urena Torres, P.A.; Bover, J.; Tartaglione, L.; Pasquali, M.; La Manna, G. Bone, inflammation and the bone marrow niche in chronic kidney disease: What do we know? *Nephrol. Dial. Transpl.* **2018**, *33*, 2092–2100. [CrossRef] [PubMed]
25. Yao, D.; Wang, S.; Wang, M.; Lu, W. Renoprotection of dapagliflozin in human renal proximal tubular cells via the inhibition of the high mobility group box 1-receptor for advanced glycation end products-nuclear factor-κB signaling pathway. *Mol. Med. Rep.* **2018**, *18*, 3625–3630. [CrossRef] [PubMed]
26. Lee, W.-C.; Chau, Y.-Y.; Ng, H.-Y.; Chen, C.-H.; Wang, P.-W.; Liou, C.-W.; Lin, T.-K.; Chen, J.-B. Empagliflozin Protects HK-2 Cells from High Glucose-Mediated Injuries via a Mitochondrial Mechanism. *Cells* **2019**, *8*, 1085. [CrossRef]
27. Panchapakesan, U.; Pegg, K.; Gross, S.; Komala, M.G.; Mudaliar, H.; Forbes, J.; Pollock, C.; Mather, A. Effects of SGLT2 inhibition in human kidney proximal tubular cells—Renoprotection in diabetic nephropathy? *PLoS ONE* **2013**, *8*, e54442. [CrossRef]
28. Kim, J.H.; Ko, H.Y.; Wang, H.J.; Lee, H.; Yun, M.; Kang, E.S. Effect of Dapagliflozin, a Sodium-glucose Cotransporter-2 Inhibitor, on Gluconeogenesis in Proximal Renal Tubules. *Diabetes Obes. Metab.* **2019**. [CrossRef]
29. Smith, J.D.; Huang, Z.; Escobar, P.A.; Foppiano, P.; Maw, H.; Loging, W.; Yu, H.; Phillips, J.A.; Taub, M.; Ku, W.W. A Predominant Oxidative Renal Metabolite of Empagliflozin in Male Mice Is Cytotoxic in Mouse Renal Tubular Cells but not Genotoxic. *Int. J. Toxicol.* **2017**, *36*, 440–448. [CrossRef]
30. Uthman, L.; Homayr, A.; Juni, R.P.; Spin, E.L.; Kerindongo, R.; Boomsma, M.; Hollmann, M.W.; Preckel, B.; Koolwijk, P.; van Hinsbergh, V.W.M.; et al. Empagliflozin and Dapagliflozin Reduce ROS Generation and

Restore NO Bioavailability in Tumor Necrosis Factor α-Stimulated Human Coronary Arterial Endothelial Cells. *Cell. Physiol. Biochem.* **2019**, *53*, 865–886. [CrossRef]
31. Chen, Y.-Y.; Wu, T.-T.; Ho, C.-Y.; Yeh, T.-C.; Sun, G.-C.; Kung, Y.-H.; Wong, T.-Y.; Tseng, C.-J.; Cheng, P.-W. Dapagliflozin Prevents NOX- and SGLT2-Dependent Oxidative Stress in Lens Cells Exposed to Fructose-Induced Diabetes Mellitus. *Int. J. Mol. Sci.* **2019**, *20*, 4357. [CrossRef]
32. Arora, M.K.; Singh, U.K. Oxidative stress: Meeting multiple targets in pathogenesis of diabetic nephropathy. *Curr. Drug Targets* **2014**, *15*, 531–538. [CrossRef]
33. Andreadou, I.; Efentakis, P.; Balafas, E.; Togliatto, G.; Davos, C.H.; Varela, A.; Dimitriou, C.A.; Nikolaou, P.-E.; Maratou, E.; Lambadiari, V.; et al. Empagliflozin Limits Myocardial Infarction in Vivo and Cell Death in Vitro: Role of STAT3, Mitochondria, and Redox Aspects. *Front. Physiol.* **2017**, *8*, 1077. [CrossRef] [PubMed]
34. Ninčević, V.; Omanović Kolarić, T.; Roguljić, H.; Kizivat, T.; Smolić, M.; Bilić Ćurčić, I. Renal Benefits of SGLT 2 Inhibitors and GLP-1 Receptor Agonists: Evidence Supporting a Paradigm Shift in the Medical Management of Type 2 Diabetes. *Int. J. Mol. Sci.* **2019**, *20*, 5831. [CrossRef] [PubMed]
35. Komala, M.G.; Panchapakesan, U.; Pollock, C.; Mather, A. Sodium glucose cotransporter 2 and the diabetic kidney. *Curr. Opin. Nephrol. Hypertens.* **2013**, *22*, 113–119. [CrossRef]
36. Secker, P.F.; Beneke, S.; Schlichenmaier, N.; Delp, J.; Gutbier, S.; Leist, M.; Dietrich, D.R. Canagliflozin mediated dual inhibition of mitochondrial glutamate dehydrogenase and complex I: An off-target adverse effect. *Cell Death Dis.* **2018**, *9*, 226. [CrossRef] [PubMed]
37. Dekkers, C.C.J.; Petrykiv, S.; Laverman, G.D.; Cherney, D.Z.; Gansevoort, R.T.; Heerspink, H.J.L. Effects of the SGLT-2 inhibitor dapagliflozin on glomerular and tubular injury markers. *Diabetes Obes. Metab.* **2018**, *20*, 1988–1993. [CrossRef] [PubMed]
38. Gonzalez-Vicente, A.; Cabral, P.D.; Hong, N.J.; Asirwatham, J.; Saez, F.; Garvin, J.L. Fructose reabsorption by rat proximal tubules: Role of Na+-linked cotransporters and the effect of dietary fructose. *Am. J. Physiol. Renal Physiol.* **2019**, *316*, F473–F480. [CrossRef]
39. Nakayama, T.; Kosugi, T.; Gersch, M.; Connor, T.; Sanchez-Lozada, L.G.; Lanaspa, M.A.; Roncal, C.; Perez-Pozo, S.E.; Johnson, R.J.; Nakagawa, T. Dietary fructose causes tubulointerstitial injury in the normal rat kidney. *Am. J. Physiol. Renal Physiol.* **2010**, *298*, F712–F720. [CrossRef]
40. Davies, M.J.; Trujillo, A.; Vijapurkar, U.; Damaraju, C.V.; Meininger, G. Effect of canagliflozin on serum uric acid in patients with type 2 diabetes mellitus. *Diabetes Obes. Metab.* **2015**, *17*, 426–429. [CrossRef]
41. Baer, P.C.; Nockher, W.A.; Haase, W.; Scherberich, J.E. Isolation of proximal and distal tubule cells from human kidney by immunomagnetic separation. Technical note. *Kidney Int.* **1997**, *52*, 1321–1331. [CrossRef]
42. Baer, P.C.; Bereiter-Hahn, J.; Schubert, R.; Geiger, H. Differentiation status of human renal proximal and distal tubular epithelial cells in vitro: Differential expression of characteristic markers. *Cells Tissues Organs* **2006**, *184*, 16–22. [CrossRef]
43. Baer, P.C.; Koch, B.; Hickmann, E.; Schubert, R.; Cinatl, J.; Hauser, I.A.; Geiger, H. Isolation, Characterization, Differentiation and Immunomodulatory Capacity of Mesenchymal Stromal/Stem Cells from Human Perirenal Adipose Tissue. *Cells* **2019**, *8*, 1346. [CrossRef] [PubMed]
44. EMA. Assessment Report-Empagliflozin-EMA/CHMP/137741/2014. Available online: https://www.ema.europa.eu/en/documents/assessment-report/jardiance-epar-public-assessment-report_en.pdf (accessed on 25 November 2019).
45. EMA. Assessment Report-Dapagliflozin-EMA/689976/2012. Available online: https://www.ema.europa.eu/en/documents/assessment-report/forxiga-epar-public-assessment-report_en.pdf (accessed on 25 November 2019).
46. Leira, F.; Louzao, M.C.; Vieites, J.M.; Botana, L.M.; Vieytes, M.R. Fluorescent microplate cell assay to measure uptake and metabolism of glucose in normal human lung fibroblasts. *Toxicol. In Vitro* **2002**, *16*, 267–273. [CrossRef]
47. Pfaffl, M.W. A new mathematical model for relative quantification in real-time RT-PCR. *Nucleic Acids Res.* **2001**, *29*, e45. [CrossRef] [PubMed]

3

Change in Renal Glomerular Collagens and Glomerular Filtration Barrier-Related Proteins in a Dextran Sulfate Sodium-Induced Colitis Mouse Model

Chia-Jung Chang [1,2], Pi-Chao Wang [3], Tzou-Chi Huang [4] and Akiyoshi Taniguchi [1,2,*]

1 Cellular Functional Nanobiomaterials Group, Research Center for Functional Materials, National Institute for Materials Science, 1-1 Namiki, Tsukuba, Ibaraki 305-0044, Japan; CHANG.Chiajung@nims.go.jp
2 Graduate School of Advanced Science and Engineering, Waseda University, 3-4-1 Okubo, Shinjuku-ku, Tokyo 169-8555, Japan
3 Graduate School of Life and Environmental Sciences, University of Tsukuba, 1-1-1 Tennoudai, Tsukuba, Ibaraki 305-8572, Japan; wangpicao@gmail.com
4 Department of Biological Science and Technology, National Pingtung University of Science and Technology, Neipu, Pingtung 912-01, Taiwan; tchuang@mail.npust.edu.tw
* Correspondence: taniguchi.akiyoshi@nims.go.jp

Abstract: Renal disease is not rare among patients with inflammatory bowel disease (IBD) and is gaining interest as a target of research. However, related changes in glomerular structural have rarely been investigated. This study was aimed at clarifying the changes in collagens and glomerular filtration barrier (GFB)-related proteins of glomeruli in a dextran sulfate sodium (DSS)-induced colitis mouse model. Acute colitis was induced by administering 3.5% DSS in Slc:ICR strain mice for eight days. Histological changes to glomeruli were examined by periodic acid-Schiff (PAS) and Masson's trichrome staining. Expressions of glomerular collagens and GFB-related proteins were analyzed by immunofluorescent staining and Western blot analysis. DSS-colitis mice showed an elevated disease activity index (DAI), colon shortening, massive cellular infiltration and colon damage, confirming that DSS-colitis mice can be used as an IBD animal model. DSS-colitis mice showed increased glycoprotein and collagen deposition in glomeruli. Interestingly, we observed significant changes in glomerular collagens, including a decrease in type IV collagen, and an increment in type I and type V collagens. Moreover, declined GFB-related proteins expressions were detected, including synaptopodin, podocalyxin, nephrin and VE-cadherin. These results suggest that renal disease in DSS-colitis mice might be associated with changes in glomerular collagens and GFB-related proteins. These findings are important for further elucidation of the clinical pathological mechanisms underlying IBD-associated renal disease.

Keywords: inflammatory bowel disease (IBD); DSS-colitis; glomerular filtration barrier (GFB); type IV collagen; type I collagen; type V collagen

---

1. Introduction

Inflammatory bowel disease (IBD) is a chronic, remitting and relapsing inflammatory disease of the gastrointestinal tract characterized by inflammation and mucosal tissue damage and is associated with significant morbidity. Ulcerative colitis and Crohn's disease are the two most common forms of IBD. Ulcerative colitis and Crohn's disease differ from each other in physiology, but show similar symptoms such as severe diarrhea, rectal bleeding, abdominal pain, fever, and weight loss [1,2].

Clinical and epidemiological evidence suggests that IBD is a systemic disorder that can affect almost every organ [2,3]. Renal manifestations and complications in patients with IBD are not rare, and numerous clinical studies have reported that 4–23% of IBD patients experience renal disease such as tubulointerstitial nephritis, nephrolithiasis, and glomerulonephritis [4–11], which eventually induce renal disease. The appropriate experimental animal model of IBD-associated renal disease thus has clinical importance for related studies, including pathological mechanisms, prevention and treatment strategies for IBD.

Dextran sulfate sodium (DSS) is a water-soluble sulfated polysaccharide. Oral administration of DSS to trigger acute colitis has been widely used in experimental animal models for preclinical studies of IBD, because the pathophysiology resembles human Ulcerative colitis [12–14]. Recent studies have reported that mice with colitis induced by DSS show renal tubular injury that might be associated with increased neutrophil infiltration and expressions of cytokines and chemokines in both intestines and kidneys [15,16]. However, these studies of DSS-related renal injury have not mentioned structural changes to the glomeruli. On the other hand, the renal glomerulus is included in the nephron with the tubule, and tubular necrosis has been reported to potentially lead to declines in glomerular function [17,18], suggesting that glomerular damage might be accompanied by tubular injury. The glomerulus contains a highly specialized filtration barrier structure that is essential for maintaining normal plasma ultrafiltration, and loss of glomerular filtration function can lead to poor blood filtration, resulting in renal disease [19,20]. The electively permeable glomerular filtration barrier (GFB) is a three-layered structure that separates the capillaries and Bowman's space, and comprises the interdigitating foot processes of the podocytes, the intervening glomerular basement membrane (GBM), and the fenestrated endothelium [21,22]. The GBM is constituted of specialized extracellular matrix (ECM) components, namely type IV collagen, laminin and other proteoglycans, which are essential for providing a complete structural scaffold to the glomeruli, and important for establishing and maintaining the integrity of the GFB [23,24]. Disrupted GBM has been demonstrated to lead to filtration barrier damage and eventual glomerular disease [24,25]. However, whether GFB-related proteins changes are involved in IBD associated renal disease has not yet been clarified. Herein, we hypothesized that DSS induces renal structural changes, particularly to the glomerular structure.

In this study, we investigated glomerular structural changes focusing on specific types of glomerular collagens and GFB-related proteins after DSS administration, to demonstrate the coexistence of glomerular structural changes and IBD in a DSS-induced colitis mouse model. This study should help establish an experimental animal model for further elucidation of the clinical pathological mechanisms of IBD-associated renal disease.

2. Results

2.1. Progression of DSS-Colitis

After DSS administration (Figure 1), significant body weight loss was observed on Days 4–8 as compared to those of controls (water only) ($p < 0.05$) (Figure 2A). DAI scores showed elevating values after three days of DSS administration, reaching a peak on Day 8 (Figure 2B). Colon shortening, a marker of the severity of colorectal inflammation [14], was significantly greater in DSS-colitis mice as compared to the control group by Day 8 (Figure 2C). Histological observation of the colon was subsequently performed using HE staining, which showed a normal morphology of crypts, abundant goblet cells, muscular layer, submucosa and mucosa in the control mice. However, DSS-colitis mice revealed severe epithelial damage with mucosa thickening, massive cellular infiltration into the lamina propria and colon mucosa, crypt distortion, goblet cells loss, and complete destruction of the architecture (Figure 2D). These histological changes indicated severe inflammatory colitis.

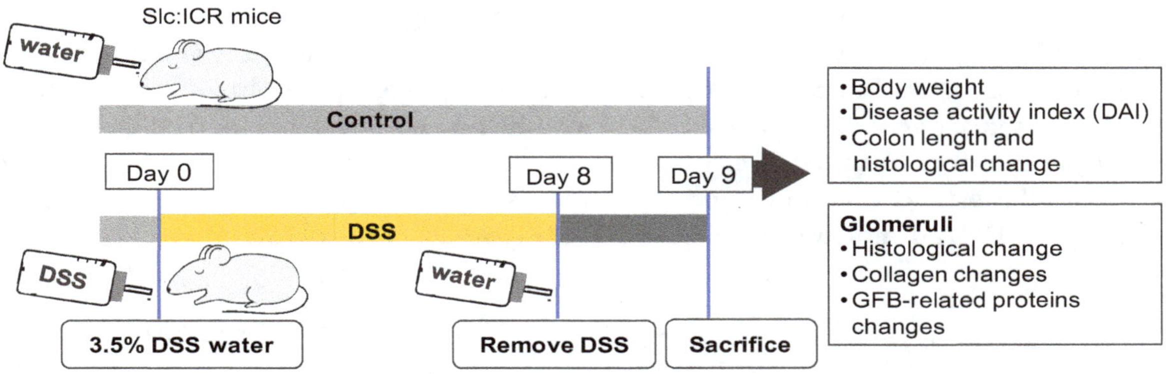

Figure 1. Investigating mouse glomerular structural changes associated with dextran sulfate sodium (DSS)-induced colitis. Slc:ICR mice were administered 3.5% DSS in drinking water for eight days, then allowed intake of filtered water on Day 8. Control mice were given filtered water. All mice were sacrificed on Day 9 and further assessments were performed. Abbreviation: GFB, glomerular filtration barrier.

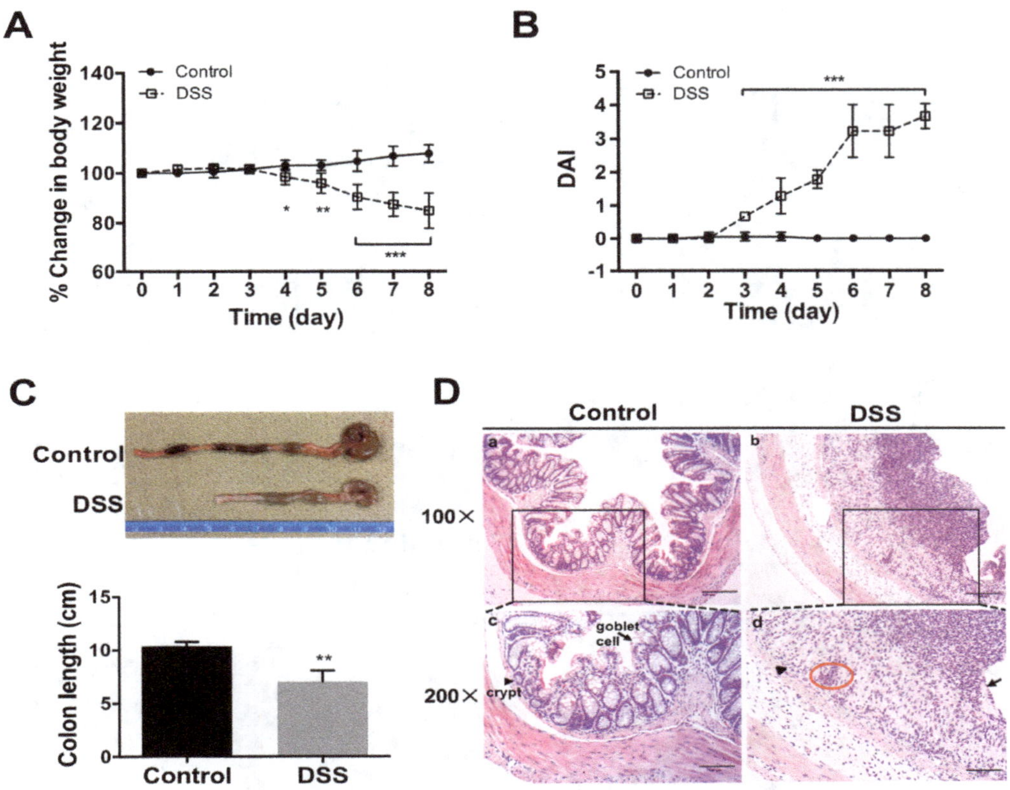

Figure 2. Macro- and microscopic changes to bowel in mice with DSS-induced colitis. Changes in body weight (**A**) and disease activity index (DAI) (**B**) were evaluated daily. Colon length was measured after sacrifice (**C**). Hematoxylin and eosin (HE) staining (**D**) showed distortion of crypts (arrowhead), loss of goblet cells (arrow), and infiltration of inflammatory cells (red circle) in colon sections from DSS-treated mice. All values are given as mean ± SEM (n = 6 mice); * $p < 0.05$, ** $p < 0.01$, and *** $p < 0.001$ vs. control. Scale bars: 200 μm (**a**,**b**); and 100 μm (**c**,**d**).

2.2. Renal Morphology and Histological Changes in DSS-Colitis Mice

Human and mouse studies have indicated the involvement of non-intestinal organs in IBD [4–9]. We therefore investigated renal changes in DSS-colitis mice. Kidney size and weight of DSS-colitis mice were decreased in mice after eight days of treatment as compared to those in controls (Figure 3A,B). To detect structural histological damage, glomerular morphology was examined in tissue sections by PAS and Masson's trichrome staining. Deep pink color (PAS-positive matrix) representing deposition of matrix glycoprotein was apparent at the GBM and mesangium, confirming increased matrix in the glomeruli of DSS-colitis mice (Figure 3C). Masson's trichrome staining was performed to detect the collagen deposition and fibrosis associated with renal disease, and blue to blue-violet staining indicated the presence of collagen in tissues. The result showed lightly stained collagen in the GBM and tubular basement membrane. On the other hand, significant collagen deposition among the glomerular capillaries and surrounding the Bowman's capsules were observed in DSS-colitis mice after eight days of DSS administration (Figure 3D) compared to control mice.

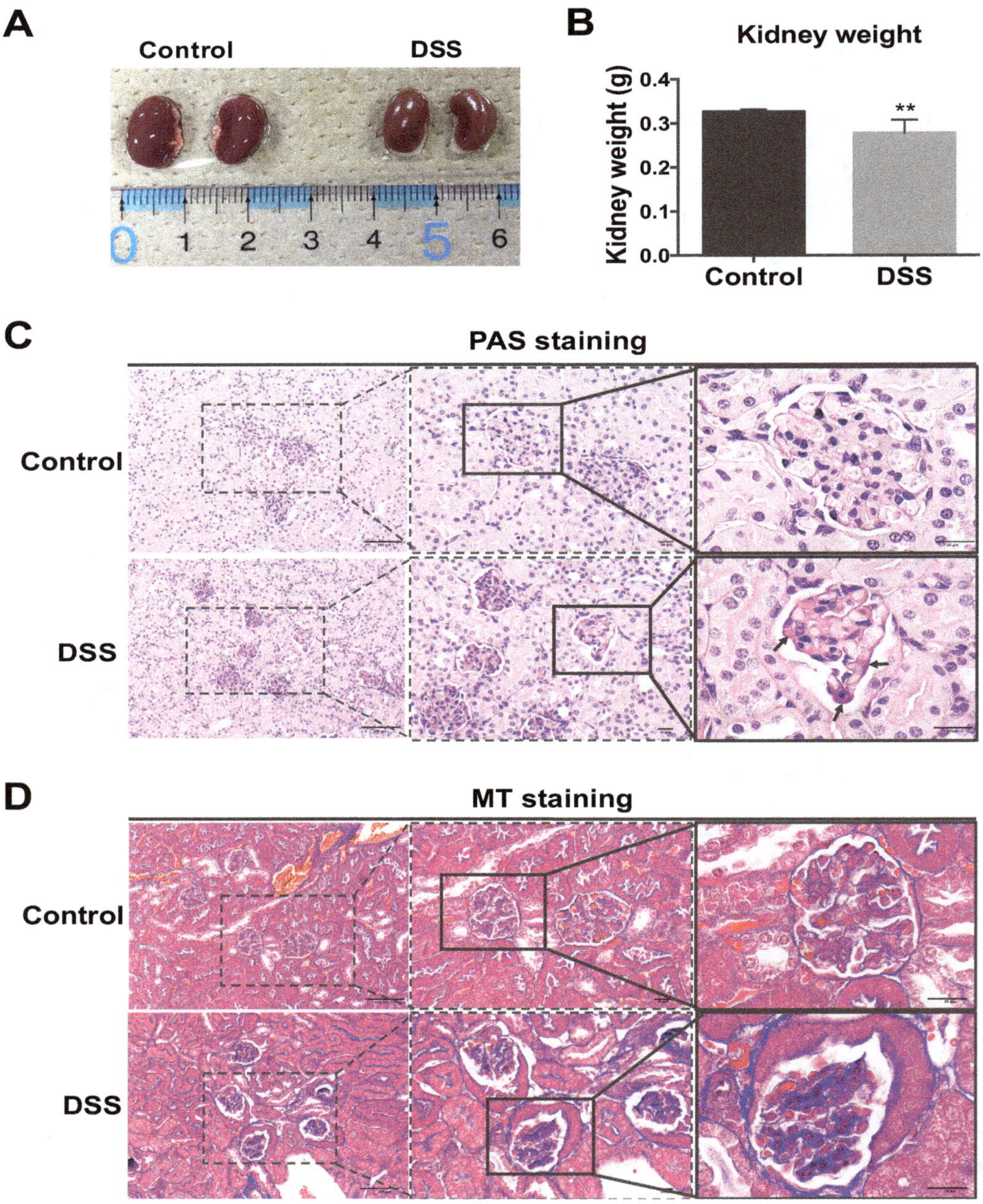

Figure 3. Macro- and microscopic changes to the kidney and glomeruli in mice after DSS administration. Mouse kidney appearance (**A**) and weight (**B**) were determined at harvest. Histological manifestations were determined by staining with periodic acid-Schiff (PAS) to assess the basement membrane of glomeruli (**C**), and Masson's trichrome (MT) staining to assess collagen deposition (**D**), respectively. Compared to control mice, glomerular accumulation of PAS-positive matrix (arrow) was prominent in DSS-treated mice (**C**). Blue staining indicates the presence of collagen fibers in tissues (**D**). All values are given as mean ± SEM (n = 6 mice); ** $p < 0.01$ vs. control. Scale bars: 100 μm and 20 μm.

2.3. Collagen Changes in Glomeruli

Glomerular collagens including type IV collagen (a typical collagen of the basement membrane matrix), type I collagen (an interstitial matrix collagen) and type V collagen (an atypical collagen that only appears at kidney development and in kidney diseases such as collagenofibrotic glomerulopathy) [26,27] were investigated by immunofluorescent microscopy and Western blot analysis. The results showed decreased type IV collagen in GBM and Bowman's capsules (Figure 4A-a′) in DSS-colitis mice as compared to controls (Figure 4A-a). In contrast to type IV collagen, type I and V collagens increased in the glomerular and renal interstitium (Figure 4A-b′,-c′) of DSS-colitis mice as compared to those in controls (Figure 4A-b,-c). Consistent with immunofluorescent microscopy results, Western blotting analysis also showed declining expressions of type IV collagen (Figure 4B-a), and increasing expressions of type I and V collagens (Figure 4B-b,-c) in the renal cortex of DSS-administered mice, indicating the influence of DSS on changes in glomerular collagens. The above results are illustrated in Figure 4C.

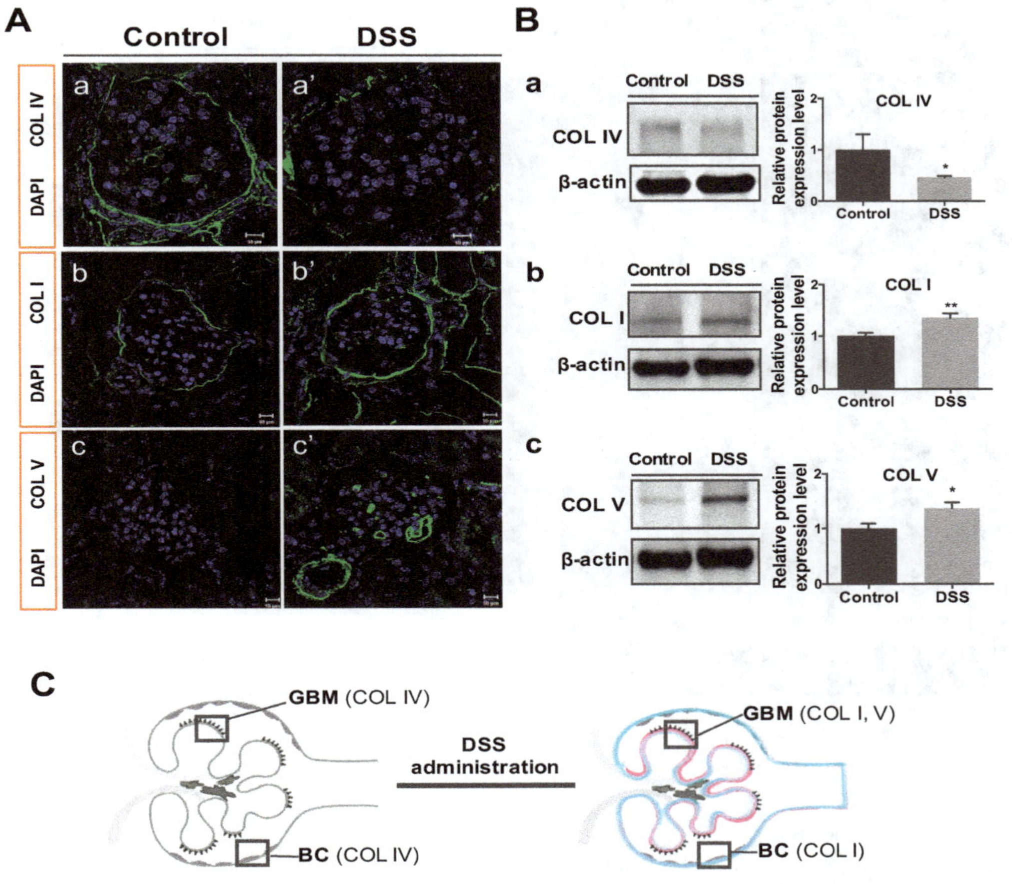

Figure 4. Changes in glomerular collagens in mice after DSS administration. Immunofluorescent microscopy (**A**) and Western blot analysis of protein expression (**B**) for type IV collagen (COL IV; A-a, A-a′; B-a; 160–190 kDa), type I collagen (COL I; A-b, A-b′; B-b; 150 kDa), and type V collagen (COL V; A-c, A-c′; B-c; 220 kDa) were conducted for control and DSS-colitis mice. Representative bands (**B**, left) and relative band intensity ratios were analyzed (**B**, right). (**C**) Illustration of glomerular collagens changes in this study. All values are means ± SEM ($n = 6$); * $p < 0.05$ and ** $p < 0.01$ vs. control. Scale bars = 10 μm. Abbreviations: GBM, glomerular basement membrane; BC, Bowman's capsule.

2.4. Changes in GFB-Related Proteins

The GFB comprises glomerular endothelial cells, the GBM and podocytes [22,23]. Podocytes and glomerular endothelial cells are located on opposite side of the GBM. Immunofluorescent investigation of podocyte-associated proteins in glomeruli (including synaptopodin, podocalyxin, and nephrin) were performed to detect changes in podocytes. The results showed that synaptopodin, podocalyxin, and nephrin were significantly expressed at capillary tufts of normal glomeruli in the control mice (Figure 5A-a, -b, -c), but declined in DSS-colitis mice after DSS administration (Figure 5A-a′, -b′, -c′). Similarly, the vascular-specific junctional molecule VE-cadherin in endothelial cells on the GBM, which is associated with the regulation of vascular permeability and glomerular filtration, showed lower immunofluorescence and discontinuous expression in DSS-colitis mice (Figure 5A-d′) as compared to that in controls (Figure 5A-d).

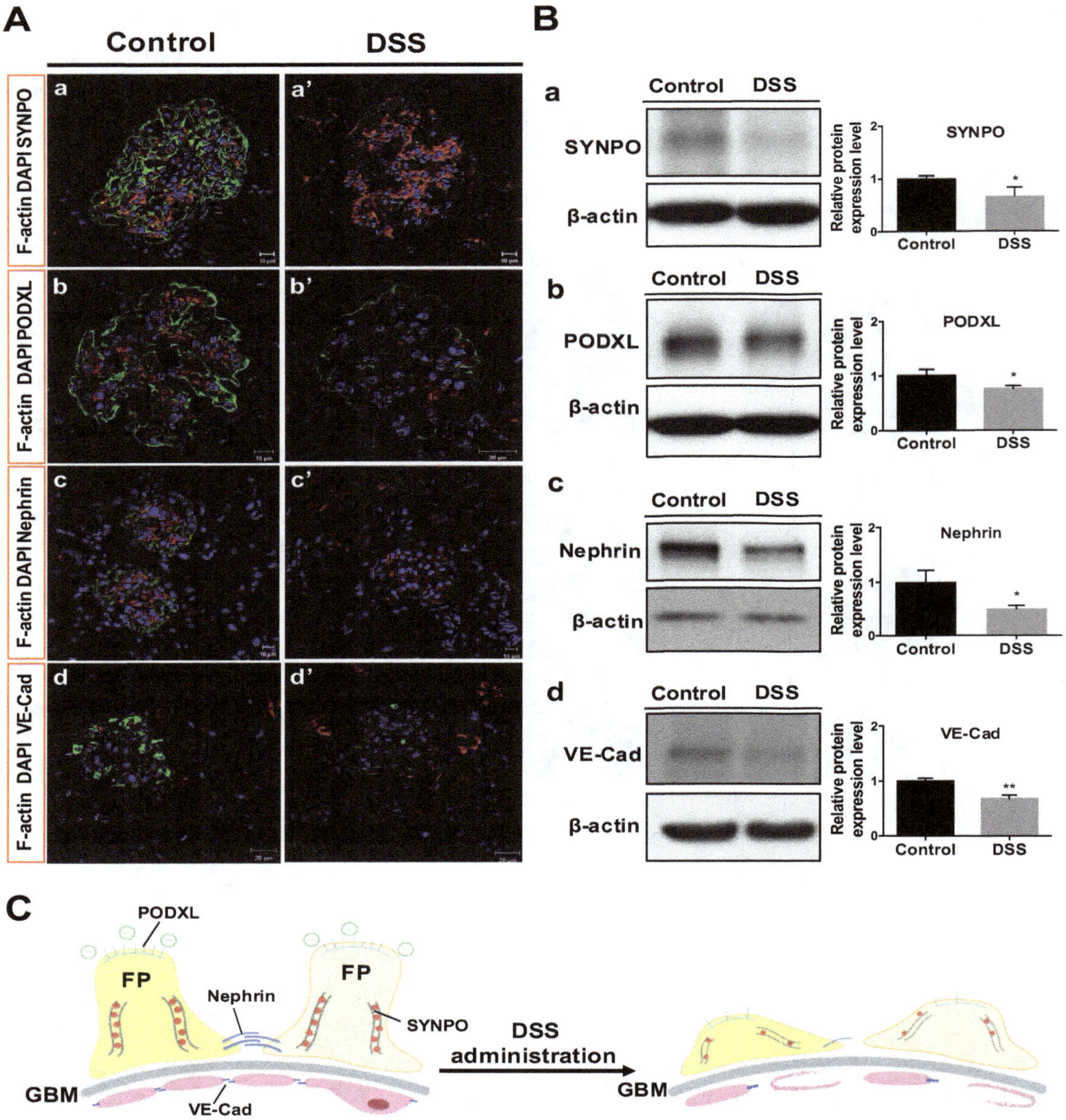

Figure 5. Changes in GFB-related proteins in mice after DSS administration. Immunofluorescent microscopy (**A**) and Western blot analysis of protein expression (**B**) against synaptopodin (A-a, A-a′; B-a; 100 kDa), podocalyxin (A-b, A-b′; B-b; 130 kDa), nephrin (A-c, A-c′; B-c; 185 kDa) and VE-cadherin (A-d, A-d′; B-d; 130 kDa) in glomeruli were conducted for control and DSS-colitis mice. (**B**) Representative bands (left), and relative band intensity ratios (right) were analyzed. (**C**) Illustration of GFB-related proteins changes in this study. All values are means ± SEM (n = 6), * $p < 0.05$ and ** $p < 0.01$ vs. control. Scale bars = 10 μm (A-a, A-a′, A-b, A-c, A-c′); 20 μm (A-b′, A-d, A-d′). Abbreviation: SYNPO, synaptopodin; PODXL, podocalyxin; VE-Cad, VE-cadherin; FP, foot processes.

Western blot analysis of these four proteins in glomeruli showed declines in all proteins (Figure 5B), consistent with the results from immunofluorescence (Figure 5A).

These findings confirmed that DSS administration caused podocyte damage (reductions in synaptopodin, podocalyxin and nephrin) and changes to endothelial adherens junctions in glomerular endothelium (reductions in VE-cadherin). These results are shown in Figure 5C.

3. Discussion

Renal manifestations and complications in patients with IBD have been reported in several clinical and experimental studies from recent years [4–11,28]. However, the coexistence of renal disease and IBD, and the related glomerular structural changes in particular, have rarely been discussed. This study provided novel data showing not only the changes in renal glomerular collagen types in a DSS-induced colitis mouse model, but also revealed the interesting fact that proteins located on both the glomerular podocyte slit diaphragm and endothelial junction declined in expression in DSS-colitis mice, reflecting GFB damage.

This study adopted the DSS-induced colitis mouse model and confirmed symptoms of DSS-induced colitis such as body weight loss, diarrhea, gross bleeding and colon architecture destruction (Figures 1 and 2), similar to IBD symptoms in humans [12,29]. Although some previous reports have mentioned that DSS might influence kidney function in mice after observing acute inflammatory responses associated with pro-inflammatory cytokine and chemokine expression in both intestines and kidneys, as well as renal tubular injury [15,16], the glomerular damage, especially the GFB damage in this DSS model still lack detailed evidence. In this study, we conducted detailed investigations into changes in the renal glomerular histology, GBM, and GFB-related protein expression, to illustrate renal damage in the DSS-induced colitis mouse model.

We noticed that kidney size and weight were decreased in DSS-colitis mice after DSS administration (Figure 3), since kidney size and weight are important indicators of renal pathology during disease development [30]. The decreased kidney size may correlate with body weight loss [30,31], and this phenomenon has been found in human patients with IBD [32]. Moreover, PAS staining revealed increasing deposition of glycoprotein matrix in GBM and mesangium, and Masson's trichome staining revealed collagen deposition was markedly increased around the glomerulus and Bowman's capsules in DSS-colitis mice. Such matrix and collagen depositions in glomeruli were also found in glomerular impairment, implicating excess ECM production as a factor in glomerular disease [27,33,34]. These observations suggest the DSS mice might show some glomerular abnormality.

To clarify the assumption that DSS induces renal structural change, we investigated the changes in specific types of collagens in the glomeruli. Our results showed that type IV collagen was decreased in the GBM, whereas type I and V collagens increased in the renal glomerular capillary loops and interstitium of DSS-colitis mice (Figure 4). Type IV collagen is well known to be the major component of the ECM in GBM, Bowman's capsule and tubular basement membranes in normal kidneys [35]. Decreased expression of type IV collagen in GBM has been reported with the increased GBM degradation associated with kidney dysfunction [35–38]. On the other hand, type I and V collagens belong to interstitial ECM and excessive deposition is known to form scar tissue in the interstitial space during fibrosis [39,40]. In fact, type I collagen seldom appears in renal vessels and glomeruli under normal conditions, but is deposited in the early stage of renal fibrosis [27,39]. Type V collagen has been reported to spread widely in glomeruli during glomerulopathy, wound healing and kidney development [26,41,42]. Our result of a decrement in type IV collagen in GBM and increments in both type I and type V collagens in renal glomerular capillary loops and interstitium suggested that DSS administration could cause these collagens changes, which may lead to glomerular structure damage.

Renal disease has been reported in human IBD patients, but GFB-related protein changes have not been closely investigated. The present study investigated four proteins (synaptopodin, podocalyxin, nephrin and VE-cadherin) to clarify GFB damage, because these proteins have not been investigated in the kidneys of DSS-colitis mice, and the relevance of GBM damage in the DSS-induced colitis mouse model has not been reported yet. Our results showed declined expression of all four proteins in glomeruli after DSS administration (Figure 5). Podocytes locating on the GBM are known to serve as the final filtration barriers of glomeruli and contain the special proteins synaptopodin, podocalyxin and nephrin. These proteins have been suggested to represent important biomarkers of podocyte deficiency [43]. Synaptopodin is known to maintain podocyte foot processes and downregulation of the podocyte actin cytoskeleton has been observed in human and rodent glomerular diseases [43]. Decreased synaptopodin expression in podocytes reflects the foot processes are associated with a loss of cytoskeletal destruction [44]. Podocalyxin is a highly electronegative sialoglycoprotein located at the apical surface of podocyte foot processes and functions to maintain the negative charge of the glomerular filtration slit diaphragm and podocyte shape by linking to the actin cytoskeleton [45]. In vivo and in vitro studies have reported that decreased podocaylxin is associated with reduced adhesiveness of cells to the GBM [43,45]. Moreover, the loss of nephrin, a structural protein located between the podocyte foot processes, causes decreased podocyte integrity of slit diaphragms, resulting in eventual damage to the GFB [19,46]. Furthermore, glomerular endothelial cells serve as the first filtration barrier through their tight adhesion to the basement membrane, and a decrease in endothelial cells can therefore worsen renal failure [20,21]. VE-cadherin is an adherens junction protein between endothelial cells that maintains vascular integrity and decreased VE-cadherin expression has been observed in the glomerular endothelium of end-stage renal disease patients [47–49].

Taken together, our results imply that DSS administration could cause the glomerular collagen changes, including decreased type IV collagen as a supporting ECM of GBM structure and deposition of type I and type V collagens in renal interstitium. These collagen changes might lead to structural damage to podocytes such as a loss of polarity and detachment from the GBM, as well as loss of endothelial cell junctions, eventually causing renal disease. Loss of the podocyte cytoskeletal proteins synaptopodin and podocalyxin and the slit diaphragms protein nephrin, as well as the defective endothelial cells adherens junction protein (VE-cadherin) which may be associated with podocyte damage.

Based on our findings, the lack or insufficiency of these GFB-related proteins in DSS-colitis mice might cause glomerular structural damage, and consequently lead to damage not only to podocytes, but also to adherens junctions in the vasculature, which might result in GFB damage.

In conclusion, this study used the DSS-induced colitis mouse model, a very common experimental model of colitis, to clarify changes in glomerular collagens and GFB-related proteins after DSS administration. These findings on glomerular structural change in experimental mice with DSS-induced colitis should lead to novel uses of the animal model for further investigations into IBD-associated renal disease.

4. Materials and Methods

4.1. Laboratory Animals

Seven-week-old male Slc:ICR strain mice weighing 28–30 g (Japan SLC, Hamamatsu, Japan) were housed in the Central Animal House at the University of Tsukuba under climate-controlled conditions (room temperature, 22 ± 2 °C; 12-h light/dark cycle; relative humidity, 65%). Cages were cleaned and sterilized every week. All mice were given free access to food and water. Animal experiments were conducted in strict accordance with the recommendations of the Guide for the Care and Use of Laboratory Animals of the Science Council of Japan and Ministry of Education, Culture, Sports, Science and Technology of Japan. The protocol was approved by the Committee on the Ethics of Animal Experiments of the University of Tsukuba (Permit Number: 14-047; May 2016) based on the Institutional Animal Care and Use Committee (IACUC). All surgery was performed under sodium pentobarbital anesthesia, and all efforts were made to minimize suffering.

4.2. *Induction of DSS-Colitis in Mice*

As a widely used model of IBD, the DSS-induced colitis mouse model was used in this study to investigate changes to renal glomerular collagens and GFB-related proteins. This mouse model was established by inducing colitis with the administration of DSS in drinking water for eight days (Figure 1), following the previously described method [15]. Briefly, mice were administered 3.5% (w/v) DSS (MW 36,000–50,000 Da; MP Biomedicals, Solon, OH, USA) dissolved in drinking water for eight days. Six mice per group were used in each experiment, and were not allowed to access to any other source of water. Mouse weights were monitored daily to quantify the systemic consequences of colitis. Mice were fed with normal water in place of DSS water on Day 8 and euthanized on Day 9. Colon length and kidney weight were measured for each mouse at harvest, then fixed in 10% neutral buffered formalin (Wako, Osaka, Japan) or stored at −80 °C for further use. Mice receiving only distilled water were used as controls.

4.3. *Disease Activity Index (DAI)*

Weight loss, stool consistency, and rectal bleeding were recorded daily to assess the severity of DSS-colitis. DAI was determined based on the methods described previously [50]. Briefly, DAI was scored from 0 to 4 for each parameter, and then averaged for each group. Parameters were body weight loss (0 = no weight loss; 1 = 1–5% weight loss; 2 = 6–10% weight loss; 3 = 11–15% weight loss; and 4 = $\geq$ 15% weight loss), stool consistency (0 = normal stools; 2 = loose stools; 4 = diarrhea) and gross bleeding (0 = negative, 2 = positive occult blood in stools, 4 = rectal bleeding). DAI was calculated as the sum of the weight loss, stool consistency and gross bleeding scores.

4.4. *Histological Investigation*

To detect injury to the colon and renal tissues, prepared tissues were cut into 2-μm thick sections using a microtome (Thermo Fisher Scientific, Waltham, MA, USA) and stained with hematoxylin and eosin (HE) for histological investigations. To assess the GBM, periodic acid-Schiff (PAS) was used to estimate the glomerular deposition of matrix glycoprotein [51]. Briefly, 3-μm-thick sections were stained using a PAS staining kit (Merck, Darmstadt, Germany) and counterstained with hematoxylin according to the instructions from the manufacturer. To detect collagen fiber deposition [52], 3-μm sections were stained with a Masson's trichrome staining kit (Muto Pure Chemicals, Tokyo, Japan) according to the manufacturer's instruction. Microscopic images were acquired using a light microscope with a charge-coupled device camera (Olympus, Tokyo, Japan).

4.5. *Immunofluorescence Staining and Confocal Imaging*

Immunofluorescence staining was performed by following the method described previously [53]. Briefly, kidneys were embedded in optimal cutting temperature compound (Sakura Finetek, Tokyo, Japan), and frozen in liquid nitrogen. Sections of 5-μm thickness were cut by a cryostat (CM3050; Leica, Wetzlar, Germany); then incubated with primary antibodies against type I collagen (Acris Antibodies, Germany), type IV collagen, type V collagen, synaptopodin, VE-cadherin (Santa Cruz Biotechnology, Santa Cruz, CA, USA), nephrin, and podocalyxin (R&D Systems, Minneapolis, MN, USA), respectively, at 4 °C overnight, and followed by secondary antibodies conjugated to Alexa Fluor® 488 or 568 (Invitrogen, Carlsbad, CA, USA); double-stained with rhodamine-conjugated phalloidin (Life Technologies, Gaithersburg, MD, USA) for F-actin; and finally submerged in fluoroshield mounting medium containing 4′,6-diamidino-2-phenylindole (DAPI) (Abcam, Cambridge, UK). Confocal imaging was performed according to the method described previously [26] with a confocal microscope (LSM700; Carl Zeiss, Jena, Germany). Alexa Fluor® 488, and 568 signals were detected at laser excitation wavelengths of 488 nm and 543 nm, respectively.

4.6. Renal Glomerular Isolation

Kidney cortex tissue from each mouse was removed, glomeruli were isolated using a serial sieving method described previously [54], and then washed with PBS to remove small tubular fragments. The isolated glomeruli were re-suspended by PBS for further use or dissolved in lysis buffer for protein extraction.

4.7. Protein Isolation and Western Blot Analysis

Kidney cortices (~50 mg) or isolated glomeruli from kidney cortices of each mouse were homogenized in lysis buffer (50 mM Tris pH 7.4, 250 mM NaCl, 5 mM EDTA, 2 mM Na_3VO_4, 1 mM NaF, 20 mM $Na_4P_2O_7$, 0.02% NaN_3, 1% Triton X-100, 0.1% SDS and 1 mM PMSF) with 1% protease inhibitor cocktail (Sigma-Aldrich, St. Louis, MO, USA) by sonication (Qsonica, Newtown, CT, USA), followed by incubation on ice for 10 min and centrifugation at 10,000 rpm for 10 min. Supernatant was collected and protein concentration was quantitated using the Micro BCA Protein Assay kit (Thermo Fisher Scientific, Waltham, MA, USA) according to the instructions from the manufacturer. Thirty micrograms of total protein were loaded per lane and separated by 7.5% polyacrylamide gels, followed by transferring onto methanol-activated PVDF membrane (Millipore, Billerica, MA, USA). Protein-transferred membranes were incubated with primary antibodies against type I collagen, type IV collagen, type V collagen, synaptopodin, VE-cadherin, nephrin, podocalyxin and β-actin, respectively, at 4 °C overnight, followed by incubation with horseradish peroxidase-conjugated secondary antibody for 2 h at room temperature. Blots were visualized with chemiluminescence substrate for 1 min and detected using a luminescent image analyzer (LAS-4000 mini; Fujifilm, Tokyo, Japan). Band density was quantitated densitometrically with Image J software (National Institutes of Health, MD, USA) by calculating the average optical density in each band. Relative and normalized protein expressions were calculated using the ratio of each protein density to β-actin density.

4.8. Statistical Analysis

Statistical analyses were performed using Prism software (GraphPad, San Diego, CA, USA). All data are expressed as mean ± standard error of the mean (SEM) from 6 replicates ($n = 6$ mice per group) in at least 3 independent experiments. The significance of differences between groups were analyzed using Student's t-test. A probability level of $p < 0.05$ was considered significant.

Author Contributions: P.-C.W. and T.-C.H. conceived the presented idea. C.-J.C. designed the study, acquired data, and drafted the manuscript. C.-J.C. and P.-C.W. analyzed and interpreted data. P.-C.W. provided critical revision. All authors discussed the results and contributed to the final manuscript. A.T. carried out final approval of the version to be published.

Acknowledgments: We wish to thank Tony Hsiang-Kuang Liang for valuable medical advice, and Yusuke Murasawa, Nishimura Yusuke and Airi Akatsuka for their technical assistance.

Abbreviations

IBD	Inflammatory bowel disease
GFB	Glomerular filtration barrier
DSS	Dextran sulfate sodium
PAS	Periodic acid-Schiff
DAI	Disease activity index
GBM	Glomerular basement membrane
ECM	Extracellular matrix

References

1. Sartor, R.B. Current concepts of the etiology and pathogenesis of ulcerative colitis and Crohn's disease. *Gastroenterol. Clin. N. Am.* **1995**, *24*, 475–507.
2. Ricart, E.; Panaccione, R.; Loftus, E.V.; Tremaine, W.J.; Harmsen, W.S.; Zinsmeister, A.R.; Sandborn, W.J. Autoimmune disorders and Extraintestinal manifestations in First-degree familial and sporadic inflammatory bowel disease. *Inflamm. Bowel Dis.* **2004**, *10*, 207–214. [CrossRef] [PubMed]
3. Christodoulou, D.K.; Katsanos, K.H.; Kitsanou, M.; Stergiopoulou, C.; Hatzis, J.; Tsianos, E.V. Frequency of extraintestinal manifestations in patients with inflammatory bowel disease in northwest Greece and review of the literature. *Dig. Liver Dis.* **2002**, *34*, 781–786. [CrossRef]
4. Ambruzs, J.M.; Walker, P.D.; Larsen, C.P. The histopathologic spectrum of kidney biopsies in patients with inflammatory bowel disease. *Clin. J. Am. Soc. Nephrol.* **2014**, *9*, 265–270. [CrossRef] [PubMed]
5. Ambruzs, J.M.; Larsen, C.P. Renal Manifestations of Inflammatory Bowel Disease. *Rheum. Dis. Clin. N. Am.* **2018**, *44*, 699–714. [CrossRef] [PubMed]
6. Rabin, B.S.; Rogers, S. Pathologic changes in the liver and kidney produced by immunization with intestinal antigens. *Am. J. Pathol.* **1972**, *84*, 201–210.
7. Kreisel, W.; Wolf, L.M.; Grotz, W.; Grieshaber, M. Renal tubular damage: An extraintestinal manifestation of chronic inflammatory bowel disease. *Eur. J. Gastroenterol. Hepatol.* **1996**, *8*, 461–468.
8. Khosroshahi, H.T.; Shoja, M.M. Tubulointerstitial disease and ulcerative colitis. *Nephrol. Dial. Transplant.* **2006**, *21*, 2340. [CrossRef]
9. Corica, D.; Romano, C. Renal Involvement in Inflammatory Bowel Diseases. *J. Crohns Colitis* **2016**, *10*, 226–235. [CrossRef]
10. Fraser, J.S.; Muller, A.F.; Smith, D.J.; Newman, D.J.; Lamb, E.J. Renal tubular injury is present in acute inflammatory bowel disease prior to the introduction of drug therapy. *Aliment. Pharmacol. Ther.* **2001**, *15*, 1131–1137. [CrossRef]
11. Tokuyama, H.; Wakino, S.; Konishi, K.; Hashiguchi, A.; Hayashi, K.; Itoh, H. Acute interstitial nephritis associated with ulcerative colitis. *Clin. Exp. Nephrol.* **2010**, *14*, 483–486. [CrossRef] [PubMed]
12. Chassaing, B.; Aitken, J.D.; Malleshappa, M.; Vijay-Kumar, M. Dextran Sulfate sodium (DSS)-induced Colitis in mice. *Trends Pharmacol. Sci.* **2014**, *104*. [CrossRef]
13. de Lange, K.M.; Barrett, J.C. Understanding inflammatory bowel disease via immunogenetics. *J. Autoimmun.* **2015**, *64*, 91–100. [CrossRef]
14. Eichele, D.D.; Kharbanda, K.K. Dextran sodium sulfate colitis murine model: An indispensable tool for advancing our understanding of inflammatory bowel diseases pathogenesis. *World J. Gastroenterol.* **2017**, *23*, 6016–6029. [CrossRef] [PubMed]
15. Ranganathan, P.; Jayakumar, C.; Santhakumar, M.; Ramesh, G. Netrin-1 regulates colon-kidney cross talk through suppression of IL-6 function in a mouse model of DSS-colitis. *Am. J. Physiol. Renal Physiol.* **2013**, *304*, 1187–1197. [CrossRef]
16. Ranganathan, P.; Jayakumar, C.; Manicassamy, S.; Ramesh, G. CXCR2 knockout mice are protected against DSS-colitis-induced acute kidney injury and inflammation. *Am. J. Physiol. Renal Physiol.* **2013**, *305*, 1422–1427. [CrossRef]
17. Meyer, T.W. Tubular injury in glomerular disease. *Kidney Int.* **2003**, *63*, 774–787. [CrossRef] [PubMed]
18. Kriz, W.; LeHir, M. Pathways to nephron loss starting from glomerular diseases-Insights from animal models. *Kidney Int.* **2005**, *67*, 404–419. [CrossRef] [PubMed]
19. Lennon, R.; Randles, M.J.; Humphries, M.J. The Importance of Podocyte Adhesion for a Healthy Glomerulus. *Front. Endocrinol.* **2014**, *5*, 160. [CrossRef] [PubMed]
20. Arif, E.; Nihalani, D. Glomerular Filtration Barrier Assembly: An insight. *Postdoc. J.* **2013**, *1*, 33–45. [CrossRef] [PubMed]
21. Scott, R.P.; Quaggin, S.E. The cell biology of renal filtration. *J. Cell Biol.* **2015**, *209*, 199–210. [CrossRef]
22. Miner, J.H. Glomerular basement membrane composition and the filtration barrier. *Pediatr. Nephrol.* **2011**, *26*, 1413–1417. [CrossRef]
23. Byron, A.; Randles, M.J.; Humphries, J.D.; Mironov, A.; Hamidi, H.; Harris, S.; Mathieson, P.W.; Saleem, M.A.; Satchell, S.C.; Zent, R.; et al. Glomerular Cell Cross-Talk Influences Composition and Assembly of Extracellular Matrix. *J. Am. Soc. Nephrol.* **2014**, *25*, 953–966. [CrossRef]

24. Chen, Y.M.; Miner, J.H. Glomerular basement membrane and related glomerular disease. *Transl. Res.* **2012**, *160*, 291–297. [CrossRef]
25. Chew, C.; Lennon, R. Basement Membrane Defects in Genetic Kidney Diseases. *Front. Pediatr.* **2018**, *6*, 11. [CrossRef] [PubMed]
26. Hsu, H.H.; Murasawa, Y.; Qi, P.; Nishimura, Y.; Wang, P.C. Type V collagen fibrils in mouse metanephroi. *Biochem. Biophys. Res. Commun.* **2013**, *441*, 649–654. [CrossRef]
27. Genovese, F.; Manresa, A.A.; Leeming, D.; Karsdal, M.; Boor, P. The extracellular matrix in the kidney: A source of novel non-invasive biomarkers of kidney fibrosis. *Fibrogenes. Tissue Repair* **2014**, *7*, 4. [CrossRef]
28. Levine, J.S.; Burakoff, R. Extraintestinal manifestations of inflammatory bowel disease. *Gastroenterol. Hepatol.* **2011**, *7*, 235–241.
29. Da Silva, A.P.; Pollett, A.; Rittling, S.R.; Denhardt, D.T.; Sodek, J.; Zohar, R. Exacerbated tissue destruction in DSS-induced acute colitis of OPN-null mice is associated with downregulation of TNF-α expression and non-programmed cell death. *J. Cell Physiol.* **2006**, *208*, 629–639. [CrossRef] [PubMed]
30. Sandilands, E.A.; Dhaun, N.; Dear, J.W.; Webb, D.J. Measurement of renal function in patients with chronic kidney disease. *Br. J. Clin. Pharmacol.* **2013**, *76*, 504–515. [CrossRef]
31. Emamian, S.A.; Nielsen, M.B.; Pedersen, J.F.; Ytte, L. Kidney dimensions at sonography: Correlation with age, sex, and habitus in 665 adult volunteers. *Am. J. Roentgenol.* **1993**, *160*, 83–86. [CrossRef] [PubMed]
32. Lauritzen, D.; Andreassen, B.U.; Heegaard, N.H.H.; Klinge, L.G.; Walsted, A.M.; Neland, M.; Nielsen, R.G.; Wittenhagen, P. Pediatric Inflammatory Bowel Diseases: Should We Be Looking for Kidney Abnormalities? *Inflamm. Bowel Dis.* **2018**, *24*, 2599–2605. [CrossRef]
33. Kashgarian, M.; Sterze, B. The pathobiology of the mesangium. *Kidney Int.* **1992**, *41*, 524–529. [CrossRef]
34. Duffield, J.S. Cellular and molecular mechanisms in kidney fibrosis. *J. Clin. Investig.* **2014**, *124*, 2299–2306. [CrossRef] [PubMed]
35. Miner, J.H. Renal basement membrane components. *Kidney Int.* **1999**, *56*, 2016–2024. [CrossRef] [PubMed]
36. Niu, H.; Li, Y.; Li, H.; Chi, Y.; Zhuang, M.; Zhang, T.; Liu, M.; Nie, L. Matrix metalloproteinase 12 modulates high-fat-diet induced glomerular fibrogenesis and inflammation in a mouse model of obesity. *Sci. Rep.* **2016**, *6*, 20171. [CrossRef]
37. Tamsma, J.T.; van den Born, J.; Bruijn, J.A.; Assmann, K.J.; Weening, J.J.; Berden, J.H.; Wieslander, J.; Schrama, E.; Hermans, J.; Veerkamp, J.H. Expression of glomerular extracellular matrix components in human diabetic nephropathy: Decrease of heparan sulphate in the glomerular basement membrane. *Diabetologia* **1994**, *37*, 313–320. [CrossRef]
38. Morita, M.; Uchigata, Y.; Hanai, K.; Ogawa, Y.; Iwamoto, Y. Association of urinary type IV collagen with GFR decline in young patients with type 1 diabetes. *Am. J. Kidney Dis.* **2011**, *58*, 915–920. [CrossRef] [PubMed]
39. Yoshioka, K.; Tohda, M.; Takemura, T.; Akano, N.; Matsubara, K.; Ooshima, A.; Maki, S. Distribution of type I collagen in human kidney diseases in comparison with type III collagen. *J. Pathol.* **1990**, *162*, 141–148. [CrossRef] [PubMed]
40. Sumiyoshi, H.; Kitamura, H.; Matsuo, N.; Tatsukawa, S.; Ishikawa, K.; Okamoto, O.; Fujikura, Y.; Fujiwara, S.; Yoshioka, H. Transient expression of mouse Pro-α3(V) collagen gene (Col5a3) in wound healing. *Connect. Tissue Res.* **2012**, *5*, 313–317. [CrossRef] [PubMed]
41. Morita, H.; Hasegawa, T.; Minamoto, T.; Oda, Y.; Inui, K.; Tayama, H.; Nakao, N.; Nakamoto, Y.; Ideura, T.; Yoshimura, A. Collagenofibrotic glomerulopathy with a widespread expression of type-v collagen. *Virchows Arch.* **2003**, *442*, 163–168. [PubMed]
42. Murasawa, Y.; Hayashi, T.; Wang, P.C. The role of type V collagen fibril as an ECM that induces the motility of glomerular endothelial cells. *Exp. Cell Res.* **2008**, *314*, 3638–3653. [CrossRef] [PubMed]
43. Sekulic, M.; Pichler, S. A compendium of urinary biomarkers indicative of glomerular podocytopathy. *Pathol. Res. Int.* **2013**, *2013*, 782395. [CrossRef] [PubMed]
44. Kwon, S.K.; Kim, S.J.; Kim, H.Y. Urine synaptopodin excretion is an important marker of glomerular disease progression. *Korean J. Intern Med.* **2016**, *31*, 938–943. [CrossRef] [PubMed]
45. Nielsen, J.S.; McNagny, K.M. The role of podocalyxin in health and disease. *J. Am. Soc. Nephrol.* **2009**, *20*, 1669–1676. [CrossRef] [PubMed]
46. Greka, A.; Mundel, P. Cell biology and pathology of podocytes. *Annu. Rev. Physiol.* **2012**, *74*, 299–323. [CrossRef]
47. Spagnuolo, R.; Corada, M.; Orsenigo, F.; Zanetta, L.; Deuschle, U.; Sandy, P.; Schneider, C.; Drake, C.J.; Breviario, F.; Dejana, E. Gas1 is induced by VE-cadherin and vascular endothelial growth factor and inhibits

endothelial cell apoptosis. *Blood* **2004**, *103*, 3005–3012. [CrossRef] [PubMed]

48. Giannotta, M.; Trani, M.; Dejana, E. VE-Cadherin and endothelial Adherens Junctions: Active guardians of vascular integrity. *Dev. Cell* **2013**, *26*, 441–454. [CrossRef]
49. Hernandez, N.M.; Casselbrant, A.; Joshi, M.; Johansson, B.R.; Sumitran-Holgersson, S. Antibodies to kidney endothelial cells contribute to a "leaky" glomerular barrier in patients with chronic kidney diseases. *Am. J. Physiol. Renal Physiol.* **2012**, *302*, F884–F894. [CrossRef]
50. Murthy, S.N.; Cooper, H.S.; Shim, H.; Shah, R.S.; Ibrahim, S.A.; Sedergran, D.J. Treatment of dextran sulfate sodium-induced murine colitis by intracolonic cyclosporine. *Dig. Dis. Sci.* **1993**, *38*, 1722–1734. [CrossRef]
51. McManus, J.F. The Periodic Acid Routine Applied to the Kidney. *Am. J. Pathol.* **1948**, *24*, 643–653. [PubMed]
52. Cohen, A.H. Masson's trichrome stain in the evaluation of renal biopsies. An appraisal. *Am. J. Clin. Pathol.* **1976**, *65*, 631–643. [CrossRef] [PubMed]
53. Nishimura, Y.; Hsu, H.H.; Wang, P.C. Detection of initial angiogenesis from dorsal aorta into metanephroi and elucidation of its role in kidney development. *Regener. Ther.* **2016**, *4*, 27–35. [CrossRef]
54. Nagao, T.; Suzuki, K.; Utsunomiya, K.; Matsumura, M.; Saiga, K.; Wang, P.C.; Minamitani, H.; Aratani, Y.; Nakayama, T.; Suzuki, K. Direct activation of glomerular endothelial cells by anti-moesin activity of anti-myeloperoxidase antibody. *Nephrol. Dial. Transplant.* **2011**, *26*, 2752–2760. [CrossRef] [PubMed]

4

Long Non-Coding RNAs in Kidney Disease

Michael Ignarski [1,2], Rashidul Islam [1,2] and Roman-Ulrich Müller [1,2,3,*]

1 Department II of Internal Medicine and Center for Molecular Medicine, University of Cologne, Faculty of Medicine and University Hospital Cologne, 50931 Cologne, Germany
2 Cologne Excellence Cluster on Cellular Stress Responses in Aging-Associated Diseases, University of Cologne, Faculty of Medicine and University Hospital Cologne, 50931 Cologne, Germany
3 Systems Biology of Ageing Cologne, University of Cologne, 50931 Cologne, Germany
* Correspondence: roman-ulrich.mueller@uk-koeln.de

Abstract: Non-coding RNA species contribute more than 90% of all transcripts and have gained increasing attention in the last decade. One of the most recent members of this group are long non-coding RNAs (lncRNAs) which are characterized by a length of more than 200 nucleotides and a lack of coding potential. However, in contrast to this simple definition, lncRNAs are heterogenous regarding their molecular function—including the modulation of small RNA and protein function, guidance of epigenetic modifications and a role as enhancer RNAs. Furthermore, they show a highly tissue-specific expression pattern. These aspects already point towards an important role in cellular biology and imply lncRNAs as players in development, health and disease. This view has been confirmed by numerous publications from different fields in the last years and has raised the question as to whether lncRNAs may be future therapeutic targets in human disease. Here, we provide a concise overview of the current knowledge on lncRNAs in both glomerular and tubulointerstitial kidney disease.

Keywords: lncRNA; long non-coding RNA; miRNA; kidney; glomerulus; podocyte; acute kidney injury; AKI; diabetic nephropathy

---

1. Introduction

Most of the human genome is actively transcribed but less than 2% contains protein coding transcripts (mRNA). The other transcripts produced show no or low coding potential and have, therefore, been summarized in the large group of non-coding RNAs (ncRNA). This group contains the long known ribosomal RNAs (rRNAs) and transfer RNAs (tRNAs) involved in protein synthesis as well as two very diverse classes of ncRNAs mainly divided by their length: the class of small non-coding RNAs containing transcripts with lengths of less than 200 nucleotides consists of small interfering RNAs (siRNAs), small nuclear RNAs (snRNA), small nucleolar RNAs (snoRNAs), PIWI-interacting RNAs (piRNAs) and microRNAs (miRNAs). The role of miRNAs in kidney disease has been investigated extensively and reviewed multiple times over the last decades [1,2], therefore, we focus on the class of long non-coding RNAs (lncRNAs) with lengths of over 200 nucleotides. Like mRNAs most lncRNAs have their own promoters, are RNA polymerase II transcribed, 5′-capped, polyadenylated and subjected to splicing [3]. LncRNA genes are dispersed throughout the genome, they can be inter- or intragenic, in the latter case positioned in sense or antisense direction, inside exons, introns or overlapping both. Intergenic lncRNAs can be located at great distance from proteins coding genes, in close proximity or divergently transcribed from protein coding gene promoters. They can also be expressed from silencer, enhancer and insulator loci. For details on genomic location of lncRNAs refer to Laurent et al. [4]. So far, there is no formal classification with respect to lncRNA localization or function. Many lncRNAs were shown to act as nucleo- or cytoplasmic scaffolds providing platforms for interactions between other cellular components (e.g., DNA, proteins and other RNA species), which implies lncRNAs as central players in epigenetic processes and chromatin regulation. Another superordinate function of lncRNAs is the competition for binding sites, this can be the competitive binding to open chromatin leading to displacement of transcription factors or the sequestration of miRNAs leading to reduced inhibition of the target mRNA. Likewise, lncRNAs can act similarly to miRNAs to enhance or decrease the stability of mRNA. The great variety of lncRNA cellular functions was recently reviewed by Yao et al. [5].

Due to their generally low expression levels the vast majority of the 215,008 annotated human lncRNAs (RNAcentral, 5 May 2019) was only discovered within the last decade [6]. Whilst the existence of lncRNAs as a biotype is well conserved in mammals, identifying the actual homologues between species is more challenging than for protein-coding transcripts. LncRNAs are often not well-conserved on the sequence level but rather regarding structure and/or genomic position [7]. The expression pattern of lncRNA genes was shown to be far more tissue- and cell-type specific than is the case for protein coding genes [8,9]. Quantitative studies based mainly on RNA sequencing have led to a rapid growth of this field and have shown dysregulation of lncRNAs in many diseases [10]. Whilst before 2010 only few studies on this topic were published each year, this changed tremendously in the last decade and several thousand publications on lncRNAs are found for the year 2018. As to lncRNAs in the kidney, this rise in publication numbers occurred around five years later and resulted in about 100 studies in the year 2018. However, especially in the beginning much of this work was merely descriptive and did not focus on kidney disease but rather renal cell carcinoma due to the ease of analyses regarding RNA expression changes in tumors. Taking this into consideration, the aim of this review is filling the gap towards non-tumorous kidney diseases to lay a foundation for future studies building on existing data.

2. LncRNAs in Glomerular Disease

As to glomerular disease by far most publications have analyzed the role of lncRNAs in diabetic nephropathy (Figure 1). Consequently, this review contains a focused paragraph on diabetic nephropathy but also provides an insight into the publications on other glomerular disease entities such as focal segmental glomerulosclerosis and membranous nephropathy (Table 1).

2.1. Diabetic Nephropathy—The Link between MicroRNAs and LncRNAs

With the incidence of diabetes mellitus rising and diabetic nephropathy (DN) being a leading cause of end-stage renal disease in Western societies [11,12], it is clear that researchers chose this entity as a key topic to elucidate the role of lncRNAs in kidney disease. Most of the work that goes beyond a mere description of non-coding RNA expression in DN focused on miRNAs and a few annotated lncRNAs the function of which had been addressed in other diseases/organs before. Despite the fact that miRNAs are not the topic of this review, it is important to note the intricate connection between miRNAs and lncRNAs. Firstly, the latter can impact miRNA function, e.g., by serving as miRNA sponges that inhibit their binding to the actual mRNA targets [13]. This has been described in the context of DN for a number of miRNA—lncRNA interactions including work on the lncRNAs TUG1, NEAT1 and MALAT1 [14–16]. Furthermore, lncRNA genes can harbor miRNAs that are set free by posttranscriptional cleavage. Prominent examples are the lncRNA PVT1 serving as a host of miRNA 1207-5p and both non-coding RNAs having been implicated in DN [17]. Importantly, miRNAs are often organized as clusters with four more miRNAs having been localized to the *PVT1* locus [18] all of which are upregulated by high glucose levels and impact extracellular matrix (ECM) formation. MiRNA clusters contained in lncRNAs can get very large as demonstrated by a megacluster of more than 40 miRNAs harbored in lnc-MGC. This cluster is induced in the glomeruli of several mouse models of diabetic nephropathy through endoplasmic reticulum (ER) stress signaling and responds to both high glucose and TGFβ-activation [19]. Inhibition of lnc-MGC using a "Gapmers"—antisense oligonucleotides that induce the RNaseH-mediated degradation of their targets often used in the lncRNA field—ameliorates several histological signs of diabetic nephropathy in a mouse model pointing towards a therapeutic potential of these findings.

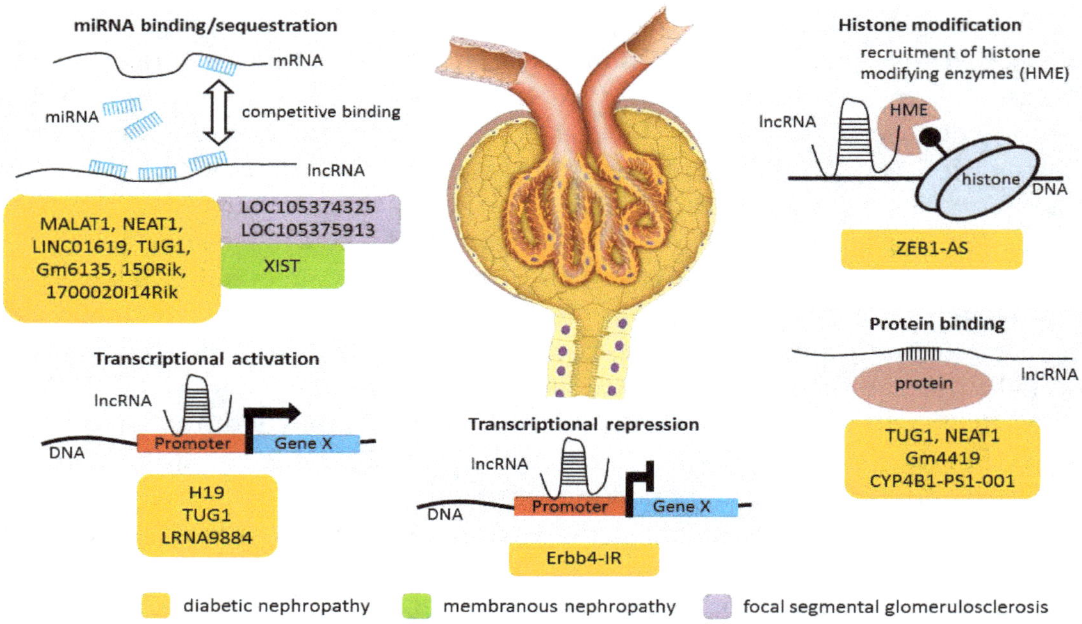

Figure 1. Long non-coding RNAs (lncRNAs) in glomerular disease and their reported molecular functions. Grey colored boxes depict the molecular mechanisms of lncRNA function (enhancer RNA, transcriptional repression, transcription activation, protein binding, miRNA binding/sequestration and histone modification) reported to play a role in glomerular disease. Orange, green and purple colored boxes indicate the disease: diabetic nephropathy, membranous nephropathy and focal segmental glomerulosclerosis, respectively. The lncRNAs associated with the particular mechanism and disease are specified by name. Glomerulus image obtained from: Aldona Griskieviciene/shutterstock.com.

2.2. Diabetic Nephropathy—Tthe Role of Specific Long Non-Coding RNAs (LncRNAs)

Regarding the involvement of specific lncRNAs we will focus on genes that have been implicated in DN by evidence from several publications.

The plasmacytoma variant translocation gene *PVT1* had been linked to diabetic nephropathy by the finding that variants in this gene are associated with the development of end-stage renal disease (ESRD) in both type 1 and 2 diabetes mellitus [20,21]. Soon after, it was noted that PVT1 was a non-coding RNA the expression of which was induced by high glucose in mesangial cells. Knockdown of PVT1 significantly decreased the upregulation of both ECM proteins and their transcriptional regulators PAI-1 and TGFβ1 [22], providing a functional link between the genomic data and the pathogenesis of DN. As described above, PVT1 hosts several miRNAs, one of which—miR-1207-5p—could be shown to regulate ECM formation in parallel to the lncRNA itself [17]. Zhang et al. provided further evidence on the role of PVT1 with a component from traditional Chinese medicine (Danggui Buxue Tang) alleviating glucose-indcued proliferation and ECM formation in mesangial cells through targeting PVT1 [23].

MALAT1 is another important example of an lncRNA involved in DN. MALAT1 is induced in the streptozocin-induced diabetic nephropathy mouse model [24]. Based on this finding and further work using cultured podocytes, Hu and colleagues hypothesized MALAT1 to play a role in high-glucose associated podocyte damage involving a feedback loop with beta-catenin employing the MALAT1-binding protein SRSF1 [24]. Furthermore, MALAT1 has been implicated in the damage of other renal cell types in DN. Regarding glomerular endothelial cells MALAT1 induction was accompanied by an epigenetically mediated decrease of Klotho expression [25]. The upregulation of this lncRNA upon glucose exposure led to increased IL1 and TNF-α levels suggesting this lncRNA to be involved in inflammatory processes of the endothelium [26]. In renal tubular epithelial cells MALAT1 induction by high glucose leads to increased pyroptosis by targeting miR-23c and consecutive upregulation of ELAVL1 and NLRP3 [16].

Mitochondrial dysfunction is one of the hallmarks in DN [27]. The modulation of mitochondrial metabolism was linked to the lncRNA TUG1 by an important study in 2016 [28]. TUG1 was differentially expressed in a murine DN model (db/db mice). Its podocyte-specific overexpression in this mouse model improved the glomerular phenotype both regarding albuminuria and histological changes. Mechanistically, TUG1 was linked to mitochondrial bioenergetics by showing that this lncRNA recruits PGC-1α to its own promoter [28]. Further studies corroborate the link of TUG1 to diabetic glomerulopathy. TUG1 both alleviated ECM deposition by acting as a sponge for miR-377 [14] and protected from podocyte apoptosis by modulating ER stress signaling, PGC-1α and TRAF5 [29,30] in different models of DN.

Besides, several lines of evidence point towards a functionally important involvement of the lncRNA NEAT1 in diabetic nephropathy. NEAT1 is induced in a streptozocin-mediated diabetic rat model and murine mesangial cells treated with high-glucose [15,31]. Increased expression of NEAT1 led to the activation of AKT/mTOR signalling accompanied by increased cellular proliferation and fibrosis [31]. Interestingly, this phenotype could be alleviated by knockdown of NEAT1, providing a therapeutic prospective. Additionally, NEAT1 served as a sponge for miR-27b-3p relieving ZEB1—a zinc finger transcription factor associated with epithelial-mesenchymal transition and ECM deposition—from miRNA-mediated repression [15].

CYP4B1-PS1-001 was first described in diabetic nephropathy in a microarray based-screen for dysregulated lncRNAs in the db/db mouse model [32]. Whilst this intergenic lncRNA was strongly downregulated in early phases of DN, its overexpression alleviated the increased proliferative tone in mesangial cells. This effect of CYP4B1-PS1-001 could later on be shown to be mediated by the proteasomal degradation of Nucleolin—a nucleolar ribosome biogenesis factor [33].

More than 20 additional lncRNAs have been implicated in diabetic nephropathy by single publications. Here, we summarize the most important findings. Several of these lncRNAs interact directly with miRNAs and inhibit their function. As examples, LINC01619 induces oxidative podocyte damage by serving as a sponge for miR-27a [34], Gm6135 protects from increased proliferation and apoptosis through impairing the miR-203-3p mediated downregulation of Toll-like receptor 4 [35], lincRNA1700020I14Rik reduces cellular proliferation via inhibition of miR-34-a-5p [36] and lncRNA 150Rik promotes proliferation by sponging miR-451 [37]. Apart from the inhibitory direct binding as described for these examples, lncRNA H19 induces the expression of miR-675 modulating vitamin D receptor expression [38] and lncRNA Erbb4-IR suppresses miR-29b on the transcriptional level [39]. The latter publication is a very good examples of a study taking lncRNAs in diabetic nephropathy beyond a mere description of expression changes by elucidating both the factor driving its expression (Smad3) as well as its downstream effects through mir-29b and by proving the therapeutic potential of Erbb4-IR inhibition in the db/db mouse model. Another lncRNA regulated by Smad3—LRNA9884—promotes DN through the stimulation of inflammation [40]. Similarly, lincRNA Gm4419 promotes inflammation in DN through the NLRP3 inflammasome [41]. Another layer of regulation through lncRNAs that has been found in other systems is epigenetic modifications. As to DN, lncRNA ZEB1-AS1 has been shown to enhance the expression of ZEB1 by promoting H3K4me3 histone modification on its promoter during high glucose treatment with increased ZEB1 exerting an anti-fibrotic role [42]. Importantly, since all of these data were primarily obtained in mouse models, a number of expression screens in DN have been able to show evolutionary conservation of lncRNA modulation in human datasets [43–45] indicating the future potential of data obtained in mouse models for the patient setting.

Table 1. LncRNAs involved in glomerular diseases.

		Diabetic Nephropathy		
lncRNA	main disease model	suggested function	target	reference
TUG1	diabetic mice (db/db)	transcriptional activation	Ppargc1a promoter	[28]
	diabetic mice (db/db)	miRNA binding	miR-377	[14]
	streptozotocin treated rats	protein binding	TRAF5	[29]
MALAT1	streptozotocin treated rats	miRNA binding	miR-23	[16]
	streptozotocin treated mice	expression changed	IL-6 and TNF-α	[26]
	streptozotocin treated mice	expression changed	β-catenin, SRSF1	[24]
NEAT1	streptozotocin treated rats	miRNA binding	miR-27b-3p	[15]
	streptozotocin treated rats	expression changed	Akt/mTOR signaling	[31]
PVT1	high glucose treated CIHP-1	expression changed	ECM-related proteins	[22]
ZEB1-AS	streptozotocin treated mice	recruitment of histone modifications	ZEB1 promoter	[42]
LRNA9884	diabetic mice (db/db)	transcriptional activation	MCP-1	[40]
LINC01619	streptozotocin treated rats	miRNA binding	miR-27a	[34]
Gm6135	diabetic mice (db/db)	miRNA binding	miR-203-3p	[35]
CYP4B1-PS1-001	diabetic mice (db/db)	protein binding	NCL	[33]
1700020I14Rik	diabetic mice (db/db)	miRNA binding	miR-34	[36]
150Rik	diabetic mice (db/db)	miRNA binding	miR-451	[37]
H19	vitamin D3 treated CIHP-1	expression changed	miR-675	[38]
Erbb4-IR	diabetic mice (db/db)	transcriptional repression	miR-29b	[39]
Gm4419	high glucose treated mouse MCs	protein binding	p50	[41]
		Focal-Segmental Glomerulosclerosis		
lncRNA	main disease model	suggested function	target	reference
LOC105374325	adriamycin treated podocytes	miRNA binding	miR-34c and miR-196a/b	[46]
LOC105375913	FSGS patient serum treated HK-2	miRNA binding	miR-27b	[47]
		Membranous Nephropathy		
lncRNA	main disease model	suggested function	target	reference
XIST	angiotensin II treated AB8/13	miRNA binding	miR-217	[48]
		Lupus Nephritis		
lncRNA	main disease model	suggested function	target	reference
RP11-2B6.2	IFN-I treated HeLa and HK-2	epigenetic inhibition	SOCS1	[49]

2.3. *LncRNAs in Other Glomerular Diseases*

In comparison to DN, little is known about the contribution of lncRNAs to other glomerular disease entitites. A Pubmed search for lncRNAs AND glomerulus revealed more than 80% of these publications to deal with DN. Fewer than 10 studies report results regarding different types of glomerulonephritis and focal-segmental glomerulosclerosis (FSGS). Due to the scarcity of data, all of these studies are discussed in the following paragraph independent from impact and approach. LncRNA LOC105375913 was found to be increased in tubular cells of 5 FSGS patients [47] and this upregulation was, based on cell culture results, induced by the C3a/p38/XBP-1s pathway. LOC105375913 exerted its profibrotic function through sequestration of miR-27b and consecutive overexpression of Snail. As to actual glomerular changes in FSGS lncRNA LOC105374325 has been described to be upregulated in podocytes of FSGS patients and to induce podocyte apoptosis. Again, the induction of this lncRNA (through p38 and C/EPBbeta) exerts its effects by serving as a sponge for two miRNAs (miR-34c, miR-196a/b) that normally regulate the expression of pro-apoptotic proteins [46]. Interestingly, the profibrotic function of LOC105375913 in the tubulointerstitium and the proapoptotic effect of LOC105374325 in podocytes could also be recapitulated in mouse models overexpressing the respective lncRNAs [46,47]. Regarding direct podocyte injury Fang et al. found the lncRNA GAS5 to be downregulated in a murine sepsis model (using lipopolysaccharide (LPS) injection) [50]. Loss of GAS5 led to a reduction of nephrin and an induction of both Snail/phosphorylated Snail and PI3K/AKT/GSK3β as potential harmful agents. In a descriptive approach Qin et al. reported 10 lncRNAs to be differentially expressed in glomeruli after treatment of mice with Adriamycin based on RNA-sequencing [51] and Gao at el. provided a similar analysis in whole kidney microarray analyses of two glomerulonephritis rat models (nephrotoxic serum nephritis and anti-glomerular basement membrane glomerulonephritis) [52]. As to human samples, two studies described the differential expression of numerous lncRNAs in either IgA-positive or -negative mesangio-proliferative glomerulonephritis [53,54]. The actual pathophysiological impact of this work remains to be determined. One of the longest-known lncRNAs—XIST, which is known for its role in the inactivation of the X-chromosome—has been linked to membranous nephropathy (MN) [48,55]. This lncRNA was found to be upregulated both in a mouse model of MN and in human samples [55]. Data in cell culture pointed towards XIST exerting its proapoptotic effect on podocytes through sequestration of miR-217 and consecutive upregulation of Toll-like receptor 4 [48]. Finally, in a recent report Liao et al. showed differential expression of lncRNAs in kidney biopsies of patients diagnosed with lupus nephritis (LN) [49]. LncRNA RP11-2B6.2 was found upregulated in kidney tissue of LN patients compared to healthy controls. Using HELA and HK-2 cell lines the authors showed that overexpression of RP11-2B6.2 led to inhibition of SOCS1, a known regulator of the IFN-1 signaling pathway and consequently increased the activity of the IFN-1 signaling pathway. They went on to evaluate chromatin accessibility of the SOCS1 locus in the presence and absence of RP11-2B6.2 and determined that downregulation of RP11-2B6.2 coincided with an open chromatin state in the promoter region of SOCS1. Based on this finding Liao et al. proposed that the inhibition of SOCS1 is conveyed by an undetermined epigenetic mechanism [49].

3. Tubulointerstitial Disease

To date, the majority of lncRNA studies on tubulointerstitial kidney disease were performed in the context of acute kidney injury (AKI) (Figure 2). Research on chronic kidney disease including genetic disorders such as autosomal dominant polycystic kidney disease (ADPKD) is still very scarce (Table 2).

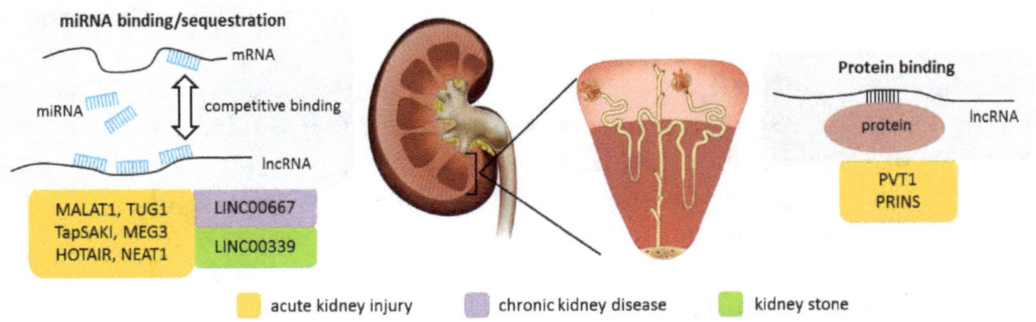

Figure 2. LncRNAs in tubulointerstitial disease and their reported molecular functions. Grey colored boxes depict the molecular mechanisms of lncRNA function (miRNA binding/sequestration and protein binding) reported to play a role in tubulointerstital disease. Orange, purple and green colored boxes indicate the disease: acute kidney injury, chronic kidney disease and kidney stone, respectively. The lncRNAs associated with the particular mechanism and disease are specified by name. Kidney image obtained from: Tefi/shutterstock.com.

3.1. *LncRNAs and Acute Kidney Injury*

AKI is a central problem in nephrology considering the high and increasing incidence associated with the demographic changes in Western societies and the lack of specific preventive and therapeutic strategies [56]. Consequently, it is crucial to gain an optimal understanding on the molecular mechanisms predisposing for and protecting from AKI and lncRNAs are an important novel layer of regulation in this context. Major triggers of AKI are sepsis, ischemia reperfusion injury and nephrotoxic agents. In recent years, based on transcriptomic data created from patient material as well as various animal models, a growing number of differentially expressed lncRNAs associated with AKI have been described. The majority of in vivo studies performed to examine AKI were carried out in mice or rats by the induction of ischemia reperfusion injury (IRI) [57–62], inflammation stimulated by lipopolysaccharide (LPS) [63,64], urine-derived sepsis [65,66] or exposure to hypoxia [67]. For in vitro models of AKI, the research community mainly relied on the HK-2 human tubular epithelial cell line either treated with LPS [64–66,68,69] or grown under hypoxic conditions [59–62,70]. However, when interpreting these data, it is important to note, that the comparability to the actual patient setting is limited especially for cell culture models. This highlights the importance of a confirmation of the findings in both rodents and especially using human biosamples.

Most evidence for an lncRNA to play a role in AKI has been presented for metastasis-associated lung adenocarcinoma transcript 1 (MALAT1). Initially identified as the most highly induced lncRNA gene in kidney and testis of hypoxic mice, MALAT1 was proposed to be hypoxia-inducible factor (HIF)-2 activated and postulated to function in renal proximal tubuli [67]. MALAT1 expression was suggested to inhibit the hypoxia-induced inflammatory response through the NF-κB pathway [57]. This idea was supported by the findings of Ding et al. who, in an LPS-induced model of AKI, found that MALAT1 interacts with mir-146a—a known regulator of the NF-κB signaling pathway [64]. In spite of these findings, no disease-specific phenotype was observed after challenging MALAT1 knockout mice with IRI-induced AKI [62]. Although the authors suggested that in vivo the impact of MALAT1 on signaling pathways might be minimal, it remains a potential biomarker of kidney IRI due to its high abundance in patient plasma and kidney biopsies [62].

Nuclear enriched abundant transcript 1 (NEAT1) was detected as significantly upregulated in the serum of patients with sepsis-induced as well as in patients with ischemia-induced AKI [71,72]. Using in vitro interaction assays both groups showed that NEAT1 interacts with several miRNAs. In the first case Chen et al. concluded that by binding to miR-204 NEAT1 reduces the cellular level of this miRNA, thereby alleviating the suppression of IL-6R and activating the NF-κB pathway with consecutive inflammation [71]. The second study conducted by Jiang et al. determined miR-27a-3p as a direct interactor of NEAT1 by RNA immunoprecipitation [72]. In knockdown and overexpression experiments the authors showed the negatively correlated influence of NEAT1 on miR-27a-3p levels leading to apoptosis.

Similar studies link the lncRNAs HOX transcript antisense RNA (HOTAIR) [66], taurine upregulated gene 1 (*TUG1*) [73], maternally expressed gene 3 (*MEG3*) [63] and transcript predicting survival in AKI (*TapSAKI*) [65] to a range of other miRNAs.

HOTAIR—known to play an important role in apoptosis—was upregulated in rats with sepsis caused by urinary tract infection [66]. The authors further observed a negative regulation of miR-22 and induction of apoptosis in HK-2 cells and related this regulation to the stabilization of high-mobility-group-protein B1 (HMGB1)—a key mediator of inflammation and a known target of miR-22. In a study using HOTAIR mimics in vivo in rats with sepsis induced AKI, Jiang et al. found that expression of HOTAIR declined serum serine—as well as blood urea nitrogen levels and reduced signs of apoptosis in kidney tissue [74]. These effects were attributed to the concomitant reduction of miR-34a and increase of B-cell leukemia/lymphoma 2 (Bcl-2) protein levels, with Bcl-2 being an anti-apoptotic factor and a target of miR-34a.

To unravel the role of the lncRNA TUG1, detected at lower levels in the serum of patients suffering from sepsis-associated AKI in comparison to healthy controls, a LPS based in vitro model was used [73]. Despite the fact that this study examined rat mesangial cells we report their results in this section due to the link to other LPS-induced AKI models. Liu et al. found that overexpression of TUG1 reversed the deteriorating effects of LPS on RMCs and showed that this was mediated by miR-142-3p. Furthermore, SIRT1 a known suppressor of the NF-κB signaling pathway, was identified as the direct target downregulated by miR-142-3p in the absence of TUG1. Consequently, these findings suggest that the lower levels of TUG1 observed in the serum of AKI patients may lead to activation of the NF-κB pathway driving inflammation. These findings are supported by a study of Xu et al. confirming the protective effect of overexpressed TUG1 on LPS-induced injury in HK-2 cells [68]. Although, the conveying factor between TUG1 and SIRT1 was found to be miR-223 in this study, the effects on the NF-κB pathway were similar. In addition, the authors suggested that the protective effects of TUG1 on renal tubular epithelial cells injury are associated with activation of the PI3K/AKT pathway.

In two individual studies MEG3 was found to be upregulated after LPS or hypoxia treatment, respectively and in both cases the authors report the sequestration of miRNAs by MEG3 [58,63]. Yang et al. showed that the higher levels of MEG3 lead to increased binding of miR-21 removing it from the pool available to inhibit the translation of programmed cell death protein 4 (PDCD4) [63]. The downregulation of MEG3 resulted in the inhibition of PDCD4 and attenuation of LPS-induced apoptosis. Likewise, data presented by Pang et al. suggested MEG3 to sequester mir-181b leading to upregulation of TNF-α in hypoxia-induced kidney injury in acute renal allografts [58].

TapSAKI, initially discovered as a circulating lncRNA upregulated in the plasma of AKI patients and their kidney tissue was proposed as a biomarker with predictive value for the survival of AKI patients [75]. Recently, Shen et al. using a urine-derived sepsis model of AKI in rats and LPS treated HK-2 cells, showed that TapSAKI interacts with miR-22 [65]. In a state of TapSAKI upregulation this interaction leads to increased levels of phosphatase and tensin homolog (PTEN) and activation of TLR4 and NF-κB pathway triggering inflammation.

In the section below we discuss lncRNAs which so far have only a single study connecting them to acute kidney injury—plasmacytoma variant translocation 1 (PVT1) [69], psoriasis-susceptibility-related RNA gene induced by stress (PRINS) [59], growth arrest-specific 5 (GAS5) [61], aspartyl-tRNA synthetase anti-sense 1 (DARS-AS1) [70], LINC00520 [60], UC.173 [76].

An involvement of PVT1 in kidney disease has been described previously for diabetic nephropathy [22] and is discussed above in the DN section. In their 2017 study on LPS-treated HK-2 cells, Huang et al. found PVT1 significantly upregulated compared to untreated control cells [69]. The authors reported PVT1 overexpression to decrease cell viability and to trigger inflammatory responses. Vice versa, downregulation of PVT1 resulted in suppression of inflammatory factors by regulation of the JNK/NF-κB signaling pathways. The authors suggested the binding of TNF-α by PVT1 to be the responsible mechanism leading to inhibition of JNK/NF-κB signaling pathways promoting inflammatory responses in sepsis-induced AKI.

The expression and secretion of RANTES/CCL5 (regulated on activation, normal T cell expressed and secreted) is known to recruit circulating leukocytes to sites of injury and to reinforce inflammatory reactions. In their report, Yu et al. showed that PRINS, a HIF-1α regulated lncRNA is potentially involved in RANTES production [59]. The study suggested a significant upregulation and direct interaction between PRINS and RANTES in hypoxic conditions leading to enhanced inflammation and AKI progression.

The hypoxia-responsive lncRNA GAS5 was reported to be upregulated in IRI treated mice by Geng et al. [61]. The increase of GAS5 was linked to induction of proapoptotic factors: p53, cIAP2 and TSP-1. Performing in vitro experiments in hypoxia treated HK-2 cells the authors confirmed this correlation for p53 and TSP-1 and in the reciprocal approach showed that knockdown of GAS5 led to downregulation of p53 and TSP-1, attenuating apoptosis.

The study conducted on HK-2 and primary renal proximal tubular epithelial cells (RPTEC) by Mimura et al. compared lncRNA expression patterns between hypoxic and normoxic cells [70]. DARS-AS1 containing hypoxia-responsive elements (HRE) in the promoter region was found upregulated as a consequence of HIF-1α binding in hypoxic conditions. The authors further showed that the expression of DARS-AS1 has inhibitory effects on cell death progression and therefore may be important for the survival of renal tubular cells during AKI.

Tian et al. observed an upregulation of LINC00520 in rat kidney tissue following IRI treatment [60]. Using HK-2 cells they determined a relation between LINC00520 and miR-27b and suggested that

LINC00520 may inhibit miR-27b by competitive binding. Reduction of miR-27b in the cellular pool resulted in the upregulation of Oncostatin M receptor (OSMR). Finally, the authors showed knockdown of LINC00520 to reduce levels of OSMR, reduction of PI3K/AKT and attenuation of renal injury in rats.

UC.173 belongs to a group of lncRNAs transcribed from an ultra-conserved region (T-UCR) shared between human, rat and mouse genomes and was initially reported as downregulated in lead-exposed human populations and animal models [77]. Qin et al. studied UC.173 in the context of lead-induced renal tubular epithelial cell apoptosis and showed that lead exposure reduced the levels of this lncRNA in HK-2 and HKC cells [76]. While the overexpression of UC.173 had no effect on cell viability, cell cycle or apoptotic factors in lead-unexposed HK-2 and HKC cells, its overexpression in lead treated cells increased cell survival and showed reduced signs of apoptosis.

Table 2. LncRNAs involved in tubulointerstitial disease.

Acute Kidney Injury				
lncRNA	main disease model	suggested function	target	reference
MEG3	IRI in renal allografts	miRNA binding	miR181b-5p	[58]
	LPS treated mice	miRNA binding	miR-21	[63]
NEAT1	LPS treated RMCs	miRNA binding	miR-204	[71]
	CoCl2 treated HK-2	miRNA binding	miR-27a-3p	[72]
MALAT1	LPS treated rats	miRNA binding	miR-146a	[64]
	hypoxia treated mice	expression changed	unknown	[67]
TapSAKI	Urine derived sepsis in rats	miRNA binding	miR-22	[65]
	AKI patients	circulating biomarker	unknown	[75]
HOTAIR	Urine derived sepsis in rats	miRNA binding	miR-22	[66]
	CLP induced sepsis in rats	expression changed	miR-34a and Bcl-2	[74]
TUG1	LPS treated RMCs	miRNA binding	miR-142-3p	[73]
	LPS treated HK-2	miRNA binding	miR-223	[68]
LINC00520	IRI in rats	miRNA binding	miR-27b-3p	[60]
PVT1	LPS treated HK-2	protein binding	TNF-α	[69]
PRINS	IRI in mice	protein binding	RANTES (CCL-5)	[59]
GAS5	IRI in mice	expression changed	mRNA of p53 and TCP1	[61]
DARS-AS1	hypoxia treated HK-2 and RPTECs	expression changed	unknown	[70]
UC.173	lead treated HK-2 and HKC	expression changed	unknown	[76]
Chronic kidney disease				
lncRNA	main disease model	suggested function	target	reference
LINC00667	CKD patients and rat model	miRNA binding	miR-19b-3p	[78]
LINC00963	CKD rat model	expression changed	mRNA of FoxO3a	[79]
Autosomal Dominant Polycystic Kidney Disease				
lncRNA	main disease model	suggested function	target	reference
Hoxb3os	Pkd1/2 knockout mice	expression changed	unknown	[80]
Kidney stone				
lncRNA	main disease model	suggested function	target	reference
LINC00339	COM treated HK-2	miRNA binding	miR-22-3p	[81]
CHCHD4P4	COM treated mice	expression changed	unknown	[82]
Uric Acid Nephropathy				
lncRNA	main disease model	suggested function	target	reference
ANRIL	uric acid treated HK-2	miRNA binding	miR-122-5p	[83]

3.2. LncRNAs Associated with Other Tubulointerstitial Diseases

In this section we give an overview of recent advances with regard to the function of lncRNAs in tubulointerstitial diseases other than acute kidney injury. We discuss the role of lncRNAs in 5/6 nephrectomy, autosomal dominant polycystic kidney disease (ADPKD) and kidney injury by crystal-formation (e.g., calcium oxalate).

To date, two lncRNAs have been associated with the transcriptional response in rat models of 5/6 nephrectomy [78,79]. LINC00963, studied by Chen et al. due to its upregulation in the context of renal interstitial fibrosis and oxidative stress, was determined to influence FoxO3a levels by an undetermined mechanism [79]. Lowered LINC00963 levels were associated with the activation of the FoxO signaling pathway, consequently leading to suppression of renal interstitial fibrosis and oxidative stress. The same group published a study investigating the role of LINC00667 [78]. LINC00667 was upregulated while miR-19b-3p was downregulated in kidney tissue of patients suffering from CKD (chronic kidney disease) of heterogenous etiology compared to normal renal tissue. The authors linked the downregulation of miR-19b-3b to a sequestration by LINC00667. In the 5/6 nephrectomy rat model used in this study, overexpression of miR-19b-3p decreased levels of TGF-β1, CTGF, α-SMA and TIMP-1 and improved the renal damage. A recent review provides a detailed view on the general role of non-coding RNAs in renal fibrosis [84].

To the best of our knowledge, so far only one lncRNA has been shown to have functional implications in ADPKD. Aboudehen et al. investigated the role of Hoxb3os, an lncRNA abundantly expressed in the kidney and evolutionary conserved with the human ortholog HOXB-AS1 [80]. The expression of HOXB-AS1 was decreased in the kidney tissue of ADPKD patients and likewise in *Pkd1* and *Pkd2* knockout mice, a genetic model of ADPKD, a downregulation of the mouse ortholog was observed. In a cell model using mIMCD3, the authors showed that knockout of Hoxb3os leads to mTORC1 activation and increase in mitochondrial respiration and that re-expression of Hoxb3os rescues this phenotype.

Recent findings have also shown that lncRNAs are associated with renal injury mediated by crystal formation. The studies - mainly based on HK-2 cell exposure to calcium oxalate monohydrate (COM), the major constituent of kidney stones [85], range from profiling changes in lncRNA expression upon COM stimulation to analysis of individual lncRNAs. Wang et al.—using the same cell model—profiled transcriptional changes by RNA sequencing and determined 25 differentially expressed lncRNAs [86]. Cao et al. used an ethylene glycol-induced rat model of kidney stone formation to profile expression changes and found 1440 lncRNAs differentially regulated in comparison to untreated controls [87]. In addition to an in vitro COM-HK-2 cell model, Zhang et al. used a mouse model of calcium oxalate-induced kidney damage and found 376 differentially regulated lncRNA in COM-treated animal in comparison to the control group. 15 of the regulated lncRNAs had homologous genes in the human genome. LncRNA AU015836 and the human homolog CHCHD4P4 were upregulated upon COM treatment in mouse kidney tissue and HK-2 cells, respectively. The authors further showed that CHCHD4P4 was involved in epithelial–mesenchymal transition (EMT) by regulation of EMT-related genes and the inhibited cell proliferation in COM-exposed HK-2 cells [82]. In their study on LINC00339 in COM-treated HK-2 cells, Song et al. linked the promotion of renal tubular epithelial pyroptosis to the activation of the NLRP3 inflammasome [81]. The inflammasome was activated due to increased levels of NLRP3 resulting from the sequestration of miR-22-3p—a regulator of NLRP3—by LINC00339. As a last example, antisense non-coding RNA in the INK4 locus ANRIL, a highly expressed lncRNA in the serum of patients suffering from uric acid nephropathy (UAN), was studied by Hu et al. in HK-2 cells and a rat model of UAN [83]. The authors report that downregulation of ANRIL in the animal model resulted in reduced signs of renal injury. According to the results from the in vitro studies in HK-2 cells this improvement was conveyed through the reduced sequestering of miR-122-5p by ANRIL, which in turn led to the downregulation of the BRCA1-BRCA2-containing complex subunit 3 (BRCC3) and as a consequence suppressed the activation of NLRP3 inflammasome.

4. Systemic Kidney Biomarkers

Regarding glomerular disease there are no reports on circulating lncRNAs as potential biomarkers. For membranous nephropathy lncRNA XIST has been hypothesized to be a potential urinary biomarker [55]. However, the increase of urinary XIST—which was originally described in kidneys of a mouse model of MN—was not specific to MN but rather reflected injury in different types of glomerulonephritis. Besides, the lncRNA TapSAKI was identified as a circulating factor with the potential to predict mortality among a cohort of 109 patients suffering from acute kidney injury [75]. A potential implementation of lncRNAs as biomarkers for standardized clinical use will require studies in larger cohorts including questions on specificity and predictive value regarding clinical outcome. Since for most renal disorders little is known regarding the impact of lncRNAs, screening studies describing differential expression of lncRNAs using state-of-the-art methodology (e.g., RNA and single cell RNA sequencing) are still an important asset but will require further complementation by targeted analyses elucidating the molecular function of specific lncRNAs (e.g., RNAscope for visualization, quantitative polymerase chain reaction (qPCR) for quantification and CHART-MS for the identification of binding partners.

5. Conclusion and Outlook

LncRNAs provide a fascinating new layer to pathophysiological studies and the search for novel therapeutic strategies in kidney disease. However, apart from few examples such as diabetic nephropathy and acute kidney injury, little is known about their impact in renal pathologies and most studies have remained primarily descriptive. Future work will need to close this gap in order to increase our understanding of this new class of non-coding RNAs in nephrology and to eventually elucidate how we can exploit the potential of lncRNA modulation for patients suffering from kidney disease. The inhibition of lncRNAs in vivo is technically no more challenging than the inhibition of messenger RNAs; therefore, with an increasing number of antisense oligonucleotide therapies coming into clinical use at the moment (e.g., RNAi for TTR-amyloidosis or modulation of splicing for spinal muscular atrophy) this concept could be of high interest for targeting lncRNAs in kidney disease [88–90]. Regarding the cell-type specific expression of RNAs in the kidney and specifically the glomerulus single cell or single nucleus RNA sequencing (scRNAseq) studies have started to add much to our knowledge in both conditions of health and disease including DN [91–94]. Importantly, since nearly all lncRNAs are polyadenylated, the commonly used 3′end sequencing approaches in scRNAseq do capture these sequences as well if samples are sequenced at a sufficient depth (due to comparably lower transcript counts of lncRNAs compared to other RNA species). These approaches will now need to be analyzed in detail regarding lncRNAs and transferred to human kidney biopsies using either scRNAseq itself (for an example regarding a first approach in Lupus nephritis see [95]) or targeted imaging of specific lncRNAs, e.g., by single-molecule FISH. When using model organisms, the difficulties in predicting evolutionary conservation are still a major challenge, which will make innovative bioinformatics solutions an essential asset. Furthermore, the function of lncRNAs can hardly be predicted and its elucidation requires continuous development of novel techniques. Taken together, it is time for nephrologists to team up with molecular and computational biologists and unravel the full impact of lncRNAs in kidney disease.

Author Contributions: M.I. and R.-U.M. drafted, wrote and revised the manuscript; R.I. performed the literature search.

Acknowledgments: We thank Petra Kleinwächter for excellent help with figure design.

Abbreviations

CIHP-1	human podocyte cell line
MC	mesangial cells
FSGS	focal-segmental glomerulosclerosis
HK-2	human proximal tubule epithelial cell line
AB8/13	human podocyte cell line
IRI	ischemia reperfusion injury
LPS	lipopolysaccharide
RMCs	rat mesangial cell line
HK-2	human proximal tubule epithelial cell line
CLP	cecal ligation puncture
RPTECs	human renal proximal tubular epithelial cell line
HKC	human kidney proximal tubular epithelial cell line
CKD	chronic kidney disease
COM	calcium oxalate monohydrate

References

1. Zhao, H.; Ma, S.X.; Shang, Y.Q.; Zhang, H.Q.; Su, W. MicroRNAs in chronic kidney disease. *Clin. Chim. Acta* **2019**, *491*, 59–65. [CrossRef] [PubMed]
2. Ledeganck, K.J.; Gielis, E.M.; Abramowicz, D.; Stenvinkel, P.; Shiels, P.G.; Van Craenenbroeck, A.H. MicroRNAs in AKI and Kidney Transplantation. *Clin. J. Am. Soc. Nephrol.* **2019**, *14*, 454–468. [CrossRef] [PubMed]
3. Quinn, J.J.; Chang, H.Y. Unique features of long non-coding RNA biogenesis and function. *Nat. Rev. Genet.* **2016**, *17*, 47–62. [CrossRef]
4. St Laurent, G.; Wahlestedt, C.; Kapranov, P. The Landscape of long noncoding RNA classification. *Trends Genet. Tig.* **2015**, *31*, 239–251. [CrossRef] [PubMed]
5. Yao, R.W.; Wang, Y.; Chen, L.L. Cellular functions of long noncoding RNAs. *Nat. Cell. Biol.* **2019**, *21*, 542–551. [CrossRef]
6. Cabili, M.N.; Trapnell, C.; Goff, L.; Koziol, M.; Tazon-Vega, B.; Regev, A.; Rinn, J.L. Integrative annotation of human large intergenic noncoding RNAs reveals global properties and specific subclasses. *Genes Dev.* **2011**, *25*, 1915–1927. [CrossRef]
7. Johnsson, P.; Lipovich, L.; Grander, D.; Morris, K.V. Evolutionary conservation of long non-coding RNAs; sequence, structure, function. *Biochim. Et. Biophys. Acta* **2014**, *1840*, 1063–1071. [CrossRef]
8. Derrien, T.; Johnson, R.; Bussotti, G.; Tanzer, A.; Djebali, S.; Tilgner, H.; Guernec, G.; Martin, D.; Merkel, A.; Knowles, D.G.; et al. The GENCODE v7 catalog of human long noncoding RNAs: Analysis of their gene structure, evolution, and expression. *Genome Res.* **2012**, *22*, 1775–1789. [CrossRef]
9. Gloss, B.S.; Dinger, M.E. The specificity of long noncoding RNA expression. *Biochim. Et. Biophys. Acta* **2016**, *1859*, 16–22. [CrossRef]
10. Maass, P.G.; Luft, F.C.; Bähring, S. Long non-coding RNA in health and disease. *J. Mol. Med.* **2014**, *92*, 337–346. [CrossRef]
11. Nathan, D.M. Diabetes: Advances in Diagnosis and Treatment. *JAMA* **2015**, *314*, 1052–1062. [CrossRef] [PubMed]
12. Fineberg, D.; Jandeleit-Dahm, K.A.; Cooper, M.E. Diabetic nephropathy: Diagnosis and treatment. *Nat. Rev. Endocrinol.* **2013**, *9*, 713–723. [CrossRef] [PubMed]
13. Paraskevopoulou, M.D.; Hatzigeorgiou, A.G. Analyzing MiRNA-LncRNA Interactions. *Methods Mol. Biol.* **2016**, *1402*, 271–286. [CrossRef] [PubMed]
14. Duan, L.J.; Ding, M.; Hou, L.J.; Cui, Y.T.; Li, C.J.; Yu, D.M. Long noncoding RNA TUG1 alleviates extracellular matrix accumulation via mediating microRNA-377 targeting of PPARgamma in diabetic nephropathy. *Biochem. Biophys. Res. Commun.* **2017**, *484*, 598–604. [CrossRef] [PubMed]
15. Wang, X.; Xu, Y.; Zhu, Y.C.; Wang, Y.K.; Li, J.; Li, X.Y.; Ji, T.; Bai, S.J. LncRNA NEAT1 promotes extracellular matrix accumulation and epithelial-to-mesenchymal transition by targeting miR-27b-3p and ZEB1 in diabetic nephropathy. *J. Cell Physiol.* **2019**, *234*, 12926–12933. [CrossRef]

16. Li, X.; Zeng, L.; Cao, C.; Lu, C.; Lian, W.; Han, J.; Zhang, X.; Zhang, J.; Tang, T.; Li, M. Long noncoding RNA MALAT1 regulates renal tubular epithelial pyroptosis by modulated miR-23c targeting of ELAVL1 in diabetic nephropathy. *Exp. Cell Res.* **2017**, *350*, 327–335. [CrossRef] [PubMed]
17. Alvarez, M.L.; Khosroheidari, M.; Eddy, E.; Kiefer, J. Role of microRNA 1207-5P and its host gene, the long non-coding RNA Pvt1, as mediators of extracellular matrix accumulation in the kidney: Implications for diabetic nephropathy. *PLoS ONE* **2013**, *8*, e77468. [CrossRef]
18. Huppi, K.; Volfovsky, N.; Runfola, T.; Jones, T.L.; Mackiewicz, M.; Martin, S.E.; Mushinski, J.F.; Stephens, R.; Caplen, N.J. The identification of microRNAs in a genomically unstable region of human chromosome 8q24. *Mol. Cancer Res.* **2008**, *6*, 212–221. [CrossRef]
19. Kato, M.; Wang, M.; Chen, Z.; Bhatt, K.; Oh, H.J.; Lanting, L.; Deshpande, S.; Jia, Y.; Lai, J.Y.; O'Connor, C.L.; et al. An endoplasmic reticulum stress-regulated lncRNA hosting a microRNA megacluster induces early features of diabetic nephropathy. *Nat. Commun.* **2016**, *7*, 12864. [CrossRef]
20. Millis, M.P.; Bowen, D.; Kingsley, C.; Watanabe, R.M.; Wolford, J.K. Variants in the plasmacytoma variant translocation gene (PVT1) are associated with end-stage renal disease attributed to type 1 diabetes. *Diabetes* **2007**, *56*, 3027–3032. [CrossRef]
21. Hanson, R.L.; Craig, D.W.; Millis, M.P.; Yeatts, K.A.; Kobes, S.; Pearson, J.V.; Lee, A.M.; Knowler, W.C.; Nelson, R.G.; Wolford, J.K. Identification of PVT1 as a candidate gene for end-stage renal disease in type 2 diabetes using a pooling-based genome-wide single nucleotide polymorphism association study. *Diabetes* **2007**, *56*, 975–983. [CrossRef] [PubMed]
22. Alvarez, M.L.; DiStefano, J.K. Functional characterization of the plasmacytoma variant translocation 1 gene (PVT1) in diabetic nephropathy. *PLoS ONE* **2011**, *6*, e18671. [CrossRef] [PubMed]
23. Zhang, R.; Li, J.; Huang, T.; Wang, X. Danggui buxue tang suppresses high glucose-induced proliferation and extracellular matrix accumulation of mesangial cells via inhibiting lncRNA PVT1. *Am. J. Transl. Res.* **2017**, *9*, 3732–3740. [PubMed]
24. Hu, M.; Wang, R.; Li, X.; Fan, M.; Lin, J.; Zhen, J.; Chen, L.; Lv, Z. LncRNA MALAT1 is dysregulated in diabetic nephropathy and involved in high glucose-induced podocyte injury via its interplay with beta-catenin. *J. Cell. Mol. Med.* **2017**, *21*, 2732–2747. [CrossRef] [PubMed]
25. Li, Y.; Ren, D.; Xu, G. Long noncoding RNA MALAT1 mediates high glucose-induced glomerular endothelial cell injury by epigenetically inhibiting klotho via methyltransferase G9a. *IUBMB Life* **2019**, *71*, 873–881. [CrossRef] [PubMed]
26. Puthanveetil, P.; Chen, S.; Feng, B.; Gautam, A.; Chakrabarti, S. Long non-coding RNA MALAT1 regulates hyperglycaemia induced inflammatory process in the endothelial cells. *J. Cell. Mol. Med.* **2015**, *19*, 1418–1425. [CrossRef]
27. Higgins, G.C.; Coughlan, M.T. Mitochondrial dysfunction and mitophagy: The beginning and end to diabetic nephropathy? *Br. J. Pharmacol.* **2014**, *171*, 1917–1942. [CrossRef]
28. Long, J.; Badal, S.S.; Ye, Z.; Wang, Y.; Ayanga, B.A.; Galvan, D.L.; Green, N.H.; Chang, B.H.; Overbeek, P.A.; Danesh, F.R. Long noncoding RNA Tug1 regulates mitochondrial bioenergetics in diabetic nephropathy. *J. Clin. Investig.* **2016**, *126*, 4205–4218. [CrossRef]
29. Lei, X.; Zhang, L.; Li, Z.; Ren, J. Astragaloside IV/lncRNA-TUG1/TRAF5 signaling pathway participates in podocyte apoptosis of diabetic nephropathy rats. *Drug Des. Devel.* **2018**, *12*, 2785–2793. [CrossRef]
30. Shen, H.; Ming, Y.; Xu, C.; Xu, Y.; Zhao, S.; Zhang, Q. Deregulation of long noncoding RNA (TUG1) contributes to excessive podocytes apoptosis by activating endoplasmic reticulum stress in the development of diabetic nephropathy. *J. Cell Physiol.* **2019**, *234*, 15123–15133. [CrossRef]
31. Huang, S.; Xu, Y.; Ge, X.; Xu, B.; Peng, W.; Jiang, X.; Shen, L.; Xia, L. Long noncoding RNA NEAT1 accelerates the proliferation and fibrosis in diabetic nephropathy through activating Akt/mTOR signaling pathway. *J. Cell Physiol.* **2019**, *234*, 11200–11207. [CrossRef] [PubMed]
32. Wang, M.; Wang, S.; Yao, D.; Yan, Q.; Lu, W. A novel long non-coding RNA CYP4B1-PS1-001 regulates proliferation and fibrosis in diabetic nephropathy. *Mol. Cell Endocrinol.* **2016**, *426*, 136–145. [CrossRef] [PubMed]
33. Wang, S.; Chen, X.; Wang, M.; Yao, D.; Chen, T.; Yan, Q.; Lu, W. Long Non-Coding RNA CYP4B1-PS1-001 Inhibits Proliferation and Fibrosis in Diabetic Nephropathy by Interacting with Nucleolin. *Cell Physiol. Biochem.* **2018**, *49*, 2174–2187. [CrossRef] [PubMed]
34. Bai, X.; Geng, J.; Li, X.; Wan, J.; Liu, J.; Zhou, Z.; Liu, X. Long Noncoding RNA LINC01619 Regulates MicroRNA-27a/Forkhead Box Protein O1 and Endoplasmic Reticulum Stress-Mediated Podocyte Injury in

Diabetic Nephropathy. *Antioxid. Redox Signal* **2018**, *29*, 355–376. [CrossRef] [PubMed]

35. Ji, T.T.; Wang, Y.K.; Zhu, Y.C.; Gao, C.P.; Li, X.Y.; Li, J.; Bai, F.; Bai, S.J. Long noncoding RNA Gm6135 functions as a competitive endogenous RNA to regulate toll-like receptor 4 expression by sponging miR-203-3p in diabetic nephropathy. *J. Cell Physiol.* **2019**, *234*, 6633–6641. [CrossRef] [PubMed]
36. Li, A.; Peng, R.; Sun, Y.; Liu, H.; Peng, H.; Zhang, Z. LincRNA 1700020I14Rik alleviates cell proliferation and fibrosis in diabetic nephropathy via miR-34a-5p/Sirt1/HIF-1alpha signaling. *Cell Death Dis.* **2018**, *9*, 461. [CrossRef] [PubMed]
37. Zhang, Y.; Sun, Y.; Peng, R.; Liu, H.; He, W.; Zhang, L.; Peng, H.; Zhang, Z. The Long Noncoding RNA 150Rik Promotes Mesangial Cell Proliferation via miR-451/IGF1R/p38 MAPK Signaling in Diabetic Nephropathy. *Cell Physiol. Biochem.* **2018**, *51*, 1410–1428. [CrossRef]
38. Fan, W.; Peng, Y.; Liang, Z.; Yang, Y.; Zhang, J. A negative feedback loop of H19/miR-675/EGR1 is involved in diabetic nephropathy by downregulating the expression of the vitamin D receptor. *J. Cell Physiol.* **2019**, *234*, 17505–17513. [CrossRef]
39. Sun, S.F.; Tang, P.M.K.; Feng, M.; Xiao, J.; Huang, X.R.; Li, P.; Ma, R.C.W.; Lan, H.Y. Novel lncRNA Erbb4-IR Promotes Diabetic Kidney Injury in db/db Mice by Targeting miR-29b. *Diabetes* **2018**, *67*, 731–744. [CrossRef]
40. Zhang, Y.Y.; Tang, P.M.-K.; Tang, P.C.-T.; Xiao, J.; Huang, X.R.; Yu, C.; Ma, R.C.; Lan, H.Y. LRNA9884, a Novel Smad3-Dependent LncRNA, Promotes Diabetic Kidney Injury in db/db Mice Via Enhancing MCP-1-Dependent Renal Inflammation. *Diabetes* **2019**, *68*, 1485–1498. [CrossRef]
41. Yi, H.; Peng, R.; Zhang, L.Y.; Sun, Y.; Peng, H.M.; Liu, H.D.; Yu, L.J.; Li, A.L.; Zhang, Y.J.; Jiang, W.H.; et al. LincRNA-Gm4419 knockdown ameliorates NF-kappaB/NLRP3 inflammasome-mediated inflammation in diabetic nephropathy. *Cell Death Dis.* **2017**, *8*, e2583. [CrossRef] [PubMed]
42. Wang, J.; Pang, J.; Li, H.; Long, J.; Fang, F.; Chen, J.; Zhu, X.; Xiang, X.; Zhang, D. lncRNA ZEB1-AS1 Was Suppressed by p53 for Renal Fibrosis in Diabetic Nephropathy. *Mol. Ther. Nucleic Acids* **2018**, *12*, 741–750. [CrossRef] [PubMed]
43. Shang, J.; Wang, S.; Jiang, Y.; Duan, Y.; Cheng, G.; Liu, D.; Xiao, J.; Zhao, Z. Identification of key lncRNAs contributing to diabetic nephropathy by gene co-expression network analysis. *Sci. Rep.* **2019**, *9*, 3328. [CrossRef] [PubMed]
44. Wang, Y.Z.; Zhu, D.Y.; Xie, X.M.; Ding, M.; Wang, Y.L.; Sun, L.L.; Zhang, N.; Shen, E.; Wang, X.X. EA15, MIR22, LINC00472 as diagnostic markers for diabetic kidney disease. *J. Cell Physiol.* **2019**, *234*, 8797–8803. [CrossRef] [PubMed]
45. Tang, W.; Zhang, D.; Ma, X. RNA-sequencing reveals genome-wide long non-coding RNAs profiling associated with early development of diabetic nephropathy. *Oncotarget* **2017**, *8*, 105832–105847. [CrossRef] [PubMed]
46. Hu, S.; Han, R.; Shi, J.; Zhu, X.; Qin, W.; Zeng, C.; Bao, H.; Liu, Z. The long noncoding RNA LOC105374325 causes podocyte injury in individuals with focal segmental glomerulosclerosis. *J. Biol. Chem.* **2018**, *293*, 20227–20239. [CrossRef] [PubMed]
47. Han, R.; Hu, S.; Qin, W.; Shi, J.; Zeng, C.; Bao, H.; Liu, Z. Upregulated long noncoding RNA LOC105375913 induces tubulointerstitial fibrosis in focal segmental glomerulosclerosis. *Sci. Rep.* **2019**, *9*, 716. [CrossRef]
48. Jin, L.W.; Pan, M.; Ye, H.Y.; Zheng, Y.; Chen, Y.; Huang, W.W.; Xu, X.Y.; Zheng, S.B. Down-regulation of the long non-coding RNA XIST ameliorates podocyte apoptosis in membranous nephropathy via the miR-217-TLR4 pathway. *Exp. Physiol.* **2019**, *104*, 220–230. [CrossRef]
49. Liao, Z.; Ye, Z.; Xue, Z.; Wu, L.; Ouyang, Y.; Yao, C.; Cui, C.; Xu, N.; Ma, J.; Hou, G.; et al. Identification of Renal Long Non-coding RNA RP11-2B6.2 as a Positive Regulator of Type I Interferon Signaling Pathway in Lupus Nephritis. *Front Immunol.* **2019**, *10*, 975. [CrossRef]
50. Fang, Y.; Hu, J.F.; Wang, Z.H.; Zhang, S.G.; Zhang, R.F.; Sun, L.M.; Cui, H.W.; Yang, F. GAS5 promotes podocyte injury in sepsis by inhibiting PTEN expression. *Eur. Rev. Med. Pharm. Sci.* **2018**, *22*, 8423–8430. [CrossRef]
51. Qin, X.J.; Gao, J.R.; Xu, X.J.; Jiang, H.; Wei, L.B.; Jiang, N.N. LncRNAs expression in adriamycin-induced rats reveals the potential role of LncRNAs contributing to chronic glomerulonephritis pathogenesis. *Gene* **2019**, *687*, 90–98. [CrossRef] [PubMed]
52. Gao, J.R.; Qin, X.J.; Jiang, H.; Gao, Y.C.; Guo, M.F.; Jiang, N.N. Potential role of lncRNAs in contributing to pathogenesis of chronic glomerulonephritis based on microarray data. *Gene* **2018**, *643*, 46–54. [CrossRef] [PubMed]
53. Sui, W.; Li, H.; Ou, M.; Tang, D.; Dai, Y. Altered long non-coding RNA expression profile in patients with

IgA-negative mesangial proliferative glomerulonephritis. *Int. J. Mol. Med.* **2012**, *30*, 173–178. [CrossRef] [PubMed]

54. Zuo, N.; Li, Y.; Liu, N.; Wang, L. Differentially expressed long noncoding RNAs and mRNAs in patients with IgA nephropathy. *Mol. Med. Rep.* **2017**, *16*, 7724–7730. [CrossRef] [PubMed]
55. Huang, Y.S.; Hsieh, H.Y.; Shih, H.M.; Sytwu, H.K.; Wu, C.C. Urinary Xist is a potential biomarker for membranous nephropathy. *Biochem. Biophys. Res. Commun.* **2014**, *452*, 415–421. [CrossRef] [PubMed]
56. Mehta, R.L.; Cerda, J.; Burdmann, E.A.; Tonelli, M.; Garcia-Garcia, G.; Jha, V.; Susantitaphong, P.; Rocco, M.; Vanholder, R.; Sever, M.S.; et al. International Society of Nephrology's 0by25 initiative for acute kidney injury (zero preventable deaths by 2025): A human rights case for nephrology. *Lancet* **2015**, *385*, 2616–2643. [CrossRef]
57. Tian, H.; Wu, M.; Zhou, P.; Huang, C.; Ye, C.; Wang, L. The long non-coding RNA MALAT1 is increased in renal ischemia-reperfusion injury and inhibits hypoxia-induced inflammation. *Ren. Fail.* **2018**, *40*, 527–533. [CrossRef] [PubMed]
58. Pang, X.; Feng, G.; Shang, W.; Liu, L.; Li, J.; Feng, Y.; Xie, H.; Wang, J. Inhibition of lncRNA MEG3 protects renal tubular from hypoxia-induced kidney injury in acute renal allografts by regulating miR-181b/TNF-α signaling pathway. *J. Cell Biochem.* **2019**, *120*, 12822–12831. [CrossRef] [PubMed]
59. Yu, T.M.; Palanisamy, K.; Sun, K.T.; Day, Y.J.; Shu, K.H.; Wang, I.K.; Shyu, W.C.; Chen, P.; Chen, Y.L.; Li, C.Y. RANTES mediates kidney ischemia reperfusion injury through a possible role of HIF-1α and LncRNA PRINS. *Sci. Rep.* **2016**, *6*, 18424. [CrossRef]
60. Tian, X.; Ji, Y.; Liang, Y.; Zhang, J.; Guan, L.; Wang, C. LINC00520 targeting miR-27b-3p regulates OSMR expression level to promote acute kidney injury development through the PI3K/AKT signaling pathway. *J. Cell Physiol.* **2019**, *234*, 14221–14233. [CrossRef]
61. Geng, X.; Xu, X.; Fang, Y.; Zhao, S.; Hu, J.; Xu, J.; Jia, P.; Ding, X.; Teng, J. Effect of long non-coding RNA growth arrest-specific 5 on apoptosis in renal ischaemia/reperfusion injury. *Nephrology* **2019**, *24*, 405–413. [CrossRef] [PubMed]
62. Kolling, M.; Genschel, C.; Kaucsar, T.; Hubner, A.; Rong, S.; Schmitt, R.; Sorensen-Zender, I.; Haddad, G.; Kistler, A.; Seeger, H.; et al. Hypoxia-induced long non-coding RNA Malat1 is dispensable for renal ischemia/reperfusion-injury. *Sci. Rep.* **2018**, *8*, 3438. [CrossRef] [PubMed]
63. Yang, R.; Liu, S.; Wen, J.; Xue, L.; Zhang, Y.; Yan, D.; Wang, G.; Liu, Z. Inhibition of maternally expressed gene 3 attenuated lipopolysaccharide-induced apoptosis through sponging miR-21 in renal tubular epithelial cells. *J. Cell Biochem.* **2018**, *119*, 7800–7806. [CrossRef] [PubMed]
64. Ding, Y.; Guo, F.; Zhu, T.; Li, J.; Gu, D.; Jiang, W.; Lu, Y.; Zhou, D. Mechanism of long non-coding RNA MALAT1 in lipopolysaccharide-induced acute kidney injury is mediated by the miR-146a/NF-kappaB signaling pathway. *Int. J. Mol. Med.* **2018**, *41*, 446–454. [CrossRef] [PubMed]
65. Shen, J.; Liu, L.; Zhang, F.; Gu, J.; Pan, G. LncRNA TapSAKI promotes inflammation injury in HK-2 cells and urine derived sepsis-induced kidney injury. *J. Pharm. Pharm.* **2019**, *71*, 839–848. [CrossRef] [PubMed]
66. Shen, J.; Zhang, J.; Jiang, X.; Wang, H.; Pan, G. LncRNA HOX transcript antisense RNA accelerated kidney injury induced by urine-derived sepsis through the miR-22/high mobility group box 1 pathway. *Life Sci.* **2018**, *210*, 185–191. [CrossRef] [PubMed]
67. Lelli, A.; Nolan, K.A.; Santambrogio, S.; Goncalves, A.F.; Schonenberger, M.J.; Guinot, A.; Frew, I.J.; Marti, H.H.; Hoogewijs, D.; Wenger, R.H. Induction of long noncoding RNA MALAT1 in hypoxic mice. *Hypoxia* **2015**, *3*, 45–52. [CrossRef]
68. Xu, Y.; Deng, W.; Zhang, W. Long non-coding RNA TUG1 protects renal tubular epithelial cells against injury induced by lipopolysaccharide via regulating microRNA-223. *Biomed. Pharmacother* **2018**, *104*, 509–519. [CrossRef]
69. Huang, W.; Lan, X.; Li, X.; Wang, D.; Sun, Y.; Wang, Q.; Gao, H.; Yu, K. Long non-coding RNA PVT1 promote LPS-induced septic acute kidney injury by regulating TNFalpha and JNK/NF-kappaB pathways in HK-2 cells. *Int. Immunopharmacol.* **2017**, *47*, 134–140. [CrossRef]
70. Mimura, I.; Hirakawa, Y.; Kanki, Y.; Kushida, N.; Nakaki, R.; Suzuki, Y.; Tanaka, T.; Aburatani, H.; Nangaku, M. Novel lnc RNA regulated by HIF-1 inhibits apoptotic cell death in the renal tubular epithelial cells under hypoxia. *Physiol. Rep.* **2017**, *5*. [CrossRef]
71. Chen, Y.; Qiu, J.; Chen, B.; Lin, Y.; Xie, G.; Tong, H.; Jiang, D. Long non-coding RNA NEAT1 plays an important role in sepsis-induced acute kidney injury by targeting miR-204 and modulating the NF-kappaB pathway. *Int. Immunopharmacol.* **2018**, *59*, 252–260. [CrossRef] [PubMed]

72. Jiang, X.; Li, D.; Shen, W.; Shen, X.; Liu, Y. LncRNA NEAT1 promotes hypoxia-induced renal tubular epithelial apoptosis through downregulating miR-27a-3p. *J. Cell Biochem.* **2019**. [CrossRef]
73. Liu, X.; Hong, C.; Wu, S.; Song, S.; Yang, Z.; Cao, L.; Song, T.; Yang, Y. Downregulation of lncRNA TUG1 contributes to the development of sepsis-associated acute kidney injury via regulating miR-142-3p/sirtuin 1 axis and modulating NF-kappaB pathway. *J. Cell Biochem.* **2019**. [CrossRef] [PubMed]
74. Jiang, Z.J.; Zhang, M.Y.; Fan, Z.W.; Sun, W.L.; Tang, Y. Influence of lncRNA HOTAIR on acute kidney injury in sepsis rats through regulating miR-34a/Bcl-2 pathway. *Eur Rev. Med. Pharm. Sci.* **2019**, *23*, 3512–3519. [CrossRef]
75. Lorenzen, J.M.; Schauerte, C.; Kielstein, J.T.; Hübner, A.; Martino, F.; Fiedler, J.; Gupta, S.K.; Faulhaber-Walter, R.; Kumarswamy, R.; Hafer, C.; et al. Circulating long noncoding RNATapSaki is a predictor of mortality in critically ill patients with acute kidney injury. *Inj. Clin. Chem.* **2015**, *61*, 191–201. [CrossRef] [PubMed]
76. Qin, J.; Ning, H.; Zhou, Y.; Hu, Y.; Huang, B.; Wu, Y.; Huang, R. LncRNA Uc.173 is a key molecule for the regulation of lead-induced renal tubular epithelial cell apoptosis. *Biomed. Pharm.* **2018**, *100*, 101–107. [CrossRef] [PubMed]
77. Nan, A.; Zhou, X.; Chen, L.; Liu, M.; Zhang, N.; Zhang, L.; Luo, Y.; Liu, Z.; Dai, L.; Jiang, Y. A transcribed ultraconserved noncoding RNA, Uc.173, is a key molecule for the inhibition of lead-induced neuronal apoptosis. *Oncotarget* **2016**, *7*, 112–124. [CrossRef]
78. Chen, W.; Zhou, Z.Q.; Ren, Y.Q.; Zhang, L.; Sun, L.N.; Man, Y.L.; Wang, Z.K. Effects of long non-coding RNA LINC00667 on renal tubular epithelial cell proliferation, apoptosis and renal fibrosis via the miR-19b-3p/LINC00667/CTGF signaling pathway in chronic renal failure. *Cell Signal.* **2019**, *54*, 102–114. [CrossRef]
79. Chen, W.; Zhang, L.; Zhou, Z.Q.; Ren, Y.Q.; Sun, L.N.; Man, Y.L.; Ma, Z.W.; Wang, Z.K. Effects of Long Non-Coding RNA LINC00963 on Renal Interstitial Fibrosis and Oxidative Stress of Rats with Chronic Renal Failure via the Foxo Signaling Pathway. *Cell Physiol. Biochem.* **2018**, *46*, 815–828. [CrossRef]
80. Aboudehen, K.; Farahani, S.; Kanchwala, M.; Chan, S.C.; Avdulov, S.; Mickelson, A.; Lee, D.; Gearhart, M.D.; Patel, V.; Xing, C.; et al. Long noncoding RNA Hoxb3os is dysregulated in autosomal dominant polycystic kidney disease and regulates mTOR signaling. *J. Biol. Chem.* **2018**, *293*, 9388–9398. [CrossRef]
81. Song, Z.; Zhang, Y.; Gong, B.; Xu, H.; Hao, Z.; Liang, C. Long noncoding RNA LINC00339 promotes renal tubular epithelial pyroptosis by regulating the miR-22-3p/NLRP3 axis in calcium oxalate-induced kidney stone. *J. Cell Biochem.* **2019**, *120*, 10452–10462. [CrossRef] [PubMed]
82. Zhang, C.; Yuan, J.; Hu, H.; Chen, W.; Liu, M.; Zhang, J.; Sun, S.; Guo, Z. Long non-coding RNA CHCHD4P4 promotes epithelial-mesenchymal transition and inhibits cell proliferation in calcium oxalate-induced kidney damage. *Braz. J. Med. Biol. Res.* **2017**, *51*, e6536. [CrossRef] [PubMed]
83. Hu, J.; Wu, H.; Wang, D.; Yang, Z.; Dong, J. LncRNA ANRIL promotes NLRP3 inflammasome activation in uric acid nephropathy through miR-122-5p/BRCC3 axis. *Biochimie* **2019**, *157*, 102–110. [CrossRef] [PubMed]
84. Van der Hauwaert, C.; Glowacki, F.; Pottier, N.; Cauffiez, C. Non-Coding RNAs as New Therapeutic Targets in the Context of Renal Fibrosis. *Int. J. Mol. Sci.* **2019**, *20*, 1977. [CrossRef] [PubMed]
85. Moe, O.W. Kidney stones: Pathophysiology and medical management. *Lancet* **2006**, *367*, 333–344. [CrossRef]
86. Wang, Z.; Zhang, J.W.; Zhang, Y.; Zhang, S.P.; Hu, Q.Y.; Liang, H. Analyses of long non-coding RNA and mRNA profiling using RNA sequencing in calcium oxalate monohydrate-stimulated renal tubular epithelial cells. *Urolithiasis* **2019**, *47*, 225–234. [CrossRef] [PubMed]
87. Cao, Y.; Gao, X.; Yang, Y.; Ye, Z.; Wang, E.; Dong, Z. Changing expression profiles of long non-coding RNAs, mRNAs and circular RNAs in ethylene glycol-induced kidney calculi rats. *BMC Genom.* **2018**, *19*, 660. [CrossRef]
88. Wan, L.; Dreyfuss, G. Splicing-Correcting Therapy for SMA. *Cell* **2017**, *170*, 5. [CrossRef]
89. Benson, M.D.; Waddington-Cruz, M.; Berk, J.L.; Polydefkis, M.; Dyck, P.J.; Wang, A.K.; Plante-Bordeneuve, V.; Barroso, F.A.; Merlini, G.; Obici, L.; et al. Inotersen Treatment for Patients with Hereditary Transthyretin Amyloidosis. *N. Engl. J. Med.* **2018**, *379*, 22–31. [CrossRef]
90. Adams, D.; Gonzalez-Duarte, A.; O'Riordan, W.D.; Yang, C.C.; Ueda, M.; Kristen, A.V.; Tournev, I.; Schmidt, H.H.; Coelho, T.; Berk, J.L.; et al. Patisiran, an RNAi Therapeutic, for Hereditary Transthyretin Amyloidosis. *N. Engl. J. Med.* **2018**, *379*, 11–21. [CrossRef]
91. Park, J.; Shrestha, R.; Qiu, C.; Kondo, A.; Huang, S.; Werth, M.; Li, M.; Barasch, J.; Susztak, K. Single-cell transcriptomics of the mouse kidney reveals potential cellular targets of kidney disease. *Science* **2018**, *360*, 758–763. [CrossRef] [PubMed]

92. Karaiskos, N.; Rahmatollahi, M.; Boltengagen, A.; Liu, H.; Hoehne, M.; Rinschen, M.; Schermer, B.; Benzing, T.; Rajewsky, N.; Kocks, C.; et al. A Single-Cell Transcriptome Atlas of the Mouse Glomerulus. *J. Am. Soc. Nephrol.* **2018**, *29*, 2060–2068. [CrossRef] [PubMed]

93. Fu, J.; Akat, K.M.; Sun, Z.; Zhang, W.; Schlondorff, D.; Liu, Z.; Tuschl, T.; Lee, K.; He, J.C. Single-Cell RNA Profiling of Glomerular Cells Shows Dynamic Changes in Experimental Diabetic Kidney Disease. *J. Am. Soc. Nephrol.* **2019**, *30*, 533–545. [CrossRef] [PubMed]

94. Wu, H.; Kirita, Y.; Donnelly, E.L.; Humphreys, B.D. Advantages of Single-Nucleus over Single-Cell RNA Sequencing of Adult Kidney: Rare Cell Types and Novel Cell States Revealed in Fibrosis. *J. Am. Soc. Nephrol.* **2019**, *30*, 23–32. [CrossRef] [PubMed]

95. Der, E.; Ranabothu, S.; Suryawanshi, H.; Akat, K.M.; Clancy, R.; Morozov, P.; Kustagi, M.; Czuppa, M.; Izmirly, P.; Belmont, H.M.; et al. Single cell RNA sequencing to dissect the molecular heterogeneity in lupus nephritis. *JCI Insight* **2017**, *2*. [CrossRef] [PubMed]

5

Unraveling the Role of Inflammation in the Pathogenesis of Diabetic Kidney Disease

Keiichiro Matoba [1,*], Yusuke Takeda [1], Yosuke Nagai [1], Daiji Kawanami [2], Kazunori Utsunomiya [3] and Rimei Nishimura [1]

1 Division of Diabetes, Metabolism, and Endocrinology, Department of Internal Medicine, The Jikei University School of Medicine, Tokyo 105-8461, Japan
2 Department of Endocrinology and Diabetes Mellitus, Fukuoka University School of Medicine, Fukuoka 814-0180, Japan
3 Center for Preventive Medicine, The Jikei University School of Medicine, Tokyo 105-8461, Japan
* Correspondence: matoba@jikei.ac.jp

Abstract: Diabetic kidney disease (DKD) remains the leading cause of end-stage renal disease (ESRD) and is therefore a major burden on the healthcare system. Patients with DKD are highly susceptible to developing cardiovascular disease, which contributes to increased morbidity and mortality rates. While progress has been made to inhibit the acceleration of DKD, current standards of care reduce but do not eliminate the risk of DKD. There is growing appreciation for the role of inflammation in modulating the process of DKD. The focus of this review is on providing an overview of the current status of knowledge regarding the pathologic roles of inflammation in the development of DKD. Finally, we summarize recent therapeutic advances to prevent DKD, with a focus on the anti-inflammatory effects of newly developed agents.

Keywords: diabetic kidney disease; diabetic nephropathy; inflammation; signaling cascade

---

1. Introduction

The pandemic of diabetes has become a global health burden. Despite accumulating evidence supporting the prevention of obesity and related metabolic disorders, this knowledge has not translated into action that strongly reduces the prevalence of diabetes, especially in middle- and low-income countries. The International Diabetes Federation (IDF) estimates that diabetes affects 425 million people globally, and the number of diabetic patients will increase to 630 million in 2045.

Such an increase also means that the prevalence of diabetic kidney disease (DKD) continues to rise. DKD is the leading cause of end-stage renal disease (ESRD) and is associated with increased mortality due to cardiovascular disease in subjects with diabetes. Evidence is mounting that albuminuria is not only a hallmark of DKD but also an independent risk factor of coronary disease. The UK Prospective Diabetes Study (UKPDS) demonstrated that annual cardiovascular mortality rates increase to 3%, 4.6%, and 19.2% with the progression to microalbuminuria, macroalbuminuria, and renal failure, respectively [1]. Indeed, patients with DKD are more likely to die from coronary disease than to ever reach ESRD. Due to its high morbidity and mortality, the socioeconomic costs of DKD are staggering. It is therefore urgent that we establish effective and safe therapeutic strategies against DKD in order to improve the prognosis of diabetic patients. To this end, a detailed understanding of the molecular mechanisms that drive DKD is required.

The current understanding of the mechanisms responsible for the progression of DKD recognizes the involvement of metabolic abnormalities (e.g., hyperglycemia, hypertension, and dyslipidemia), hemodynamic changes, renin–angiotensin system (RAS) activation, and oxidative stress. While several approaches have been clinically implemented in order to slow the acceleration of DKD, the current management of DKD is insufficient, both for preventing DKD and for halting its progression.

Given the limitations of therapeutic regimens for inhibiting DKD, there has been an ongoing effort to elucidate the molecular basis responsible for the renal damage and to develop novel drugs. Recent research is characterized by a variety of investigations exploring the inflammatory regulators of DKD. Circulating levels of inflammatory mediators and macrophage infiltration into renal tissue have been found to be increased in both animal models and patients with DKD. Furthermore, adhesion molecules and chemokines are upregulated in diabetic kidneys. These findings highlight the importance of inflammatory mechanisms in facilitating renal damage in the setting of diabetes.

We herein review the inflammatory mediators of diabetes and their contribution to renal injury and describe the potential of anti-diabetic medications as well as drug candidates for inhibiting renal inflammation in the progression of DKD.

2. Inflammatory Mediators in Diabetic Kidney Disease (DKD)

Low-grade inflammation is defined as an activation of the innate immune system response. This is clinically considered an increase in circulating levels of pro-inflammatory cytokines and other mediators that activate the immune system. Chronic low-grade inflammation plays a causal role in the progression of obesity and insulin resistance. Deficits in specific genes critical for inflammation are known to be protective against the initiation and development of metabolic diseases in animal models. Therefore, inflammation is considered to be a trigger rather than a result of chronic underlying conditions.

Inflammation is increasingly postulated to be central to the progression of atherogenic changes and microvascular complications in the setting of diabetes [2]. For example, the activation of inflammatory pathways, especially E-selectin and other adhesion molecules, is linked to the pathogenesis of diabetic retinopathy [3]. These adhesion mediators stimulate the migration of retinal capillary endothelium and angiogenesis in the progression of diabetic retinopathy. In addition, evidence of the role of inflammatory signals in the development of diabetic neuropathy has been shown in experimental models of diabetes [4,5] and in clinical studies [6,7]. Diabetic patients with painful peripheral neuropathy have higher levels of inflammatory markers than subjects without pain, and the elevation of interleukin (IL)-1, IL-6, and tumor necrosis factor α (TNF-α) are correlated with the progression of degenerative changes in the peripheral nerves. The expression of nuclear factor-2 erythroid related factor 2 (Nrf2), a regulator of endogenous anti-oxidant production, is decreased in patients with diabetic peripheral neuropathy, which can result in inflammation, exacerbated oxidative stress, nerve injury, and an insufficient blood supply [8]. As with retinopathy and neuropathy, the infiltration of inflammatory cells and expression of adhesion molecules and cytokines are detected in renal tissue obtained from subjects with DKD.

2.1. *Macrophages*

Blood monocytes and tissue macrophages are key members of the mononuclear phagocyte system, a component of innate immunity. Recently, intensive research has shown that the influx of macrophages is a prominent feature during the progression of chronic kidney disease [9] and is tightly correlated with the decline in the glomerular filtration rate (GFR), histological changes, and a poor outcome in this condition [10]. Macrophage-derived products, including reactive oxygen species (ROS), pro-inflammatory factors, metalloproteinases, and growth factors, can induce further renal damage in the setting of diabetes. Macrophage-depletion studies in rodent models have shown a causal role for macrophages in the progression of DKD. For instance, the deletion of a macrophage scavenger receptor protected diabetic mice from albuminuria, mesangial matrix expansion, and the overproduction of transforming growth factor β (TGF-β) [11]. The gene expression of pro-inflammatory factors was strongly suppressed in this diabetic mouse model.

Macrophages are classified into classically-activated M1 and alternatively-activated M2 states [12]. M1 macrophages promote the inflammatory process by elaborating pro-inflammatory factors and ROS, whereas M2 macrophages resolve inflammation and induce tissue remodeling with the release of growth factors. In simple inflammatory reactions, such as acute arthritis, macrophages progress linearly through the M1 and M2 phases. However, under chronic inflammatory conditions, such as atherosclerosis and DKD, both M1 and M2 macrophages coexist, and this imbalance in the M1/M2 macrophage phenotype may be a key point of DKD.

Notably, an experimental study showed that macrophages in streptozotocin-induced DKD are predominantly of the M1 phenotype [9,13]. Furthermore, RAW264.7 macrophages switch to the M1 phenotype when cultured in a high-glucose milieu. Consistent with these results, the glomerular expression of inducible nitric oxide and TNF-α is increased in insulin-deficient diabetic mouse models, suggesting the presence of M1 macrophages. The deletion of the Toll-like receptor-2 gene significantly induces a macrophage M1 to M2 polarization shift in the diabetic kidney, attenuates urinary albumin excretion, and protects podocytes from apoptosis and morphological changes [13]. The mechanisms by which M2 macrophages promote kidney repair and attenuate DKD progression are still under debate and merit further investigation.

2.2. *Adhesion Molecules and Chemokines*

While the precise molecular mechanisms that direct monocyte homing into the sites of renal inflammation are not fully understood, endothelial-leukocyte adhesion molecules, including vascular cell adhesion molecule 1 (VCAM1) and intercellular adhesion molecule 1 (ICAM1), have been considered to play important roles in the initiation of renal inflammation. Several studies provide compelling evidence supporting the importance of these molecules in monocyte recruitment. For example, these adhesion molecules are abundantly expressed in renal biopsy specimens obtained from patients with DKD. Furthermore, circulating levels of VCAM1 and ICAM1 are independently associated with DKD progression [14,15].

VCAM1, also known as CD106, is a transmembrane glycoprotein expressed in activated endothelium under a variety of pathologic conditions, including atherosclerosis and DKD. VCAM1 binds to $\alpha4\beta1$ integrin, which is constitutively expressed on lymphocytes, monocytes, and eosinophils. The renal filtration function declines and urinary albumin excretion levels increase progressively with the elevation in VCAM1 levels in serum [16]. ICAM1, also known as CD54, is expressed structurally on endothelial cells and works as a ligand for lymphocyte function-associated antigen 1 (LFA-1) on monocytes. Its expression is also upregulated in endothelial cells in a diabetic milieu, and genetic polymorphisms in its gene are associated with DKD progression [17]. The deletion of the ICAM1 gene ameliorates renal inflammation in mice [18], indicating that ICAM1 contributes to the pathogenesis of DKD.

After adhering to the endothelium, monocytes migrate through endothelial cells via chemokines. Studies of DKD rodents and in human diabetic kidneys have shown that macrophages infiltrate the renal tissue in response to an upregulation of chemokines, such as monocyte chemoattractant protein 1 (MCP1), also known as CCL2. Nadkarni et al. investigated urinary MCP1 for its associations with the deterioration of the renal function in order to illuminate its potential as a urinary marker of DKD progression [19]. They reported that an increased level of urinary MCP1 was strongly associated with a decline in the renal function in patients with diabetes, suggesting that excreted MCP1 levels may be a useful biomarker for predicting progressive decline in DKD [20].

The induction of MCP1 by inflammatory cytokines in renal cells elicits the initial step of glomerular and tubular inflammation. Although a number of cytokines have been shown to be involved in the production of MCP1, there is compelling evidence that TNF-α functions as a potent inducer of MCP1 expression in the kidney. TNF-α is expressed in adipose tissue and has been implicated in the pathogenesis of insulin resistance and type 2 diabetes. In addition, it has been shown that the serum concentrations and urinary excretion of TNF-α are increased in patients with various kidney diseases, suggesting that excessive TNF-α in the systemic circulation may result in the upregulation of MCP1 in the kidney. Furthermore, elevated serum levels of TNF receptors (TNF-R) 1 or 2 are strongly associated with a risk of renal functional decline or ESRD [7,21]. Niewczas et al. investigated 194 circulating inflammatory factors in patients from three independent cohorts with type 1 and type 2 diabetes and demonstrated an extremely robust kidney risk inflammatory signature, including 17 proteins enriched in TNF-R superfamily members [22], which were associated with a 10-year risk of ESRD.

TNF-α secreted by infiltrated macrophages itself may also stimulate the local production of MCP1 in renal cells. Consequently, manipulating the MCP1 signaling axis offers an opportunity for therapeutic gain. A clinical trial is underway investigating the effectiveness of MCP1 inhibitors in patients with progressive DKD [23]. Treatment with emapticap pegol, a Spiegelmer that specifically binds and inhibits MCP1, was found to be generally safe and well tolerated. In that study, albuminuria was attenuated by treatment with emapticap pegol, and the beneficial effects were maintained even after cessation of the intervention.

Intrarenal amplification of macrophages also plays an important role in the progression of renal disease, including DKD. Colony-stimulating factor 1 (CSF1), also known as macrophage colony-stimulating factor, is a homodimer glycoprotein that governs the survival, proliferation, and differentiation of macrophages. In particular, CSF1 is required for macrophage proliferation throughout the G1 phase of the cell cycle, and this chemokine is constitutively expressed in glomerular mesangial cells, tubular epithelial cells, and endothelial cells. Experimental studies have demonstrated that the deletion of CSF1 in mice leads to the attenuation of macrophage recruitment and proliferation during renal inflammation [24]. Of interest, the implantation of CSF1-generating cells into the kidneys of autoimmune lupus mice incites local macrophage-mediated inflammation [25]. CSF1 is also upregulated in type 2 diabetic db/db mice [26]. Furthermore, the administration of an antibody against the CSF1 receptor attenuates the accumulation of macrophages in rodent models of renal diseases, including unilateral ureteric obstruction, renal allograft rejection, and DKD [27]. Given these findings, it is reasonable to suggest that CSF1 is a critical determinant of the survival and proliferation of macrophages in several kidney diseases.

Dysregulation of the immune system is an important determinant in the initiation of DKD. Studies have provided convincing evidence that T cells, B cells, and NK cells are critical drivers of inflammation. Activated T cells cause renal damage directly via cytotoxic effects and indirectly by the recruitment and activation of macrophages. It is possible that pro-inflammatory cytokines secreted by T cells activate neighboring macrophages and stimulate the production of MCP1 and CSF-1 from glomerular cells. B cells could affect the proliferation of Th17 and the production of pro-inflammatory cytokines in patients with diabetes. Both T cells and B cells were shown to infiltrate glomeruli in a diabetic mouse model of diabetes, however, the evidence for the involvement of B cells and NK cells in DKD is more limited than that for T cells [28].

Overall, these findings provide evidence that immune system components are involved in the initiation of DKD and that adhesion molecules and chemokines play an essential role in the progression of inflammation in DKD.

3. Signaling Cascade Governing Inflammatory Reactions

A variety of upstream mediators (e.g., metabolic changes, altered redox balance, and intestinal dysbiosis) have been shown to be associated with inflammation in renal tissue. Cell death is induced under hyperglycemic conditions and activates the infiltration of macrophages and other immune cells into the kidney. Furthermore, the hyperglycemia-associated generation of advanced glycation end products (AGEs) and engagement of the receptor for AGE (RAGE) with its ligands induces oxidative stress and renal inflammation, resulting in a decline in renal function. Thus, the inhibition of AGE–RAGE signaling seems to be an attractive therapeutic strategy against renal inflammation. Interestingly, recent studies have reported the beneficial effects of RAGE blockade with FPS-ZM1 and RAGE-aptamers in DKD [29]. In addition to hyperglycemia-associated factors, systemic inflammation leads to dysregulation of the microcirculation network in the kidney and contributes to the in-site production of pro-inflammatory factors and ROS. Signaling events during renal inflammation orchestrate widespread transcriptional programs that affect the functions of adhesion molecules and inflammatory immune cells. An accumulating body of evidence exists defining the important roles for several signaling cascades in the control of renal inflammation, which we review below (Figure 1).

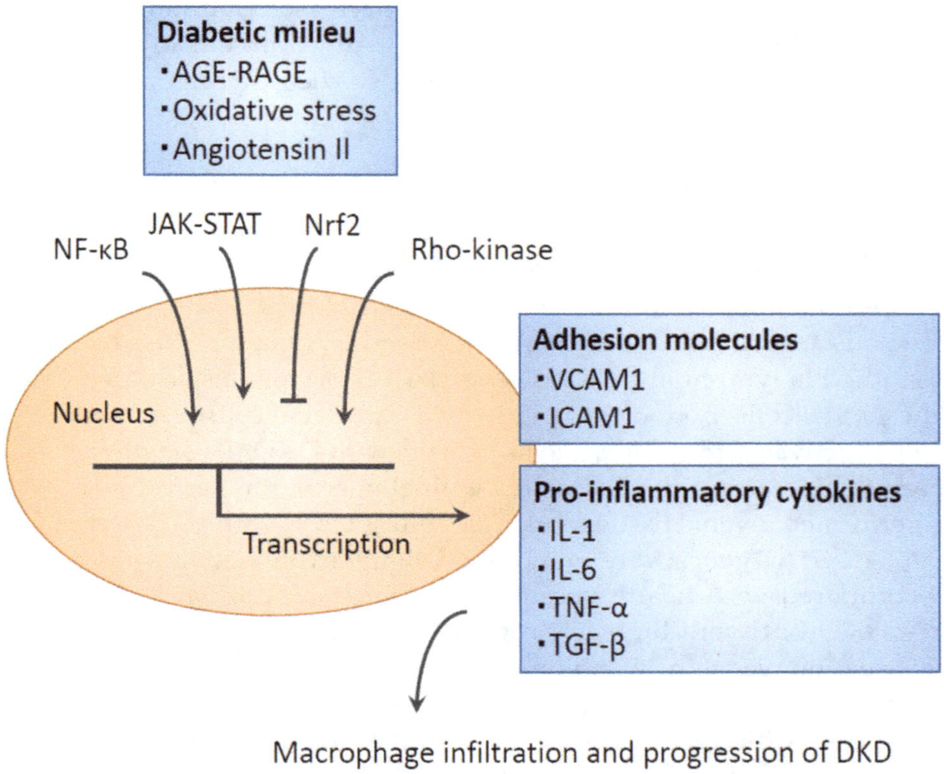

Figure 1. In the diabetic kidney, advanced glycation end products (AGEs) and oxidative stress activate a variety of signaling cascades to induce monocyte infiltration. In addition, chemokines drive inflammation, leading to macrophage-mediated tissue injury. DKD, Diabetic kidney disease; RAGE, receptor for AGE; VCAM1, vascular cell adhesion molecule 1; ICAM1, intercellular adhesion molecule 1; JAK-STAT, Janus kinase/signal transducer and activator of transcription; NF-κB, Nuclear factor Kb; Nrf2, nuclear factor-2 erythroid related factor 2; TNF-α, tumor necrosis factor α; TGF-β, transforming growth factor β.

3.1. Nuclear Factor κB (NF-κB) and Activating Protein 1 (AP1)

Nuclear factor κB (NF-κB) is a family of transcription factors central in regulating inflammatory signals. The complex of NF-κB is a dimer of two members of the Rel family of proteins: p65 and p50. In unstimulated cells, NF-κB is sequestered in the cytoplasm by IκB family proteins, the best characterized of which is IκBα. IκBα phosphorylation leads to its ubiquitination and subsequent proteasome-mediated protein degradation, which exposes its nuclear localization signal. The subsequent recognition of NF-κB by karyopherin β directs it to the nuclear pore complex, where nuclear translocation takes place. In addition, the coactivator p300 can complex with the p65/p50 heterodimer to stabilize the chromatin structure for efficient transcription.

Glucose can activate NF-κB, resulting in increased inflammatory gene expression, in part through oxidative stress, AGEs, protein kinase C, and Mitogen-activated protein kinases (MAPKs) [30]. Increased renal NF-κB levels are detected in the kidneys of diabetic experimental models, and this activates glomerular and tubular cells to induce renal injury [26,31]. Downstream targets of NF-κB include adhesion molecules and pro-inflammatory cytokines (e.g., IL-6, TNF-α, MCP1, RANTES

(Regulated on Activation, Normal T Cell Expressed and Secreted)), which all drive the development of DKD.

Similar to NF-κB, activating protein 1 (AP1) is activated by glucose and oxidative and inflammatory stimuli. AP1 regulates the TGF-β expression in mesangial cells, and the AP1 binding activity was found to be markedly enhanced by high glucose treatment [32]. PPARγ ligands are known to inhibit inflammatory gene expression via the attenuation of AP1, suggesting a potential anti-inflammatory therapeutic strategy by thiazolidine (TZD). Indeed, TZD decreases albuminuria, mesangial expansion, and the expression of TGF-β and osteopontin, a phosphor–glycoprotein adhesion molecule, in mouse models of diabetes [33]. Further clinical and mechanistic studies are required in order to validate the role of AP1 in the pathogenesis of DKD.

3.2. *Janus Kinase/Signal Transducer and Activator of Transcription (JAK-STAT)*

Experimental work over the past several years has shown the key roles of the Janus kinase/signal transducer and activator of transcription (JAK-STAT) pathway. The JAK-STAT pathway transduces signals from extracellular ligands (e.g., cytokines, chemokines, growth factors, and hormones) directly to the nucleus to activate a variety of cellular responses. Most of these reactions have been extensively studied in lymphoid cells, however, JAK-STAT signals also play critical roles in renal cells, including mesangial cells, podocytes, and tubular epithelial cells [34]. Studies have shown that JAK-STAT signaling is activated in renal tissue in patients with DKD. This pathway is activated by ROS induced by hyperglycemic states and is associated with glomerular hypertrophy [31]. A transcriptomic examination was performed in renal tissues obtained from subjects with early and progressive DKD [35]. In this analysis, all JAK-STAT genes were found to be highly expressed in the glomeruli from patients with early DKD compared with healthy controls. In contrast, tubular JAK-STAT genes were not increased in early DKD but were high in progressive DKD. Notably, the degree of induction of JAK-STAT gene expression was tightly and inversely correlated with the decline in the GFR.

A series of studies indicated that JAK family members JAK1, 2, and 3, as well as STAT1 and STAT3, are induced in DKD. In addition, Zhang et al. showed that the overexpression of JAK2 in podocytes can lead to worse renal damage in mouse models of diabetes [36]. Baricitinib, an oral inhibitor of the JAK family of protein tyrosine kinases that selectively inhibits JAK1 and JAK2, attenuates urinary albumin excretion in diabetic patients. Therefore, inhibiting JAK-STAT signaling may have potential utility for treating DKD and improving health outcomes in patients with diabetes [34].

3.3. *Nuclear Factor-2 Erythroid Related Factor (Nrf2)-Keep1*

The upregulation of Nrf2-dependent antioxidants attenuates systemic oxidative overload and renal inflammation. Beyond the resolution of oxidative stress, Nrf2 inhibits inflammation by directly regulating the transcription of pro-inflammatory cytokines (e.g., IL-1, IL-6). Kobayashi et al. reported that Nrf2 binds to the regulatory regions of inflammatory genes and thereby induces their transcription in macrophages and alleviates RNA polymerase II recruitment [37]. The pharmacological activation of Nrf2 decreases cytokine production, M1 macrophage accumulation, and the formation of an atherosclerotic plaque lipid core in the experimental model of streptozotocin-induced diabetic mice on an apolipoprotein E-deficient background [38]. Importantly, Nrf2 activation improves the pathological changes in the glomerulus of streptozotocin-injected diabetic mice through a reduction in oxidative stress, TGF-β expression, and extracellular matrix proteins [39]. Furthermore, Nrf2 attenuates mesangial hypertrophy induced by high glucose. Thus, Nrf2 activators have been suggested to prevent DKD. Bardoxolone methyl, one such Nrf2 activator, has been demonstrated in clinical trials to have reno-protective effects in patients with type 2 diabetes [40].

3.4. *Rho-Kinase Signaling*

A Rho-associated coiled-coil containing protein kinase (Rho-kinase) was initially identified as a regulator of Rho-induced stress fiber formation. Rho-kinase activation results in the phosphorylation of downstream targets, including myosin phosphatase target subunit, which has been demonstrated to mediate a wide array of cellular functions (e.g., cell proliferation, contraction, migration, and transcriptional regulation). Recent experimental studies have implicated Rho-kinase signaling in cardiovascular and kidney disease. Initial insights linking Rho-kinase to diabetes were gleaned from our studies defining Rho-kinase as a regulator of diabetic complications both in the microvasculature and large blood vessels. For example, Rho-kinase inhibition attenuates albuminuria, glomerular matrix expansion [41,42], and infiltration of macrophages [26] in mouse models of DKD. Subsequent analyses in endothelial cells identified Rho-kinase as a key molecule of vascular inflammation [43].

Of note, Rho-kinase mediates the production of MCP1 and monocyte chemotaxis toward glomerular cells. Furthermore, Rho-kinase functions as an important regulator of CSF1 production both in vitro and in vivo. From a transcriptional standpoint, there is evidence for an interaction between Rho-kinase and NF-κB activation. We recently showed that thrombin induces endothelial NF-κB activation through a molecular mechanism involving Rho-kinase [44]. Furthermore, Rho-kinase also plays an important role in the regulation of lysophosphatidic acid-induced endothelial NF-κB activation [45] and has been shown to be associated with neuropeptide-induced NF-κB activation and subsequent IL-8 induction in colonic epithelial cells [46]. Moreover, Rho exchange factor regulates NF-κB activation in monocytes, and the significance of the Rho-kinase/NF-κB axis in the kidney has been shown in mouse models of lipopolysaccharide injection [47]. These data suggest the existence of a mechanistic linkage between Rho-kinase and NF-κB signaling. CSF1 production in the glomerular mesangium is dependent on the NF-κB function, and the inhibition of Rho-kinase significantly inhibits NF-κB-mediated reporter activity via the p38 MAPK pathway. While some studies have demonstrated the direct regulation of Rho-kinase on either IκBα degradation or p65 phosphorylation, an interaction between Rho-kinase and the nuclear translocation of p65 without affecting either IκBα degradation or phosphorylation of p65 has also been reported [26].

Rho-kinase (ROCK) has two isoforms, ROCK1 and ROCK2, that share 65% sequence similarity but have different activation mechanisms. It has become increasingly clear that ROCK1 and ROCK2 play distinctive roles in regulating the cellular function. For instance, Takeda et al. showed the strong contribution of ROCK2 to the induction of E-selectin and MCP1 via NF-κB activation [48]. In vitro, ROCK2 is known to be localized in the nucleus and interacts with p300 acetyltransferase to activate p300-modulated transcription [49]. Taken together, these findings raise the possibility that targeting Rho-kinase may be a new therapeutic target against renal inflammation through a reduction in NF-κB-mediated macrophage accumulation.

4. Targeting Renal Inflammation for Prophylaxis and Therapy

With the discovery that inflammatory mediators are increased in DKD, researchers have begun to focus on therapeutic strategies targeting these inflammatory mediators. Several approaches have been proposed to treat inflammation in DKD, including lifestyle modifications, drugs, and dialysis optimization. As discussed above, the suppression of cytokine signaling with specific inhibitors, antibodies, or aptamers has the potential to reduce the risk of albuminuria and decline in the filtration function, highlighting the important role of these inflammatory mediators in DKD. In addition, novel pharmacological approaches to the management of diabetes have direct or indirect anti-inflammatory actions, the latter potentially attributable to an improvement in the metabolic status.

4.1. Sodium-Glucose Co-Transporter-2 (SGLT2) Inhibitors

SGLT2 inhibitors are now established therapies for treating hyperglycemia in patients with diabetes. By blocking SGLT2 at the proximal tubule, these agents limit the reabsorption of glucose, which in turn induces glycosuria and blood glucose reduction, independent of the insulin action [50]. Treatment with SGLT2 inhibitors leads to sustained systolic and diastolic blood pressure reductions, partially via natriuresis, which also contributes to the improvement of glomerular hyperfiltration and albuminuria through the activation of tubuloglomerular feedback [51].

Secondary outcome analyses in cardiovascular safety trials have shown the potential of SGLT2 inhibition to attenuate the risks of DKD progression and ESRD. For example, the renal composite outcomes (doubling of creatinine, renal replacement therapy, or renal death) decreased by 46% in patients with type 2 diabetes treated with empagliflozin [52]. A similar trend was reported with canagliflozin. The Canagliflozin and Renal Endpoints in Diabetes with Established Nephropathy Clinical Evaluation (CREDENCE) trial was designed to assess the efficacy and safety of canagliflozin versus placebo for reducing clinically important renal and cardiovascular outcomes in patients with diabetes and established kidney disease. This trial was restricted to participants who were taking the maximum tolerated dose of an angiotensin-converting enzyme inhibitor or angiotensin receptor blocker. Compared to a placebo, the reduction in the relative risk of renal-specific composites of ESRD, doubling of the creatinine level, or death from renal causes was greater in the canagliflozin group. An important observation from the CREDENCE trial is that the canagliflozin group also had a lower risk of cardiovascular death, myocardial infarction, or stroke and hospitalization for heart failure than the placebo group. Importantly, this trial showed no imbalance in rates of amputation or bone fracture, and no new safety concerns were identified [53]. Because few drugs are capable of preventing the progressive loss of the kidney function for this population, the current data will provide important evidence supporting the development of diabetes and nephrology guidelines.

Notably, canagliflozin reduces the plasma levels of TNF-R1 (9.2%; $p < 0.001$) and IL-6 (26.6%; $p = 0.010$) compared to glimepiride in patients with diabetes [54]. Similar effects were reported by Garvey et al. [55]. This evidence indicates that canagliflozin reverses molecular processes induced by inflammation. Experimental studies have also suggested the anti-inflammatory effects of SGLT2 inhibitors [56,57]. In diabetic Akita mice, empagliflozin inhibited albuminuria via a reduction in the levels of inflammatory cytokines, including MCP1 and IL-6 [57]. However, whether or not SGLT2 inhibitors can reduce the renal risk in patients with type 1 diabetes is unclear. This point will be investigated in a multicentre international randomized parallel group double-blind placebo-controlled clinical trial of EMPAgliflozin once daily to assess cardio-renal outcomes in patients with chronic KIDNEY disease (EMPA-KIDNEY), which will include patients with type 1 diabetes.

Basic mechanisms to explain anti-inflammatory effects may involve body weight loss and the improvement of obesity-induced insulin resistance. For instance, empagliflozin was shown to modulate energy metabolism by promoting fat utilization, browning of white adipose tissue, and blocking the infiltration of macrophages in high-fat-diet-fed obese mice [58]. Since there is a direct association between fat mass and the amount of pro-inflammatory mediators, a lower fat mass reflects less storage space for pro-inflammatory mediators and thus results in the attenuation of kidney inflammation. In addition, SGLT2 inhibitors may suppress inflammatory responses in the kidney by modulating RAS activity, hemodynamic changes, and changes in the immune system function. The increase in ketone bodies and inhibition of oxidative stress might also have contributed to the beneficial effects on renal inflammation.

Further studies are required in order to assess the inflammatory markers and elucidate the specific contribution of SGLT2 inhibition to the reduction in the DKD risk and associated mortality. When considered alongside very recent observations concerning the SGLT2-mediated oxidative pathway in mesangial cells [59], it will also be interesting to explore whether or not SGLT2 inhibitors affect glomerular inflammation directly.

4.2. Glucagon-Like Peptide 1 (GLP-1) Receptor Agonists and Dipeptidyl Peptidase 4 (DPP-4) Inhibitors

Glucagon-like peptide 1 (GLP-1) is a gut-derived peptide secreted from intestinal L-cells upon meal ingestion, that regulates glucose homeostasis by modulating the pancreatic islet cell function, food intake, and gastrointestinal motility. In addition to pancreatic β cells, GLP-1 receptor is expressed in proximal tubular cells and the kidney vasculature. GLP-1 receptor-mediated natriuresis is induced by the inhibition of sodium-hydrogen exchanger 3 (NHE3), which is located at the brush border of the renal proximal tubule. Mechanistically, GLP-1 receptor agonists (GLP-1RA) promote the phosphorylation of NHE3 at Ser552 and Ser605, which results in a decreased activity of NHE3 and natriuresis. Experimental studies in rodents and humans have shown that the activation of GLP-1 receptor leads to an increase in lithium clearance and pH, indicating the existence of NHE3-mediated regulation. Such proximal natriuresis would be expected to activate tubuloglomerular feedback and afferent vasoconstriction, leading to the downregulation of the renal blood flow and GFR. However, there were no changes in the renal hemodynamics or GFR in subjects with type 2 diabetes treated with GLP-1RA. These data are attributed to the direct nitric oxide-dependent reduction of afferent vascular resistance by GLP-1RA, which might override vasoconstriction induced by tubuloglomerular feedback [60].

GLP-1 receptors are expressed in renal tissue as well as the pancreas, heart, and intestine. Although the exact distribution of GLP-1 receptors in the kidney is not well characterized, clinical studies have shown that treatment with GLP-1RA reduces new-onset macroalbuminuria. These renal benefits may be explained by the known actions of GLP-1RA on metabolic risk factors for DKD, including reductions in blood glucose, blood pressure, and weight. However, several studies in rodents have demonstrated renoprotective effects of GLP-1RA beyond metabolic improvements in models of DKD. Aside from GLP-1RA, DPP-4 inhibitors also exert various extrapancreatic actions. DPP-4 inhibitors can attenuate inflammatory signaling pathways. For example, linagliptin exerts antioxidant and anti-inflammatory actions in endothelium, independent of its glucose-lowering effects [61,62]. In'addition, circulating levels of inflammatory cytokines and markers of inflammation were reduced in diabetic patients treated with sitagliptin or vildagliptin [63]. Experimental studies have demonstrated the renoprotective effects of DPP-4 inhibitors in the models of DKD and nondiabetic glomerular injury [64]. Some of these beneficial actions may be due to elevated GLP-1 levels. However, evidence suggests that the albuminuria-lowering effect of the DPP-4 inhibitor is weak compared to that of GLP-1RA [65,66].

The protective effect of GLP-1RA is mediated at least in part via inhibitory effects on renal inflammation, as well as NHE3-dependent sodium reabsorption [67]. For instance, exenatide was shown to inhibit albuminuria and the influx of glomerular macrophages in type 2 diabetic db/db mice [68]. Albuminuria and mesangial expansion were attenuated by treatment with exenatide in streptozotocin-injected type 1 diabetic rats through a mechanism involving inflammatory cytokines and adhesion molecules [69]. Furthermore, exenatide and dulaglutide reduced the circulating levels of C-reactive protein (CRP) in patients with type 2 diabetes [70]. Studies have shown that GLP-1RA's anti-inflammatory effects are modulated through the prevention of oxidative stress. Subsequent detailed investigations have revealed that liraglutide treatment inhibited albuminuria and nicotinamide adenine dinucleotide phosphate oxidase activity in a KK/Ta-Akita mouse model of type 1 diabetes without altering the blood glucose levels [71]. A more detailed understanding will be required to fully characterize the exact renal tissue distribution of GLP-1 receptors, as well as the associated anti-inflammatory effects and antioxidant mechanisms, in order to explain the renoprotection mediated by GLP-1RA.

4.3. Metformin

Metformin is now widely used for the treatment of type 2 diabetes as a first-line drug. Clinical studies have demonstrated that metformin not only attenuates chronic inflammation through the improvement of metabolic parameters (e.g., hyperglycemia, dyslipidemia), but also has direct anti-inflammatory properties. Metformin regulates miR-34a, a tumor-suppressor microRNA, to inhibit mesangial inflammation under high glucose conditions [72]. By activating AMPK, metformin disrupts the phosphorylation of STAT signaling and attenuates the differentiation of monocytes into macrophages [73].

4.4. Immunosuppressive Agents

Pharmacological modulation of the immune system may have beneficial effects on DKD development. For example, glucocorticoids are known to exert anti-inflammatory and immunosuppressive actions by genomic and nongenomic effects. Glucocorticoids have been extensively used in nephrotic syndrome. Cell-based studies suggest that glucocorticoids may have protective effects on podocyte injury [74]. Mechanistically, glucocorticoids reduce podocyte apoptosis and increase the number of podocyte progenitors via key components of the glucocorticoid receptor complex (e.g., heat shock protein 90, immunophilins FK506 binding protein (FKBP) 51, and FKBP52). However, the risk and potential clinical benefits of glucocorticoids are different for each patient. It is important to consider whether the benefits outweigh the side effects.

Mycophenolate mofetil is an anti-lymphocyte agent with immunosuppressive properties. This drug is clinically used to prevent allograft rejection. Mycophenolic acid, the active metabolite of mycophenolate mofetil, attenuates lymphocyte proliferation by blocking the early phases of the cell cycle. Experimental studies have demonstrated that mycophenolate mofetil decreases proteinuria and glomerulosclerosis through the reduction of macrophage infiltration in rodent models of type 1 and type 2 diabetes [75,76]. Furthermore, podocyte apoptosis and ROS production were attenuated in mycophenolate mofetil-treated diabetic mice [77]. Clinical evidence is required before recommendations can be made for treatment against DKD.

Regulatory T-cells (Tregs) control self-tolerance and allogeneic tolerance, and the dysfunction of Tregs is supposed to mediate the progression of DKD. Recent evidence from the Treg inhibition approach with anti-CD25 antibody emphasizes the importance of Treg in DKD. Treatment with anti-CD25 accelerated kidney damage in db/db mice and the adoptive transfer of Tregs inhibited proteinuria and glomerular hypertrophy [78]. Therefore, Tregs may be an attractive target for the treatment of DKD. Since the transfer of Treg has technical limitations, approaches that enhance endogenous Tregs are likely to be beneficial for DKD patients.

5. Conclusions and Future Perspectives

It is becoming clear that DKD is associated with the increased expression of inflammation-associated mediators. Since the diagnosis of DKD is still difficult due to a lack of reliable biomarkers capable of predicting patient outcomes, especially in the early stages (albuminuria is not specific for diabetic renal damage), the levels of pro-inflammatory cytokines may be a useful marker for making a diagnosis of DKD. From this standpoint, urinary proteomics and peptidomics have gained attention as a study tool for the detection of diagnostic markers of DKD. The urinary omics studies in DKD have revealed several markers, including inflammatory mediators such as MCP1 and TGF-β [79,80]. Whether inflammation is a trigger or a result of a chronic underlying condition is an important topic. Gene manipulation studies on the impact of renal inflammation on DKD development have greatly expanded our knowledge in this field. Furthermore, studies exploring the cause of this pro-inflammatory milieu and the contribution of these pathways to DKD development will strengthen the significance of inflammatory mediators as biomarker of DKD.

Recent systems biological approaches have revealed molecular abnormalities in DKD and have directly led to the identification of potential targets for DKD. A comprehensive transcriptome analysis demonstrated that the top differentially regulated genes in DKD tissue are associated with inflammation and fibrosis [81]. In this assessment, the complement signal was the highest degree of statistical significance in both glomeruli and tubulointerstitium. Studies will be required to determine the pathological significance of the complement system in human DKD.

The cumulative data on the role of inflammation in the pathogenesis of DKD are sufficient to warrant their consideration as therapeutic targets. Targeting inflammatory cytokines or adhesion molecules will offer novel avenues for therapeutic intervention. However, a central challenge remains: how to leverage our comprehension of the inflammatory mechanism in order to establish an intervention that can prevent DKD progression and prolong the lifespan of diabetic patients. Over the past decade, new classes of anti-hyperglycemic drugs with renal benefits have been introduced for the management of diabetes, namely SGLT2 inhibitors and GLP-1RA. These agents seem to have additional pleiotropic anti-inflammatory properties mediated through distinct molecular mechanisms by both direct and indirect actions. A greater understanding of the mechanisms underlying these agents' renal benefits would facilitate the development of novel therapies for DKD and its associated sequelae.

Author Contributions: K.M. wrote the manuscript; Y.T., Y.N., D.K., K.U. and R.N. helped edit the manuscript and revised the manuscript for important intellectual content. All of the authors read and approved the final manuscript.

Acknowledgments: This work was supported by a Grant-in-Aid for Scientific Research from Japan Society for the Promotion of Science (to Keiichiro Matoba and Daiji Kawanami), the Ichiro Kanehara Foundation (to Keiichiro Matoba), the MSD Life Science Foundation (to Keiichiro Matoba), and the Yokoyama Foundation for Clinical Pharmacology (to Keiichiro Matoba).

References

1. Adler, A.I.; Stevens, R.J.; Manley, S.E.; Bilous, R.W.; Cull, C.A.; Holman, R.R.; UKPDS GROUP. Development and progression of nephropathy in type 2 diabetes: The United Kingdom Prospective Diabetes Study (UKPDS 64). *Kidney Int.* **2003**, *63*, 225–232. [CrossRef] [PubMed]
2. Goldfine, A.B.; Shoelson, S.E. Therapeutic approaches targeting inflammation for diabetes and associated cardiovascular risk. *J. Clin. Invest.* **2017**, *127*, 83–93. [CrossRef] [PubMed]
3. Simo-Servat, O.; Simo, R.; Hernandez, C. Circulating Biomarkers of Diabetic Retinopathy: An Overview Based on Physiopathology. *J. Diabetes Res.* **2016**, *2016*, 5263798. [CrossRef] [PubMed]
4. Paeschke, S.; Paeschke, S.; Baum, P.; Toyka, K.V.; Blüher, M.; Koj, S.; Klöting, N.; Bechmann, I.; Thiery, J.; Kosacka, J.; et al. The Role of Iron and Nerve Inflammation in Diabetes Mellitus Type 2-Induced Peripheral Neuropathy. *Neuroscience* **2019**, *406*, 496–509. [CrossRef] [PubMed]
5. Xu, L.; Lin, X.; Guan, M.; Zeng, Y.; Liu, Y. Verapamil Attenuated Prediabetic Neuropathy in High-Fat Diet-Fed Mice through Inhibiting TXNIP-Mediated Apoptosis and Inflammation. *Oxid Med. Cell Longev.* **2019**, *2019*, 1896041. [CrossRef]
6. Doupis, J.; Lyons, T.E.; Wu, S.; Gnardellis, C.; Dinh, T.; Veves, A. Microvascular reactivity and inflammatory cytokines in painful and painless peripheral diabetic neuropathy. *J. Clin. Endocrinol Metab.* **2009**, *94*, 2157–2163. [CrossRef] [PubMed]
7. Pop-Busui, R.; Ang, L.; Holmes, C.; Gallagher, K.; Feldman, E.L. Inflammation as a Therapeutic Target for Diabetic Neuropathies. *Curr. Diab. Rep.* **2016**, *16*, 29. [CrossRef]
8. Ganesh Yerra, V.; Negi, G.; Sharma, S.S.; Kumar, A. Potential therapeutic effects of the simultaneous targeting of the Nrf2 and NF-kappaB pathways in diabetic neuropathy. *Redox Biol.* **2013**, *1*, 394–397. [CrossRef]
9. Tian, S.; Chen, S.Y. Macrophage polarization in kidney diseases. *Macrophage (Houst)* **2015**, *2*, e679.
10. Klessens, C.Q.F.; Zandbergen, M.; Wolterbeek, R.; Bruijn, J.A.; Rabelink, T.J.; Bajema, I.M.; IJpelaar, D.H.T. Macrophages in diabetic nephropathy in patients with type 2 diabetes. *Nephrol. Dial. Transpl.* **2017**, *32*, 1322–1329. [CrossRef]
11. Usui, H.K.; Shikata, K.; Sasaki, M.; Okada, S.; Matsuda, M.; Shikata, Y.; Ogawa, D.; Kido, Y.; Nagase, R.; Yozai, K.; et al. Macrophage scavenger receptor-a-deficient mice are resistant against diabetic nephropathy through amelioration of microinflammation. *Diabetes* **2007**, *56*, 363–372. [CrossRef] [PubMed]
12. Landis, R.C.; Quimby, K.R.; Greenidge, A.R. M1/M2 Macrophages in Diabetic Nephropathy: Nrf2/HO-1 as Therapeutic Targets. *Curr. Pharm. Des.* **2018**, *24*, 2241–2249. [CrossRef] [PubMed]
13. Devaraj, S.; Tobias, P.; Kasinath, B.S.; Ramsamooj, R.; Afify, A.; Jialal, I. Knockout of toll-like receptor-2 attenuates both the proinflammatory state of diabetes and incipient diabetic nephropathy. *Arterioscler Thromb. Vasc. Biol.* **2011**, *31*, 1796–1804. [CrossRef] [PubMed]
14. Clausen, P.; Jacobsen, P.; Rossing, K.; Jensen, J.S.; Parving, H.H.; Feldt-Rasmussen, B. Plasma concentrations of VCAM-1 and ICAM-1 are elevated in patients with Type 1 diabetes mellitus with microalbuminuria and overt nephropathy. *Diabet Med.* **2000**, *17*, 644–649. [CrossRef] [PubMed]
15. Hojs, R.; Ekart, R.; Bevc, S.; Hojs, N. Markers of Inflammation and Oxidative Stress in the Development and Progression of Renal Disease in Diabetic Patients. *Nephron* **2016**, *133*, 159–162. [CrossRef] [PubMed]
16. Liu, J.J.; Yeoh, L.Y.; Sum, C.F.; Tavintharan, S.; Ng, X.W.; Liu, S.; Lee, S.B.; Tang, W.E.; Lim, S.C.; SMART2D study. Vascular cell adhesion molecule-1, but not intercellular adhesion molecule-1, is associated with diabetic kidney disease in Asians with type 2 diabetes. *J. Diabetes Complicat.* **2015**, *29*, 707–712. [CrossRef] [PubMed]

17. Lim, A.K.; Tesch, G.H. Inflammation in diabetic nephropathy. *Mediators Inflamm.* **2012**, *2012*, 146154. [CrossRef] [PubMed]
18. Okada, S.; Shikata, K.; Matsuda, M.; Ogawa, D.; Usui, H.; Kido, Y.; Nagase, R.; Wada, J.; Shikata, Y.; Makino, H. Intercellular adhesion molecule-1-deficient mice are resistant against renal injury after induction of diabetes. *Diabetes* **2003**, *52*, 2586–2593. [CrossRef]
19. Nadkarni, G.N.; Rao, V.; Ismail-Beigi, F.; Fonseca, V.A.; Shah, S.V.; Simonson, M.S.; Cantley, L.; Devarajan, P.; Parikh, C.R.; Coca, S.G. Association of Urinary Biomarkers of Inflammation, Injury, and Fibrosis with Renal Function Decline: The ACCORD Trial. *Clin. J. Am. Soc. Nephrol.* **2016**, *11*, 1343–1352. [CrossRef]
20. Satirapoj, B.; Dispan, R.; Radinahamed, P.; Kitiyakara, C. Urinary epidermal growth factor, monocyte chemoattractant protein-1 or their ratio as predictors for rapid loss of renal function in type 2 diabetic patients with diabetic kidney disease. *BMC Nephrol.* **2018**, *19*, 246. [CrossRef]
21. Niewczas, M.A.; Gohda, T.; Skupien, J.; Smiles, A.M.; Walker, W.H.; Rosetti, F.; Cullere, X.; Eckfeldt, J.H.; Doria, A.; Mayadas, T.N.; et al. Circulating TNF receptors 1 and 2 predict ESRD in type 2 diabetes. *J. Am. Soc. Nephrol.* **2012**, *23*, 507–515. [CrossRef] [PubMed]
22. Niewczas, M.A.; Pavkov, M.E.; Skupien, J.; Smiles, A.; Md Dom, Z.I.; Wilson, J.M.; Park, J.; Nair, V.; Schlafly, A.; Saulnier, P.J.; et al. A signature of circulating inflammatory proteins and development of end-stage renal disease in diabetes. *Nat. Med.* **2019**, *25*, 805–813. [CrossRef] [PubMed]
23. Menne, J.; Eulberg, D.; Beyer, D.; Baumann, M.; Saudek, F.; Valkusz, Z.; Więcek, A.; Haller, H.; Emapticap Study Group. C-C motif-ligand 2 inhibition with emapticap pegol (NOX-E36) in type 2 diabetic patients with albuminuria. *Nephrol. Dial. Transplant.* **2017**, *32*, 307–315. [CrossRef] [PubMed]
24. Lenda, D.M.; Kikawada, E.; Stanley, E.R.; Kelley, V.R. Reduced macrophage recruitment, proliferation, and activation in colony-stimulating factor-1-deficient mice results in decreased tubular apoptosis during renal inflammation. *J. Immunol.* **2003**, *170*, 3254–3262. [CrossRef] [PubMed]
25. Naito, T.; Yokoyama, H.; Moore, K.J.; Dranoff, G.; Mulligan, R.C.; Kelley, V.R. Macrophage growth factors introduced into the kidney initiate renal injury. *Mol. Med.* **1996**, *2*, 297–312. [CrossRef] [PubMed]
26. Matoba, K.; Kawanami, D.; Tsukamoto, M.; Kinoshita, J.; Ito, T.; Ishizawa, S.; Kanazawa, Y.; Yokota, T.; Murai, N.; Matsufuji, S.; et al. Rho-kinase regulation of TNF-alpha-induced nuclear translocation of NF-kappaB RelA/p65 and M-CSF expression via p38 MAPK in mesangial cells. *Am. J. Physiol. Renal Physiol.* **2014**, *307*, F571–F580. [CrossRef] [PubMed]
27. Lim, A.K.; Ma, F.Y.; Nikolic-Paterson, D.J.; Thomas, M.C.; Hurst, L.A.; Tesch, G.H. Antibody blockade of c-fms suppresses the progression of inflammation and injury in early diabetic nephropathy in obese db/db mice. *Diabetologia* **2009**, *52*, 1669–1679. [CrossRef]
28. Pichler, R.; Afkarian, M.; Dieter, B.P.; Tuttle, K.R. Immunity and inflammation in diabetic kidney disease: Translating mechanisms to biomarkers and treatment targets. *Am. J. Physiol. Renal Physiol.* **2017**, *312*, F716–F731. [CrossRef]
29. Sanajou, D.; Ghorbani Haghjo, A.; Argani, H.; Aslani, S. AGE-RAGE axis blockade in diabetic nephropathy: Current status and future directions. *Eur. J. Pharmacol.* **2018**, *833*, 158–164. [CrossRef]
30. Pérez-Morales, R.E.; Del Pino, M.D.; Valdivielso, J.M.; Ortiz, A.; Mora-Fernández, C.; Navarro-González, J.F. Inflammation in Diabetic Kidney Disease. *Nephron* **2018**, 1–5. [CrossRef]
31. Toth-Manikowski, S.; Atta, M.G. Diabetic Kidney Disease: Pathophysiology and Therapeutic Targets. *J. Diabetes Res.* **2015**, *2015*, 697010. [CrossRef] [PubMed]
32. Weigert, C.; Sauer, U.; Brodbeck, K.; Pfeiffer, A.; Häring, H.U.; Schleicher, E.D. AP-1 proteins mediate hyperglycemia-induced activation of the human TGF-beta1 promoter in mesangial cells. *J. Am. Soc. Nephrol.* **2000**, *11*, 2007–2016. [PubMed]
33. Nicholas, S.B.; Liu, J.; Kim, J.; Ren, Y.; Collins, A.R.; Nguyen, L.; Hsueh, W.A. Critical role for osteopontin in diabetic nephropathy. *Kidney Int.* **2010**, *77*, 588–600. [CrossRef] [PubMed]
34. Tuttle, K.R.; Brosius III, F.C.; Adler, S.G.; Kretzler, M.; Mehta, R.L.; Tumlin, J.A.; Tanaka, Y.; Haneda, M.; Liu, J.; Silk, M.E.; et al. JAK1/JAK2 inhibition by baricitinib in diabetic kidney disease: Results from a Phase 2 randomized controlled clinical trial. *Nephrol. Dial. Transplant.* **2018**, *33*, 1950–1959. [CrossRef] [PubMed]
35. Brosius, F.C.; Ju, W. The Promise of Systems Biology for Diabetic Kidney Disease. *Adv. Chronic Kidney Dis.* **2018**, *25*, 202–213. [CrossRef]
36. Zhang, H.; Nair, V.; Saha, J.; Atkins, K.B.; Hodgin, J.B.; Saunders, T.L.; Myers, M.G.Jr.; Werner, T.; Kretzler, M.; Brosius, F.C. Podocyte-specific JAK2 overexpression worsens diabetic kidney disease in mice. *Kidney Int.* **2017**, *92*, 909–921. [CrossRef]

37. Kobayashi, E.H.; Suzuki, T.; Funayama, R.; Nagashima, T.; Hayashi, M.; Sekine, H.; Tanaka, N.; Moriguchi, T.; Motohashi, H.; Nakayama, K.; et al. Nrf2 suppresses macrophage inflammatory response by blocking proinflammatory cytokine transcription. *Nat. Commun.* **2016**, *7*, 11624. [CrossRef]
38. Lazaro, I.; Lopez-Sanz, L.; Bernal, S.; Oguiza, A.; Recio, C.; Melgar, A.; Jimenez-Castilla, L.; Egido, J.; Madrigal-Matute, J.; Gomez-Guerrero, C. Nrf2 Activation Provides Atheroprotection in Diabetic Mice Through Concerted Upregulation of Antioxidant, Anti-inflammatory, and Autophagy Mechanisms. *Front. Pharmacol.* **2018**, *9*, 819. [CrossRef]
39. Zheng, H.; Whitman, S.A.; Wu, W.; Wondrak, G.T.; Wong, P.K.; Fang, D.; Zhang, D.D. Therapeutic potential of Nrf2 activators in streptozotocin-induced diabetic nephropathy. *Diabetes* **2011**, *60*, 3055–3066. [CrossRef]
40. Pergola, P.E.; Raskin, P.; Toto, R.D.; Meyer, C.J.; Huff, J.W.; Grossman, E.B.; Krauth, M.; Ruiz, S.; Audhya, P.; Christ-Schmidt, H.; et al. Bardoxolone methyl and kidney function in CKD with type 2 diabetes. *N. Engl. J. Med.* **2011**, *365*, 327–336. [CrossRef]
41. Matoba, K.; Kawanami, D.; Okada, R.; Tsukamoto, M.; Kinoshita, J.; Ito, T.; Ishizawa, S.; Kanazawa, Y.; Yokota, T.; Murai, N.; et al. Rho-kinase inhibition prevents the progression of diabetic nephropathy by downregulating hypoxia-inducible factor 1alpha. *Kidney Int.* **2013**, *84*, 545–554. [CrossRef] [PubMed]
42. Kawanami, D.; Matoba, K.; Utsunomiya, K. Signaling pathways in diabetic nephropathy. *Histol. Histopathol.* **2016**, *31*, 1059–1067. [PubMed]
43. Kawanami, D.; Matoba, K.; Okada, R.; Tsukamoto, M.; Kinoshita, J.; Ishizawa, S.; Kanazawa, Y.; Yokota, T.; Utsunomiya, K. Fasudil inhibits ER stress-induced VCAM-1 expression by modulating unfolded protein response in endothelial cells. *Biochem. Biophys. Res. Commun.* **2013**, *435*, 171–175. [CrossRef] [PubMed]
44. Kawanami, D.; Matoba, K.; Kanazawa, Y.; Ishizawa, S.; Yokota, T.; Utsunomiya, K. Thrombin induces MCP-1 expression through Rho-kinase and subsequent p38MAPK/NF-kappaB signaling pathway activation in vascular endothelial cells. *Biochem. Biophys. Res. Commun.* **2011**, *411*, 798–803. [CrossRef] [PubMed]
45. Shimada, H.; Rajagopalan, L.E. Rho kinase-2 activation in human endothelial cells drives lysophosphatidic acid-mediated expression of cell adhesion molecules via NF-kappaB p65. *J. Biol. Chem.* **2010**, *285*, 12536–12542. [CrossRef] [PubMed]
46. Zhao, D.; Kuhnt-Moore, S.; Zeng, H.; Wu, J.S.; Moyer, M.P.; Pothoulakis, C. Neurotensin stimulates IL-8 expression in human colonic epithelial cells through Rho GTPase-mediated NF-kappa B pathways. *Am. J. Physiol. Cell Physiol.* **2003**, *284*, C1397–C1404. [CrossRef] [PubMed]
47. Meyer-Schwesinger, C.; Dehde, S.; von Ruffer, C.; Gatzemeier, S.; Klug, P.; Wenzel, U.O.; Stahl, R.A.; Thaiss, F.; Meyer, T.N. Rho kinase inhibition attenuates LPS-induced renal failure in mice in part by attenuation of NF-kappaB p65 signaling. *Am. J. Physiol. Renal Physiol.* **2009**, *296*, F1088–F1099. [CrossRef] [PubMed]
48. Takeda, Y.; Matoba, K.; Kawanami, D.; Nagai, Y.; Akamine, T.; Ishizawa, S.; Kanazawa, Y.; Yokota, T.; Utsunomiya, K. ROCK2 Regulates Monocyte Migration and Cell to Cell Adhesion in Vascular Endothelial Cells. *Int. J. Mol. Sci.* **2019**, *20*, 1331. [CrossRef]
49. Tanaka, T.; Nishimura, D.; Wu, R.C.; Amano, M.; Iso, T.; Kedes, L.; Nishida, H.; Kaibuchi, K.; Hamamori, Y. Nuclear Rho kinase, ROCK2, targets p300 acetyltransferase. *J. Biol. Chem.* **2006**, *281*, 15320–15329. [CrossRef]
50. Thomas, M.C.; Cherney, D.Z.I. The actions of SGLT2 inhibitors on metabolism, renal function and blood pressure. *Diabetologia* **2018**, *61*, 2098–2107. [CrossRef] [PubMed]
51. Kawanami, D.; Matoba, K.; Takeda, Y.; Nagai, Y.; Akamine, T.; Yokota, T.; Sango, K.; Utsunomiya, K. SGLT2 Inhibitors as a Therapeutic Option for Diabetic Nephropathy. *Int. J. Mol. Sci.* **2017**, *18*, 1083. [CrossRef] [PubMed]
52. Wanner, C.; Inzucchi, S.E.; Lachin, J.M.; Fitchett, D.; von Eynatten, M.; Mattheus, M.; Johansen, O.E.; Woerle, H.J.; Broedl, U.C.; Zinman, B.; et al. Empagliflozin and Progression of Kidney Disease in Type 2 Diabetes. *N. Engl. J. Med.* **2016**, *375*, 323–334. [CrossRef] [PubMed]
53. Perkovic, V.; Jardine, M.J.; Neal, B.; Bompoint, S.; Heerspink, H.J.L.; Charytan, D.M.; Edwards, R.; Agarwal, R.; Bakris, G.; Bull, S.; et al. Canagliflozin and Renal Outcomes in Type 2 Diabetes and Nephropathy. *N. Engl. J. Med.* **2019**, *380*, 2295–2306. [CrossRef] [PubMed]
54. Heerspink, H.J.L.; Perco, P.; Mulder, S.; Leierer, J.; Hansen, M.K.; Heinzel, A.; Mayer, G. Canagliflozin reduces inflammation and fibrosis biomarkers: A potential mechanism of action for beneficial effects of SGLT2 inhibitors in diabetic kidney disease. *Diabetologia* **2019**, *62*, 1154–1166. [CrossRef]
55. Garvey, W.T.; Van Gaal, L.; Leiter, L.A.; Vijapurkar, U.; List, J.; Cuddihy, R.; Ren, J.; Davies, M.J. Effects of canagliflozin versus glimepiride on adipokines and inflammatory biomarkers in type 2 diabetes. *Metabolism* **2018**, *85*, 32–37. [CrossRef]

56. Tahara, A.; Takasu, T.; Yokono, M.; Imamura, M.; Kurosaki, E. Characterization and comparison of SGLT2 inhibitors: Part 3. Effects on diabetic complications in type 2 diabetic mice. *Eur. J. Pharmacol.* **2017**, *809*, 163–171. [CrossRef]
57. Vallon, V.; Gerasimova, M.; Rose, M.A.; Masuda, T.; Satriano, J.; Mayoux, E.; Koepsell, H.; Thomson, SC.; Rieg, T. SGLT2 inhibitor empagliflozin reduces renal growth and albuminuria in proportion to hyperglycemia and prevents glomerular hyperfiltration in diabetic Akita mice. *Am. J. Physiol. Renal Physiol.* **2014**, *306*, F194–F204. [CrossRef]
58. Xu, L.; Nagata, N.; Nagashimada, M.; Zhuge, F.; Ni, Y.; Chen, G.; Mayoux, E.; Kaneko, S.; Ota, T. SGLT2 Inhibition by Empagliflozin Promotes Fat Utilization and Browning and Attenuates Inflammation and Insulin Resistance by Polarizing M2 Macrophages in Diet-induced Obese Mice. *EBioMedicine* **2017**, *20*, 137–149. [CrossRef]
59. Maki, T.; Maeno, S.; Maeda, Y.; Yamato, M.; Sonoda, N.; Ogawa, Y.; Wakisaka, M.; Inoguchi, T. Amelioration of diabetic nephropathy by SGLT2 inhibitors independent of its glucose-lowering effect: A possible role of SGLT2 in mesangial cells. *Sci. Rep.* **2019**, *9*, 4703. [CrossRef]
60. Muskiet, M.H.; Tonneijck, L.; Smits, M.M.; Kramer, M.H.; Diamant, M.; Joles, J.A.; van Raalte, D.H. Acute renal haemodynamic effects of glucagon-like peptide-1 receptor agonist exenatide in healthy overweight men. *Diabetes Obes. Metab.* **2016**, *18*, 178–185. [CrossRef]
61. Kröller-Schön, S.; Knorr, M.; Hausding, M.; Oelze, M.; Schuff, A.; Schell, R.; Sudowe, S.; Scholz, A.; Daub, S.; Karbach, S.; et al. Glucose-independent improvement of vascular dysfunction in experimental sepsis by dipeptidyl-peptidase 4 inhibition. *Cardiovasc Res.* **2012**, *96*, 140–149. [CrossRef]
62. Kanasaki, K. The role of renal dipeptidyl peptidase-4 in kidney disease: Renal effects of dipeptidyl peptidase-4 inhibitors with a focus on linagliptin. *Clin. Sci.* **2018**, *132*, 489–507. [CrossRef] [PubMed]
63. Barbieri, M.; Rizzo, M.R.; Marfella, R.; Boccardi, V.; Esposito, A.; Pansini, A.; Paolisso, G. Decreased carotid atherosclerotic process by control of daily acute glucose fluctuations in diabetic patients treated by DPP-IV inhibitors. *Atherosclerosis* **2013**, *227*, 349–354. [CrossRef]
64. Higashijima, Y.; Tanaka, T.; Yamaguchi, J.; Tanaka, S.; Nangaku, M. Anti-inflammatory role of DPP-4 inhibitors in a nondiabetic model of glomerular injury. *Am. J. Physiol. Renal Physiol.* **2015**, *308*, F878–F887. [CrossRef] [PubMed]
65. Pollock, C.; Stefánsson, B.; Reyner, D.; Rossing, P.; Sjöström, C.D.; Wheeler, D.C.; Langkilde, A.M.; Heerspink, H.J.L. Albuminuria-lowering effect of dapagliflozin alone and in combination with saxagliptin and effect of dapagliflozin and saxagliptin on glycaemic control in patients with type 2 diabetes and chronic kidney disease (DELIGHT): A randomised, double-blind, placebo-controlled trial. *Lancet Diabetes Endocrinol.* **2019**, *7*, 429–441. [PubMed]
66. Rosenstock, J.; Perkovic, V.; Johansen, O.E.; Cooper, M.E.; Kahn, S.E.; Marx, N.; Alexander, J.H.; Pencina, M.; Toto, R.D.; Wanner, C.; et al. Effect of Linagliptin vs Placebo on Major Cardiovascular Events in Adults With Type 2 Diabetes and High Cardiovascular and Renal Risk: The CARMELINA Randomized Clinical Trial. *JAMA.* **2019**, *321*, 69–79. [CrossRef]
67. Kawanami, D.; Matoba, K.; Sango, K.; Utsunomiya, K. Incretin-Based Therapies for Diabetic Complications: Basic Mechanisms and Clinical Evidence. *Int. J. Mol. Sci.* **2016**, *17*, 1223. [CrossRef]
68. Park, C.W.; Kim, H.W.; Ko, S.H.; Lim, J.H.; Ryu, G.R.; Chung, H.W.; Han, S.W.; Shin, S.J.; Bang, B.K.; Breyer, M.D.; et al. Long-term treatment of glucagon-like peptide-1 analog exendin-4 ameliorates diabetic nephropathy through improving metabolic anomalies in db/db mice. *J. Am. Soc. Nephrol.* **2017**, *18*, 1227–1238. [CrossRef]
69. Kodera, R.; Shikata, K.; Kataoka, H.U.; Takatsuka, T.; Miyamoto, S.; Sasaki, M.; Kajitani, N.; Nishishita, S.; Sarai, K.; Hirota, D.; et al. Glucagon-like peptide-1 receptor agonist ameliorates renal injury through its anti-inflammatory action without lowering blood glucose level in a rat model of type 1 diabetes. *Diabetologia* **2011**, *54*, 965–978. [CrossRef]
70. Ferdinand, K.C.; White, W.B.; Calhoun, D.A.; Lonn, E.M.; Sager, P.T.; Brunelle, R.; Jiang, H.H.; Threlkeld, R.J.; Robertson, K.E.; Geiger, M.J. Effects of the once-weekly glucagon-like peptide-1 receptor agonist dulaglutide on ambulatory blood pressure and heart rate in patients with type 2 diabetes mellitus. *Hypertension* **2014**, *64*, 731–737. [CrossRef]
71. Fujita, H.; Morii, T.; Fujishima, H.; Sato, T.; Shimizu, T.; Hosoba, M.; Tsukiyama, K.; Narita, T.; Takahashi, T.; Drucker, D.J.; et al. The protective roles of GLP-1R signaling in diabetic nephropathy: Possible mechanism and therapeutic potential. *Kidney Int.* **2014**, *85*, 579–589. [CrossRef] [PubMed]
72. Wu, C.; Qin, N.; Ren, H.; Yang, M.; Liu, S.; Wang, Q. Metformin Regulating miR-34a Pathway to Inhibit Egr1 in Rat Mesangial Cells Cultured with High Glucose. *Int. J. Endocrinol.* **2018**, *2018*, 6462793. [CrossRef] [PubMed]

73. Vasamsetti, S.B.; Karnewar, S.; Kanugula, A.K.; Thatipalli, A.R.; Kumar, J.M.; Kotamraju, S. Metformin inhibits monocyte-to-macrophage differentiation via AMPK-mediated inhibition of STAT3 activation: Potential role in atherosclerosis. *Diabetes* **2015**, *64*, 2028–2041. [CrossRef]
74. Guess, A.; Agrawal, S.; Wei, C.C.; Ransom, R.F.; Benndorf, R.; Smoyer, W.E. Dose- and time-dependent glucocorticoid receptor signaling in podocytes. *Am. J. Physiol. Renal Physiol.* **2010**, *299*, F553–F845. [CrossRef] [PubMed]
75. Utimura, R.; Fujihara, C.K.; Mattar, A.L.; Malheiros, D.M.; Noronha, I.L.; Zatz, R. Mycophenolate mofetil prevents the development of glomerular injury in experimental diabetes. *Kidney Int.* **2003**, *63*, 209–216. [CrossRef] [PubMed]
76. Rodríguez-Iturbe, B.; Quiroz, Y.; Shahkarami, A.; Li, Z.; Vaziri, N.D. Mycophenolate mofetil ameliorates nephropathy in the obese Zucker rat. *Kidney Int.* **2005**, *68*, 1041–1047. [CrossRef]
77. Seo, J.W.; Kim, Y.G.; Lee, S.H.; Lee, A.; Kim, D.J.; Jeong, K.H.; Lee, K.H.; Hwang, S.J.; Woo, J.S.; Lim, S.J.; et al. Mycophenolate Mofetil Ameliorates Diabetic Nephropathy in db/db Mice. *Biomed. Res. Int.* **2015**, *2015*, 301627. [CrossRef]
78. Eller, K.; Kirsch, A.; Wolf, A.M.; Sopper, S.; Tagwerker, A.; Stanzl, U.; Wolf, D.; Patsch, W.; Rosenkranz, A.R.; Eller, P. Potential role of regulatory T cells in reversing obesity-linked insulin resistance and diabetic nephropathy. *Diabetes* **2011**, *60*, 2954–2962. [CrossRef] [PubMed]
79. Pena, M.J.; Mischak, H.; Heerspink, H.J. Proteomics for prediction of disease progression and response to therapy in diabetic kidney disease. *Diabetologia* **2016**, *59*, 1819–1831. [CrossRef]
80. Verhave, J.C.; Bouchard, J.; Goupil, R.; Pichette, V.; Brachemi, S.; Madore, F.; Troyanov, S. Clinical value of inflammatory urinary biomarkers in overt diabetic nephropathy: A prospective study. *Diabetes Res. Clin. Pract.* **2013**, *101*, 333–340. [CrossRef]
81. Woroniecka, K.I.; Park, A.S.; Mohtat, D.; Thomas, D.B.; Pullman, J.M.; Susztak, K. Transcriptome analysis of human diabetic kidney disease. *Diabetes* **2011**, *60*, 2354–2369. [CrossRef] [PubMed]

6

Noninvasive Urinary Monitoring of Progression in IgA Nephropathy

Joshua Y. C. Yang [1,2], Reuben D. Sarwal [1], Fernando C. Fervenza [3], Minnie M. Sarwal [1,2,*] and Richard A. Lafayette [4,*]

1 Department of Surgery, University of California San Francisco, San Francisco, CA 94143, USA
2 KIT Bio, 665 3rd St, Suite 280, San Francisco, CA 94107, USA
3 Division of Nephrology and Hypertension, Mayo Clinic, Rochester, MN 55905, USA
4 Division of Nephrology and Hypertension, Stanford University, Stanford, CA 94305, USA
* Correspondence: minnie.sarwal@ucsf.edu (M.M.S.); czar@stanford.edu (R.A.L.)

Abstract: Standard methods for detecting and monitoring of IgA nephropathy (IgAN) have conventionally required kidney biopsies or suffer from poor sensitivity and specificity. The Kidney Injury Test (KIT) Assay of urinary biomarkers has previously been shown to distinguish between various kidney pathologies, including chronic kidney disease, nephrolithiasis, and transplant rejection. This validation study uses the KIT Assay to investigate the clinical utility of the non-invasive detection of IgAN and predicting the progression of renal damage over time. The study design benefits from longitudinally collected urine samples from an investigator-initiated, multicenter, prospective study, evaluating the efficacy of corticosteroids versus Rituximab for preventing progressive IgAN. A total of 131 urine samples were processed for this study; 64 urine samples were collected from 34 IgAN patients, and urine samples from 64 demographically matched healthy controls were also collected; multiple urinary biomarkers consisting of cell-free DNA, methylated cell-free DNA, DMAIMO, MAMIMO, total protein, clusterin, creatinine, and CXCL10 were measured by the microwell-based KIT Assay. An IgA risk score (KIT-IgA) was significantly higher in IgAN patients as compared to healthy control (87.76 vs. 14.03, $p < 0.0001$) and performed better than proteinuria in discriminating between the two groups. The KIT Assay biomarkers, measured on a spot random urine sample at study entry could distinguish patients likely to have progressive renal dysfunction a year later. These data support the pursuit of larger prospective studies to evaluate the predictive performance of the KIT-IgA score in both screening for non-invasive diagnosis of IgAN, and for predicting risk of progressive renal disease from IgA and utilizing the KIT score for potentially evaluating the efficacy of IgAN-targeted therapies.

Keywords: IgA nephropathy; KIT assay; KIT-IgA score; noninvasive; diagnostics; prediction

---

1. Introduction

IgA nephropathy (IgAN) remains the most common type of primary chronic glomerulonephritis worldwide [1]. Its prevalence varies among different groups of people, where IgAN makes up about 20–40% of primary glomerular disease in Asia, and about 15–20% in Northern Europe [2]. The onset of

IgAN may occur at any age, but the condition most frequently develops in patients in their second and third decades of life [3]. Many patients who present with mild symptoms will not require treatment, though they will be monitored for disease progression, but up to 40% of patients with IgAN will eventually develop end-stage renal disease [1]. Trials have established the benefit of agents that antagonize the renin-angiotensin-aldosterone system (RAAS) in reducing or delaying progression, but even patients treated with RAAS blockade still face deterioration of their kidney function over time [4]. One major issue in the treatment of IgAN is that there are few biomarkers that can predict progression of disease and monitor the efficacy of treatment [5].

Currently, IgAN is diagnosed by renal biopsy which is often performed to confirm causes of mild urinary abnormalities, particularly hematuria; however, biopsies are invasive procedures [6] that carry the risk for complications such as bleeding, and the majority of cases of microscopic hematuria are not associated with any kidney pathology. Recent advances in the analysis of the urinary proteome suggest that the excreted polypeptides include disease-specific patterns [7] and as such, much of the current research has investigated urinary biomarkers of IgA-associated glomerulonephritides. Biomarkers such as urinary neutrophil gelatinase-associated lipocalin or cystatin C [8] and protein/polypeptide patterns [9] have been studied in IgAN; however, their discriminative abilities appear modest and many studies exclude patients undergoing treatment, thus limiting any determination of the monitoring utility of such biomarkers. As a result, there exists a need for a reliable and non-invasive method to diagnose and monitor IgAN, especially in the context of treatment.

Recently, the Kidney Injury Test (KIT) Assay was developed by our group as a noninvasive test to measure kidney injury and function in the context of chronic kidney disease [10], nephrolithiasis [11], and transplant rejection [12]. The KIT Assay measures a panel of urinary biomarkers in a microwell-based format that were identified through a combination of proteomics, genomics, and metabolomics approaches [13–15] to be the most sensitive indicators of various etiologies of kidney injury and functional changes. In this investigator-initiated, multicenter, prospective study, we investigated the utility of the KIT Assay, a urine-based, microwell format assay for the detection of patients with IgAN who were treated with standard of care or with Rituximab. We additionally investigated the utility of the KIT-IgA score to predict progression of renal functional decline longitudinally on a subset of these patients who had longitudinally collected samples.

2. Results

2.1. *Study Design and Patient Disposition*

Sixty-nine spot urine samples were collected from 34 enrolled patients in the IgAN clinical trial over the study follow-up of 1 year (Figure 1). Patients were randomized at study entry 1:1, to receive either standard of care (corticosteroids) or Rituximab. Patients had biopsy-confirmed IgAN at study entry and serial urine samples were collected at study entry, 6 and 12 months. Two or more samples were available from 25 patients, and a complete set of three time-points were available from 14 patients. The baseline characteristics and disposition of the 34 patients are listed in Table 1.

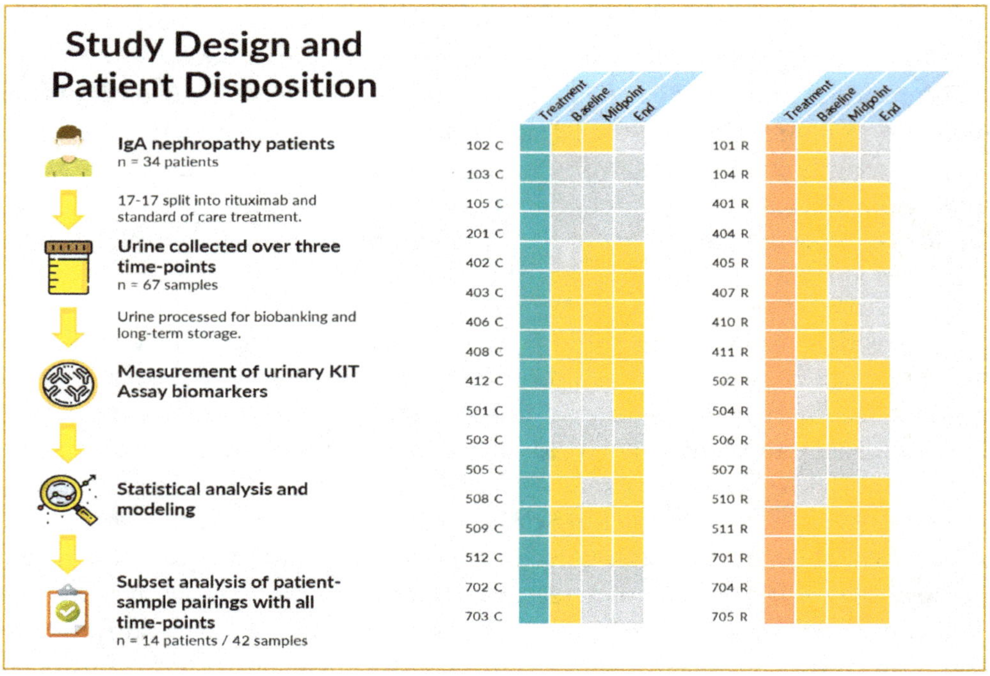

Figure 1. Study design and patient disposition. (Left) In the original trial, 34 patients met inclusion criteria and were randomized into Rituximab and standard of care treatment groups. At least one urine sample was available from 28 of the 34 patients, with 14 having urine samples at all three designated time-points. (Right) Pictorial depiction of patients, treatment, and sample availability. Patients were segregated based on treatment, either with standard of care (turquoise) or Rituximab (coral), with individual patients as rows. A yellow square indicates a urine sample was available at the indicated time-point, while gray indicates that no urine sample was available for analysis due to failure to collect or insufficient sample volume.

Table 1. Baseline characteristics of IgA nephropathy (IgAN) patients.

Baseline Characteristics	IgA Cohort (n = 34) [1]
Age, years	40 (21–63)
Sex	
• Female	9
• Male	25
Race	
• Caucasian	24
• Asian/Pacific Islander	6
• Hispanic/Latino	3
• African American	1
Weight, kg	89.7 (57–120)
eGFR, mL/min per 1.73 m^2	49 (30–122)
Treatment	
• Rituximab	17
• Standard of Care	17

[1] Data are reported as median (range) or count. n indicates the number of patients in the cohort.

As concluded by the original study, and as shown in Figure 2, there was no statistically significant difference between the change in eGFR over the course of the study by treatment with Rituximab (coral) over standard of care (teal). However, while some patients maintained or even recovered kidney function as seen in an increase in eGFR, some patients had IgAN progression with functional decline. This finding motivated us to investigate whether the KIT Assay biomarkers could be used to not only detect IgA nephropathy through urine alone, but also predict and monitor kidney function changes longitudinally.

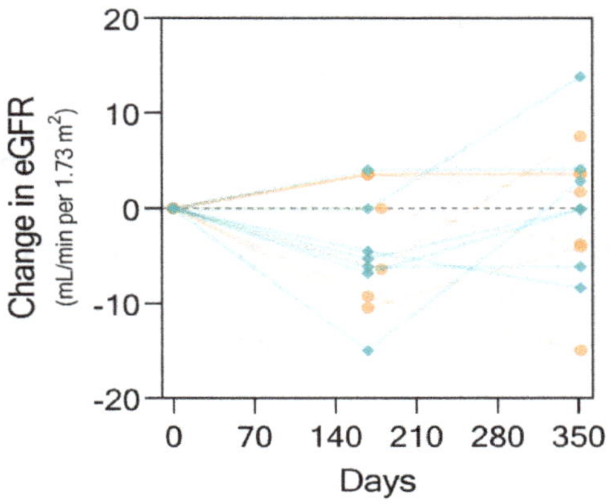

Figure 2. Changes in eGFR (by Modification of Diet in Renal Disease (MDRD) [16]) from baseline. Data shown here for the change in eGFR values over the time-course of the study for a subset of 14 patients who had complete urine samples collected at all three study time-points. Each line represents an individual patient trajectory. Trajectories in teal represent patients who received standard of care while those in salmon represent those who received Rituximab.

2.2. The KIT Assay Biomarkers Can Discriminate Healthy Controls from Patients with IgA Nephropathy

Urine samples from 64 healthy control patients were assessed and compared to those collected from the IgA nephropathy patients for the KIT biomarkers. A KIT-IgA risk score, ranging from 0 to 100, was developed on these biomarkers using a Bootstrap Forest ensemble model. The KIT-IgA scores for each of the patients in the two groups are depicted in Figure 3A. The KIT-IgA score could distinguish between healthy controls (median 14.03, 95% CI 8.94–18.52) and IgA patients (median 87.76, 95% CI 83.39–90.32) ($p < 0.0001$). Receiver–operator characteristic curves (Figure 3B) comparing the discrimination abilities of the IgA risk score and proteinuria identifies the IgA risk score (AUC 0.9935, 95% CI 0.985–1.000) as performing better than proteinuria (AUC 0.9100, 95% CI 0.855–0.965), suggesting that the KIT-IgA risk score is more sensitive and may detect IgAN earlier than proteinuria. For the KIT-IgA risk score, the sensitivity and specificity were 95.5% and 98.4% respectively.

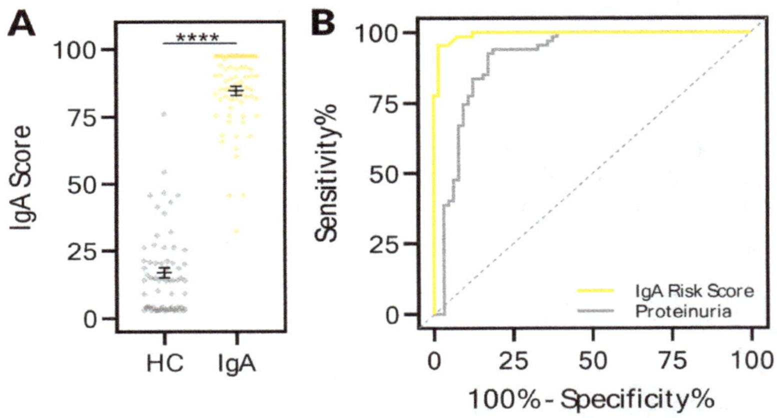

Figure 3. The urinary KIT biomarkers could segregate healthy controls from those with IgA nephropathy. (**A**) An IgA risk score ranging from 0 to 100 segregated healthy control patients from those with IgA nephropathy. Urine samples were collected from healthy controls ($n = 64$) who had no evidence of kidney disease or injury as assessed by both absence of proteinuria and eGFR greater than 120. All urine samples from IgA patients ($n = 67$) were used, as none of these patients had remission of IgA during the treatment duration. (**B**) Receiver–operator characteristic (ROC) curves of the IgA risk score with AUC of 0.994 ($p < 0.0001$) and proteinuria. For the IgA risk score, the sensitivity and specificity were 95.5% and 98.4% respectively. **** $p < 0.0001$.

2.3. The KIT Assay Biomarkers Can Discriminate Progressors from Non-Progressors and Predict Progression

We further investigated whether the KIT Assay biomarkers and the KIT-IgA score could distinguish progressors versus non-progressors. Progression was assessed based on a composite clinical evaluation of changes in proteinuria and eGFR from baseline (>50% increase in proteinuria and/or a 25% reduction in eGFR) and, as such, was dependent on both urine and serum biomarker values. We first sought to investigate whether urinary biomarkers alone could be used to classify progressor status. Looking at the 1-year endpoint biomarkers (Figure 4A), progressor status could be classified using nominal logistic regression with 100% accuracy based on urinary measurements alone ($p = 0.0154$). We then investigated whether midpoint (0.5 year prior to progression determination) and baseline (1 year prior) urinary biomarkers could predict progression status. We found that the KIT-IgA score could predict progressor status with 100% accuracy at both time-points (midpoint $p = 0.0269$, baseline $p = 0.0383$). For both the baseline and midpoint predictions, the cfDNA values were the most important predictors, with chi square likelihood ratios of 25.92 and 141.98, respectively, and with $p < 0.0001$ for both. However, neither baseline nor midpoint proteinuria alone could predict progression (Figure 4B). As the progressor definition was based on a composite of proteinuria and eGFR changes, there was no expectation that endpoint proteinuria alone could predict progressor status, as reflected in the probabilities. We further assessed the ability of the baseline urinary biomarkers to predict progression status on the entire set of patients who had baseline urine samples, regardless of the presence of additional longitudinal samples. For these 23 urine-patient pairs, the results were similar to the original analysis in that the KIT biomarkers could segregate progressors from non-progressors with 100% accuracy ($p < 0.0001$) (ROC AUC = 1.00).

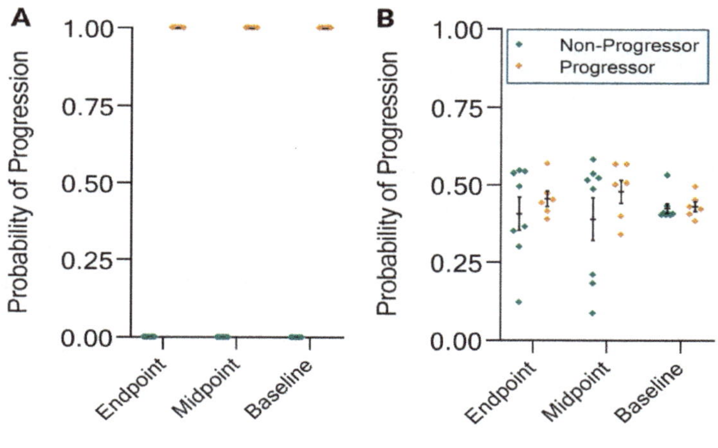

Figure 4. KIT Assay biomarker modeling of progression status after one year of treatment. Modeling was performed on endpoint, midpoint, and baseline biomarker data on either (**A**) the set of KIT Assay biomarkers or (**B**) proteinuria alone. The y-axis shows the probability of progression as determined by a nominal logistic regression model.

3. Materials and Methods

3.1. Patients and Study Characteristics

Samples were those from a study done in 2017 (NCT00498368) and the study was registered with clinicaltrials.gov [17]. Patient inclusion and exclusion criteria were as described in the previous study. Subjects included adults, ages 18–70 years old, with biopsy-proven IgAN within 2 years of enrollment were included. Patients were excluded if their biopsy showed >50% glomerular sclerosis or interstitial fibrosis or >10% glomerular crescents. Subjects were then randomly assigned to receive Rituximab or continue standard care. Baseline Oxford classification score [18] was recorded in blinded fashion by an expert renal pathologist. eGFR (by Modification of Diet in Renal Disease (MDRD) [16]) or measured creatinine clearance had to be <90 and >30 mL/min per 1.73 m^2. To establish continued risk, baseline proteinuria needed to be >1000 mg/day while on stable doses of angiotensin-converting enzyme inhibitor, angiotensin receptor blocker, or renin inhibitor therapy for at least 2 months. However, patients who were on dual therapy with agents that inhibit angiotensin II required a lower proteinuria threshold of >500 mg/day. Baseline BP was controlled to <130/80 mmHg. Patients with secondary forms of IgAN, such as cirrhosis, were excluded, although subjects with Henoch–Schönlein purpura nephritis (HSPN) could be included. Patients were excluded if they had previously received Rituximab, were receiving other immunosuppressive therapy, or had ever received >6 months of prednisone or other systemic corticosteroid therapy in the past. There was no corticosteroid exposure within 3 months of study initiation. Randomization was done centrally by a random assignment by prefilled envelopes. The protocol was approved by the institutional review board of each participating center. The study was registered with clinicaltrials.gov, protocol NCT00498368. Informed consent was obtained before all study procedures, and the study adhered to the Declaration of Helsinki.

The primary outcome measures were the change in proteinuria and the change in eGFR from baseline to 12 months. The secondary outcome was safety related, comparing overall adverse events and monitoring for potential intervention-specific complications, such as infusion-related reactions, hypogammaglobulinemia, and infections. Progression was defined as a >50% increase in proteinuria and/or a 25% reduction in eGFR at the one-year time-point. Results showed that treatment with Rituximab resulted in statistically insignificant changes in proteinuria or partial remissions that could not be distinguished from the response to supportive therapy alone.

For the healthy control cohort, urine samples were collected from healthy controls (n = 64) who had no evidence of kidney disease or injury as assessed by both absence of proteinuria and eGFR greater than 120. Demographics of this cohort include a median age of 24 (range 2 to 64), median weight of 57.5 kg (range 13.7 to 120.2), 53.1% female, 9.4% African American, and median eGFR of 132 (range 120 to 213).

3.2. Urine Sample Processing

Voided urine samples were collected in sterile containers. Urine samples were centrifuged at 2000× g for 30 min at 4 °C. The supernatant was separated from the urine pellet containing cells and cell debris. The pH of the supernatant was adjusted to 7.0 using Tris-HCl and stored at −80 °C in the UCSF Biorepository until further analysis.

3.3. KIT Assay Biomarkers

Measurement of the KIT Assay biomarkers was performed as previously described [10]. Total protein was measured using the Pierce™ Coomassie Plus Assay Kit (Thermo Fisher Scientific, Waltham, MA, USA). Urinary creatinine was measured using the Creatinine Assay Kit (BioAssay Systems, Hayward, CA, USA) as a method for urinary concentration and hydration status normalization. Briefly, cell-free DNA (cfDNA), methylated cell-free DNA (m-cfDNA), CXCL10, Clusterin, (Dimethylamino)iminomethyl-ornithine (DMAIMO), and (Methylamino)(methylimino)methyl-ornithine (MAMIMO), were measured using the KIT Assay (KIT Bio, San Francisco, CA, USA), a set of in-house developed ELISA assays. Microwell plate readings were measured using a SpectraMax iD3 Multi-Mode Microplate Reader (Molecular Devices, San Jose, CA, USA). All assays were run in duplicates.

3.4. Statistical Analysis

Comparisons involving two groups were performed using the nonparametric Mann–Whitney U test. Comparisons involving three groups were performed using the nonparametric Kruskal–Wallis test with Dunn's post-hoc multiple comparisons correction. The IgA risk score was determined using a Bootstrap Forest ensemble model by averaging numerous decision trees each fit to a bootstrap sample of the training data. The final prediction is the average of the predicted values over all the decision trees. Specifically, six trees were used in the forest, with a minimum of ten splits per tree and a minimum size split of five. The number of splits for trees 1–6 were 9, 17, 15, 7, 13, and 11 respectively. The top contributing biomarkers as based on G^2 were total protein, MAMIMO, creatinine, and DMAIMO, with G^2 values of 36.02, 21.12, 9.72, and 6.74 respectively. The overall statistics for the Entropy R^2 was 0.7422, Generalized R^2 was 0.8568, and Root Mean Square Error (RMSE) was 0.1996.

Modeling of progressor status was done using nominal logistic regression. All analyses were performed using either GraphPad Prism 8.0.2 (GraphPad Software, Carlsbad, CA, USA) or JMP 14.3 (SAS Institute, Cary, NC, USA).

4. Discussion

In this study, we used urine samples from IgA nephropathy (IgAN) patients to evaluate the predictive capacity of the KIT Assay biomarkers to discriminate IgAN from healthy controls as well as predict progression of renal functional decline. Our results show that these urinary biomarkers could distinguish between healthy control patients and those with IgAN better than urinary protein alone. Furthermore, the biomarkers could predict progressor status up to one year in advance of status determination while urinary protein could not.

Such findings are important because IgAN is the most prevalent chronic glomerular disease worldwide [19], with diagnosis historically requiring kidney biopsy. While recent studies have identified serum and urinary biomarkers that can diagnose IgAN with high accuracy [7,8,20], the clinical utility of individual biomarkers is limited by the high overlap between the healthy and diseased ranges of these biomarkers in an individual and temporal manner. Such biomarkers, while indicative of IgAN, have shown less utility in predicting progression of disease. While some studies have suggested the use of GC–MS and similar technologies to identify a panel of biomarkers, these proteomic studies are not easily transferrable to the clinical setting. Identifying biomarkers that not only can identify IgAN but can also predict progression is important for the future development and evaluation of therapies that seek to treat and prevent functional decline in IgAN.

The multi-hit hypothesis for the pathogenesis of IgA nephropathy is the leading theory behind the mechanism of progression [20]. In this hypothesis, deposition of IgA1-containing circulating immune complexes in the glomeruli induce renal injury by subsequent induction of local cytokine, growth factor, and complement system production and activation [21–24]. While currently approved therapies for IgAN are largely non-IgAN specific and consist of supportive therapy with corticosteroids and blood pressure control [25], future directed therapies targeting the specific "hits" in IgAN will address these acute causes of glomerular injury. Monitoring the efficacy of such therapies will require biomarkers that not only reflect kidney function, but also convey the acute status of kidney injury and resolution of that injury.

We had previously validated the utility of the biomarkers comprising the KIT Assay in chronic kidney disease [10], chronic lung transplant rejection [26,27], nephrolithiasis [11], and kidney transplant rejection [12,28], suggesting its utility across a range of diseases and chronicity states. The KIT Assay biomarkers are measured in a microwell format, contributing to their ease of use and deployment. Additionally, urine is a completely noninvasive biofluid that is available in virtually unlimited quantities, enabling a frequency of monitoring that can be adjusted to the functional status of the patient. Due to the acute and chronic injury mechanism present in IgAN [29], we investigated whether the KIT Assay biomarkers could also be applied to detection of IgAN as well as prediction of progression status.

We have discussed the rationale of the KIT Assay biomarkers previously [10], with selection of these biomarkers due to the various temporal and regional differences in levels as dependent upon renal injury and function. While proteinuria has been shown to be a predictor of outcome in IgAN [30] and is a commonly used endpoint, proteinuria did not perform as well as the composite IgA risk score in discriminating patients with IgAN from healthy controls, likely because many patients with IgAN present with low levels of proteinuria despite disease progression [31]. That the KIT-IgA risk score could identify IgAN more accurately is likely due to the composite integration of functional, injury, and renal-specific markers that may reflect IgAN across a spectrum of disease states.

Further, proteinuria alone was not a significant predictor for progression at one-year of treatment duration measured at either the baseline or midpoint time-points. It is notable that the cfDNA values at baseline and midpoint were the strongest predictors of progression at the one-year timepoint. Urinary cfDNA has been previously reported to be a sensitive indicator of kidney injury and reflects ongoing damage to the kidney prior to functional changes or decline [15,32,33]. This finding is in concordance with these reports, suggesting that while progression may be defined by functional measures such as eGFR and proteinuria, the underlying cause of such progression may be acute injury such as that measured by cfDNA burden. As such, measurement of cfDNA, as done in the KIT Assay, may be beneficial for measuring the efficacy of treatment in IgAN.

In summary, our data indicate that the non-invasive KIT Assay panel of urinary biomarkers can distinguish between healthy controls and patients with IgAN. Furthermore, this panel could monitor progression of disease and changes in kidney function. We believe that the KIT-IgA score would have great utility in (1) screening for IgAN in patients with hematuria, as a replacement for biopsy as done in many Asian countries; (2) diagnosis; (3) monitoring efficacy of treatment; and (4) predicting progression and monitoring disease activity. While our sample size is limited by the small size of the parent study, these results add to a growing body of evidence of the generalizability and utility of the KIT Assay biomarkers in renal disease and beyond. Additionally, while all comparisons in this study were between healthy control and IgAN patients, we have planned additional studies where we will include samples from patients with other types of renal diseases so that we can assess the performance of these and other biomarkers in discriminating IgAN from other nephropathies. Future studies using additional kidney disease cohorts will clarify whether there is a specific pattern among these biomarkers to discriminate one disease from another. Future multi-center, prospective studies are planned to further build on the clinical utility of these observations to assess serial performance of the KIT assay in IgAN patients as a non-invasive tool to monitor disease progression and evaluate the efficacy of new reno-protective therapies for IgA disease.

Author Contributions: M.M.S. and R.A.L. designed the study and experiments; J.Y.C.Y. and R.D.S. carried out experiments; J.Y.C.Y., M.M.S., and R.A.L. analyzed the data; J.Y.C.Y. made the figures; J.Y.C.Y., R.D.S., F.C.F., M.M.S., and R.A.L. drafted and revised the paper; all authors revised the manuscript critically for important intellectual content and approved the final version of the manuscript. R.A.L. had full access to all the data in the study and takes responsibility for the integrity of the data and the accuracy of the data analysis.

Acknowledgments: We are grateful for the help from physicians, clinical coordinators, research personnel, patients, and patient families.

Abbreviations

AUC	area-under-curve
BMI	body mass index
cfDNA	cell-free deoxyribonucleic acid
DMAIMO	(dimethylamino)iminomethyl-ornithine
eGFR	estimated glomerular filtration rate
GC–MS	gas chromatography–mass spectrometry
HSPN	Henoch–Schönlein purpura nephritis
IgAN	immunoglobulin alpha nephropathy
KIT	Kidney Injury Test
m-cfDNA	methylated cfDNA
MAMIMO	(methylamino)(methylimino)methyl-ornithine
MDRD	Modification of Diet in Renal Disease
RAAS	renin–angiotensin–aldosterone system
ROC	Receiver-operator characteristic

References

1. Wyatt, R.J.; Julian, B.A. IgA Nephropathy. *N. Engl. J. Med.* **2013**, *368*, 2402–2414. [CrossRef]
2. D'Amico, G. Clinical features and natural history in adults with IgA nephropathy. *Am. J. Kidney Dis.* **1988**, *12*, 353–357. [CrossRef]
3. Yap, H.K.; Quek, C.M.; Shen, Q.; Joshi, V.; Chia, K.S. Role of urinary screening programmes in children in the prevention of chronic kidney disease. *Ann. Acad. Med. Singap.* **2005**, *34*, 3–7. [PubMed]
4. Boyd, J.K.; Cheung, C.K.; Molyneux, K.; Feehally, J.; Barratt, J. An update on the pathogenesis and treatment of IgA nephropathy. *Kidney Int.* **2012**, *81*, 833–843. [CrossRef] [PubMed]
5. Maixnerova, D.; Reily, C.; Bian, Q.; Neprasova, M.; Novak, J.; Tesar, V. Markers for the progression of IgA nephropathy. *J. Nephrol.* **2016**, *29*, 535–541. [CrossRef]
6. Donadio, J.V.; Joseph, P. Grande IgA Nephropathy. *N. Engl. J. Med.* **2002**, *347*, 738–748. [CrossRef] [PubMed]
7. Julian, B.A.; Wittke, S.; Haubitz, M.; Zürbig, P.; Schiffer, E.; McGuire, B.M.; Wyatt, R.J.; Novak, J. Urinary biomarkers of IgA nephropathy and other IgA-associated renal diseases. *World J. Urol.* **2007**, *25*, 467–476. [CrossRef] [PubMed]
8. Ding, H.; He, Y.; Li, K.; Yang, J.; Li, X.; Lu, R.; Gao, W. Urinary neutrophil gelatinase-associated lipocalin (NGAL) is an early biomarker for renal tubulointerstitial injury in IgA nephropathy. *Clin. Immunol.* **2007**, *123*, 227–234. [CrossRef] [PubMed]
9. Haubitz, M.; Wittke, S.; Weissinger, E.M.; Walden, M.; Rupprecht, H.D.; Floege, J.; Haller, H.; Mischak, H. Urine protein patterns can serve as diagnostic tools in patients with IgA nephropathy. *Kidney Int.* **2005**, *67*, 2313–2320. [CrossRef]
10. Watson, D.; Yang, J.Y.C.; Sarwal, R.D.; Sigdel, T.K.; Liberto, J.M.; Damm, I.; Louie, V.; Sigdel, S.; Livingstone, D.; Soh, K.; et al. A Novel Multi-Biomarker Assay for Non-Invasive Detection and Quantitative Monitoring of Kidney Injury. *J. Clin. Med.* **2019**, *8*, 499. [CrossRef]
11. Yang, J.Y.C.; Sarwal, R.D.; Ky, K.; Dong, V.; Stoller, M.; Watson, D.; Sarwal, M.M.; Chi, T. Non-Radiologic Assessment of Kidney Stones by KIT, a Spot Urine Assay. *Br. J. of Urol. Int.* **2019**. under review.
12. Yang, J.Y.C.; Sarwal, R.D.; Sigdel, T.K.; Sarwal, M.M. Predicting Transplant Rejection by a Composite Urinary Injury Score. *Am. J. Transpl.* **2019**, *17*, 519.
13. Sigdel, T.K.; Gao, Y.; He, J.; Wang, A.; Nicora, C.D.; Fillmore, T.L.; Shi, T.; Webb-Robertson, B.-J.; Smith, R.D.; Qian, W.-J.; et al. Mining the human urine proteome for monitoring renal transplant injury. *Kidney Int.* **2016**, *89*, 1244–1252. [CrossRef] [PubMed]
14. Yang, J.Y.C.; Sigdel, T.K.; Sarwal, M.M. Self-antigens and rejection: A proteomic analysis. *Curr. Opin. Organ Transpl.* **2016**, *21*, 362–367. [CrossRef] [PubMed]
15. Yang, J.Y.C.; Sarwal, M.M. Transplant genetics and genomics. *Nat. Rev. Genet.* **2017**, *18*, 309–326. [CrossRef] [PubMed]
16. Levey, A.S.; Bosch, J.P.; Lewis, J.B.; Greene, T.; Rogers, N.; Roth, D. A more accurate method to estimate glomerular filtration rate from serum creatinine: A new prediction equation. Modification of Diet in Renal Disease Study Group. *Ann. Intern. Med.* **1999**, *130*, 461–470. [CrossRef]
17. Lafayette, R.A.; Canetta, P.A.; Rovin, B.H.; Appel, G.B.; Novak, J.; Nath, K.A.; Sethi, S.; Tumlin, J.A.; Mehta, K.; Hogan, M.; et al. A Randomized, Controlled Trial of Rituximab in IgA Nephropathy with Proteinuria and Renal Dysfunction. *J. Am. Soc. Nephrol.* **2017**, *28*, 1306–1313. [CrossRef]
18. Cattran, D.C.; Coppo, R.; Cook, H.T.; Feehally, J.; Roberts, I.S.D.; Troyanov, S.; Alpers, C.E.; Amore, A.; Barratt, J.; Berthoux, F.; et al. The Oxford classification of IgA nephropathy: Rationale, clinicopathological correlations, and classification. *Kidney Int.* **2009**, *76*, 534–545. [CrossRef]
19. Schena, F.P.; Nistor, I. Epidemiology of IgA Nephropathy: A Global Perspective. *Semin. Nephrol.* **2018**, *38*, 435–442. [CrossRef]
20. Suzuki, H. Biomarkers for IgA nephropathy on the basis of multi-hit pathogenesis. *Clin. Exp. Nephrol.* **2019**, *23*, 26–31. [CrossRef]
21. Lai, K.N. Pathogenesis of IgA nephropathy. *Nat. Rev. Nephrol.* **2012**, *8*, 275–283. [CrossRef] [PubMed]
22. Sigdel, T.K.; Woo, S.H.; Dai, H.; Khatri, P.; Li, L.; Myers, B.; Sarwal, M.M.; Lafayette, R.A. Profiling of Autoantibodies in IgA Nephropathy, an Integrative Antibiomics Approach. *J. Am Soc. Nephrol.* **2011**, *6*, 2775–2784. [CrossRef] [PubMed]
23. Woo, S.H.; Sigdel, T.K.; Dinh, V.T.; Vu, M.T.; Sarwal, M.M.; Lafayette, R.A. Mapping novel immunogenic epitopes in IgA nephropathy. *Clin. J. Am. Soc. Nephrol.* **2015**, *10*, 372–381. [CrossRef] [PubMed]

24. Rizk, D.V.; Saha, M.K.; Hall, S.; Novak, L.; Brown, R.; Huang, Z.-Q.; Fatima, H.; Julian, B.A.; Novak, J. Glomerular Immunodeposits of Patients with IgA Nephropathy Are Enriched for IgG Autoantibodies Specific for Galactose-Deficient IgA1. *J. Am. Soc. Nephrol.* **2019**, *30*, 9. [CrossRef] [PubMed]
25. Floege, J.; Eitner, F. Current Therapy for IgA Nephropathy. *J. Am. Soc. Nephrol.* **2011**, *22*, 1785–1794. [CrossRef] [PubMed]
26. Yang, J.Y.C.; Verleden, S.E.; Zarinsefat, A.; Vanaudenaerde, B.M.; Vos, R.; Verleden, G.M.; Sarwal, R.D.; Sigdel, T.K.; Liberto, J.M.; Damm, I.; et al. Cell-Free DNA and CXCL10 Derived from Bronchoalveolar Lavage Predict Lung Transplant Survival. *J. Clin. Med.* **2019**, *8*, 9. [CrossRef] [PubMed]
27. Sacreas, A.; Yang, J.Y.C.; Vanaudenaerde, B.M.; Sigdel, T.K.; Liberto, J.M.; Damm, I.; Verleden, G.M.; Vos, R.; Verleden, E.; Sarwal, M.M. The common rejection module in chronic rejection post lung transplantation. *PLoS ONE* **2018**, *13*, 1–16. [CrossRef]
28. Sigdel, T.K.; Yang, J.Y.C.; Bestard, O.; Schroeder, A.; Hsieh, S.-C.; Liberto, J.M.; Damm, I.; Geraedts, A.C.M.; Sarwal, M.M. A urinary Common Rejection Module (uCRM) score for non-invasive kidney transplant monitoring. *PLoS ONE* **2019**, *7*, 1–15. [CrossRef] [PubMed]
29. Kusano, T.; Takano, H.; Kang, D.; Nagahama, K.; Aoki, M.; Morita, M.; Kaneko, T.; Tsuruoka, S.; Shimizu, A. Endothelial cell injury in acute and chronic glomerular lesions in patients with IgA nephropathy. *Hum. Pathol.* **2016**, *49*, 135–144. [CrossRef]
30. Reich, H.N.; Troyanov, S.; Scholey, J.W.; Cattran, D.C. Remission of Proteinuria Improves Prognosis in IgA Nephropathy. *J. Am. Soc. Nephrol.* **2007**, *18*, 3177–3183. [CrossRef]
31. Gutiérrez, E. IgA nephropathy: Is a new approach beyond proteinuria necessary? *Pediatr. Nephrol.* **2019**, 921–924. [CrossRef] [PubMed]
32. Burnham, P.; Dadhania, D.; Heyang, M.; Chen, F.; Westblade, L.F.; Suthanthiran, M.; Lee, J.R.; De Vlaminck, I. Urinary cell-free DNA is a versatile analyte for monitoring infections of the urinary tract. *Nat. Commun.* **2018**, *9*, 1–10. [CrossRef] [PubMed]
33. Celec, P.; Vlková, B.; Lauková, L.; Bábíčková, J.; Boor, P. Cell-free DNA: The role in pathophysiology and as a biomarker in kidney diseases. *Expert Rev. Mol. Med.* **2018**, *20*, 1–14. [CrossRef] [PubMed]

7

Xanthine Oxidase Inhibitor Febuxostat Exerts an Anti-Inflammatory Action and Protects against Diabetic Nephropathy Development in KK-Ay Obese Diabetic Mice

Yu Mizuno [1], Takeshi Yamamotoya [1], Yusuke Nakatsu [1], Koji Ueda [1], Yasuka Matsunaga [1,2], Masa-Ki Inoue [1], Hideyuki Sakoda [3], Midori Fujishiro [4], Hiraku Ono [5], Takako Kikuchi [6], Masahiro Takahashi [7], Kenichi Morii [8], Kensuke Sasaki [8], Takao Masaki [8], Tomoichiro Asano [1,*] and Akifumi Kushiyama [7,*]

[1] Department of Medical Science, Graduate School of Medicine, University of Hiroshima, 1-2-3 Kasumi, Minami-ku, Hiroshima City, Hiroshima 734-8551, Japan; d186723@hiroshima-u.ac.jp (Y.M.); ymmty@hiroshima-u.ac.jp (T.Y.); nakatsu@hiroshima-u.ac.jp (Y.N.); urouedakouji@yahoo.co.jp (K.U.); ymatsunaga@tulane.edu (Y.M.); b131831@hiroshima-u.ac.jp (M.-K.I.)

[2] Center for Translational Research in Infection & Inflammation, School of Medicine, Tulane University, 6823 St. Charles Avenue, New Orleans, LA 70118, USA

[3] Division of Neurology, Respirology, Endocrinology, and Metabolism, Department of Internal Medicine, Faculty of Medicine, University of Miyazaki, 5200 Kihara, Kiyotake, Miyazaki 889-1692, Japan; hideyuki_sakoda@med.miyazaki-u.ac.jp

[4] Division of Diabetes and Metabolic Diseases, Nihon University School of Medicine, Itabashi, Tokyo 173-8610, Japan; fujishiro.midori@nihon-u.ac.jp

[5] Department of Clinical Cell Biology, Graduate School of Medicine, Chiba University, 1-8-1 Inohana, Chuo-ku, Chiba City, Chiba 260-8670, Japan; hono@chiba-u.jp

[6] Division of Diabetes and Metabolism, The Institute for Adult Diseases, Asahi Life Foundation, 2-2-6, Nihonbashi Bakurocho, Chuo-ku, Tokyo 103-0002, Japan; kikuchi-tk@umin.ac.jp

[7] Department of Pharmacotherapy, Meiji Pharmaceutical University, 2-522-1 Noshio, Kiyose City, Tokyo 204-8588, Japan; t-masa@my-pharm.ac.jp

[8] Department of Nephrology, Hiroshima University Hospital, 1-2-3 Kasumi, Minami-ku, Hiroshima City, Hiroshima 734-8551, Japan; kenichi_morii@yahoo.co.jp (K.M.); sasakikuma@gmail.com (K.S.); masakit@hiroshima-u.ac.jp (T.M.)

* Correspondence: tasano@hiroshima-u.ac.jp (T.A.); kushiyama@my-pharm.ac.jp (A.K.)

Abstract: Hyperuricemia has been recognized as a risk factor for insulin resistance as well as one of the factors leading to diabetic kidney disease (DKD). Since DKD is the most common cause of end-stage renal disease, we investigated whether febuxostat, a xanthine oxidase (XO) inhibitor, exerts a protective effect against the development of DKD. We used KK-Ay mice, an established obese diabetic rodent model. Eight-week-old KK-Ay mice were provided drinking water with or without febuxostat (15 μg/mL) for 12 weeks and then subjected to experimentation. Urine albumin secretion and degrees of glomerular injury judged by microscopic observations were markedly higher in KK-Ay than in control lean mice. These elevations were significantly normalized by febuxostat treatment. On the other hand, body weights and high serum glucose concentrations and glycated albumin levels of KK-Ay mice were not affected by febuxostat treatment, despite glucose tolerance and insulin tolerance tests having revealed febuxostat significantly improved insulin sensitivity and glucose tolerance. Interestingly, the IL-1β, IL-6, MCP-1, and ICAM-1 mRNA levels, which were increased in KK-Ay mouse kidneys as compared with normal controls, were suppressed by febuxostat administration. These data indicate a protective effect of XO inhibitors against the development of DKD, and the underlying mechanism likely involves inflammation suppression which is independent of hyperglycemia amelioration.

Keywords: diabetic kidney diseases; xanthine oxidase; glomerular damage

1. Introduction

Diabetic kidney disease (DKD) is currently a leading cause of end-stage renal failure [1], while treatments with renin–angiotensin–aldosterone system blockers with normalization of hyperglycemia are regarded as the gold standard [2,3]. In addition, several studies have shown hyperuricemia to be an independent factor impacting insulin resistance and also to play a significant role in the development of diabetic nephropathy [4,5]. In patients with type 1 diabetic nephropathy, usually not accompanied by insulin resistance, hyperuricemia is also shown to be an independent risk of renal dysfunction [6].

Uric acid is generated from hypoxanthine and xanthine by xanthine oxidase (XO) as the final step in the metabolism of endogenous and exogenous purines [7]. Clinical trials have proven the efficacy of XO inhibitors, including allopurinol and febuxostat, not only for lowering the serum uric acid concentration but also for protection against the progression of renal diseases [8,9]. Even for diabetic nephropathy, XO inhibition has been shown to be effective in several clinical trials [10–12]. However, whether reducing the serum uric acid level or suppression of XO activity contributes to the protective effect of XO inhibitors on renal diseases remains unclear. Therefore, elucidation of the effects and mechanisms of action of XO inhibitors is eagerly awaited.

A previous study using an insulin-deficient Type 1 diabetic model rat and XO inhibitors, including allopurinol and febuxostat, suggested the renal protective effect of febuxostat to be mediated via attenuation of oxidative and inflammatory effects [13,14]. On the other hand, a study using obese diabetic db/db mice treated with allopurinol also showed the renal protective effect of XO inhibitors to involve lowering uric acid directly [13,15]. Therefore, to date, only a few studies have focused on the mechanism, particularly that against diabetic nephropathy, underlying XO inhibitor-mediated renal protective effects.

In this study, we employed KK-Ay mice that spontaneously exhibit type 2 diabetes associated with hyperglycemia, glucose intolerance, hyperinsulinemia, obesity, and microalbuminuria [16], and investigated the effects of febuxostat on the development of diabetic nephropathy in these mice. Our observations raise the possibility that the renal protective effects of the XO inhibitor febuxostat are mediated mainly by an anti-inflammatory effect, which is independent of the effects on glycemic control.

2. Results

2.1. *Effects of XO Inhibitor Febuxostat on Glycemic Control and Serum Uric Acid Levels*

Diabetic KK-Ay mice were divided into two groups, with and without febuxostat in drinking water. After 12 weeks of treatment, while KK-Ay mice had higher body weights, blood glucose concentrations in the fed state, serum glycated albumin, and serum uric acid levels than the wild-type mice (Figure 1A–D), febuxostat treatment reduced the serum uric acid level of KK-Ay mice without significantly affecting other parameters. However, unexpectedly, glucose tolerance and insulin tolerance tests revealed treatment with febuxostat significantly ameliorated the impairments in KK-Ay mice (Figure 1E,F).

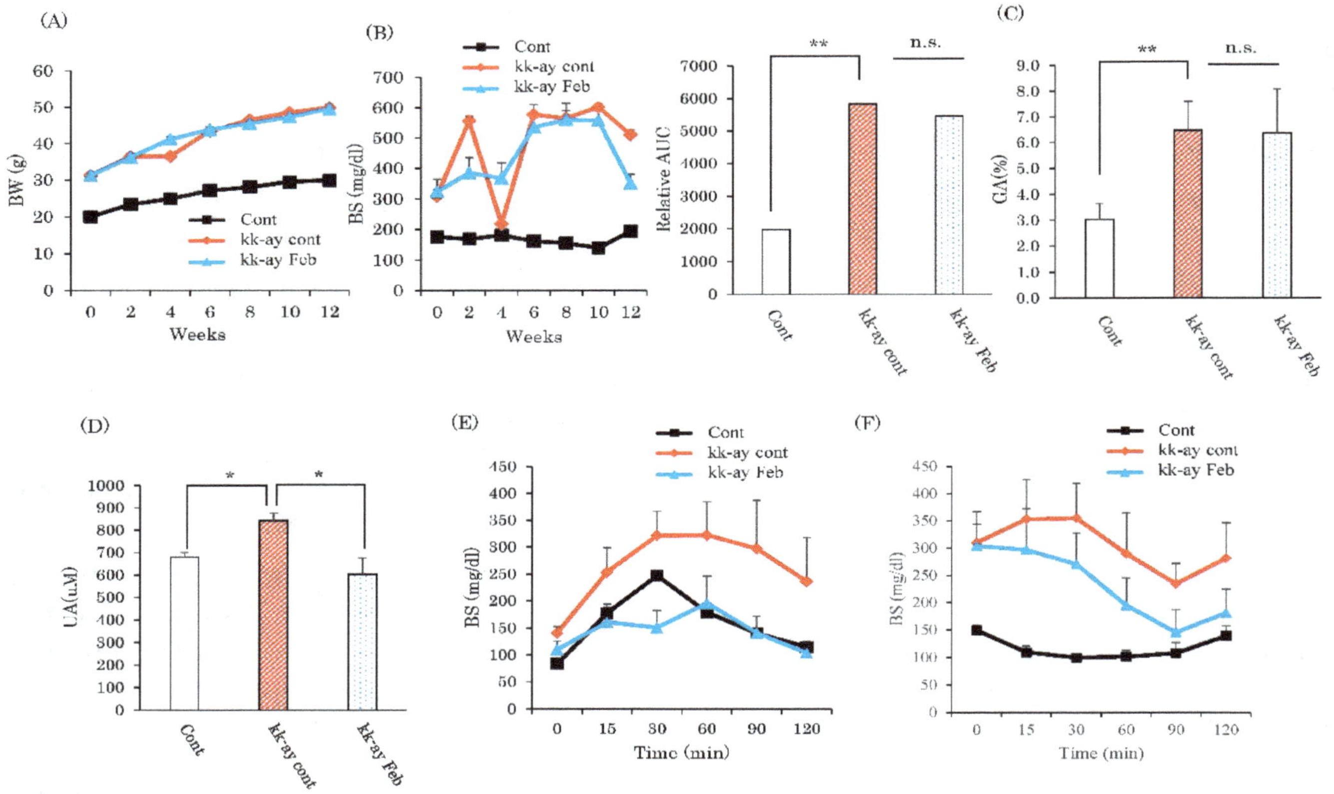

Figure 1. Inhibitory effects of xanthine oxidase inhibitor febuxostat on the progression of diabetic nephropathy. (**A**) Body weights and (**B**) blood sugar levels were measured. (**C**) Serum glycated albumin levels. (**D**) Serum uric acid levels. (**E**) Glucose tolerance test results. (**F**) Insulin tolerance test. Data are means ± SE. * $p < 0.05$, ** $p < 0.001$, n = 8 for control group, n = 10 for KK-Ay mice without febuxostat group and n = 8 for KK-Ay mice with febuxostat group.

2.2. *Effects of Febuxostat Administration on Glomerular Sclerosis*

Glomerular sclerosis is among the features of diabetic nephropathy. The degrees of glomerular sclerosis were estimated based on the findings of Hematoxylin–Eosin (HE) staining and positive peroxide acid-Schiff (PAS) staining (Figure 2A,B). PAS staining is reportedly useful for definitively demonstrating glomerular hypertrophy, an early feature of diabetic nephropathy [17]. Both HE and PAS staining showed glomerular sclerosis to be markedly advanced in KK-Ay mice as compared with wild-type mice, and that this progression showed significant attenuation in response to febuxostat treatment in KK-Ay mice (Figure 2B). Glomerular injury score (GIS) and glomerular areas calculated based on PAS-stained areas were markedly increased in KK-Ay mice than in wild-type controls, and these changes were partially but significantly normalized in febuxostat-treated KK-Ay mice (Figure 2C). While febuxostat treatment did not normalize the increased kidney weights of KK-Ay mice as compared with those of wild-type mice (Figure 2D), an approximately 10-fold increase in the urinary albumin-to-creatinine ratio (ACR) in KK-Ay mice was markedly ameliorated, to a level near that of control C57BL/6 mice, by febuxostat treatment (Figure 2E).

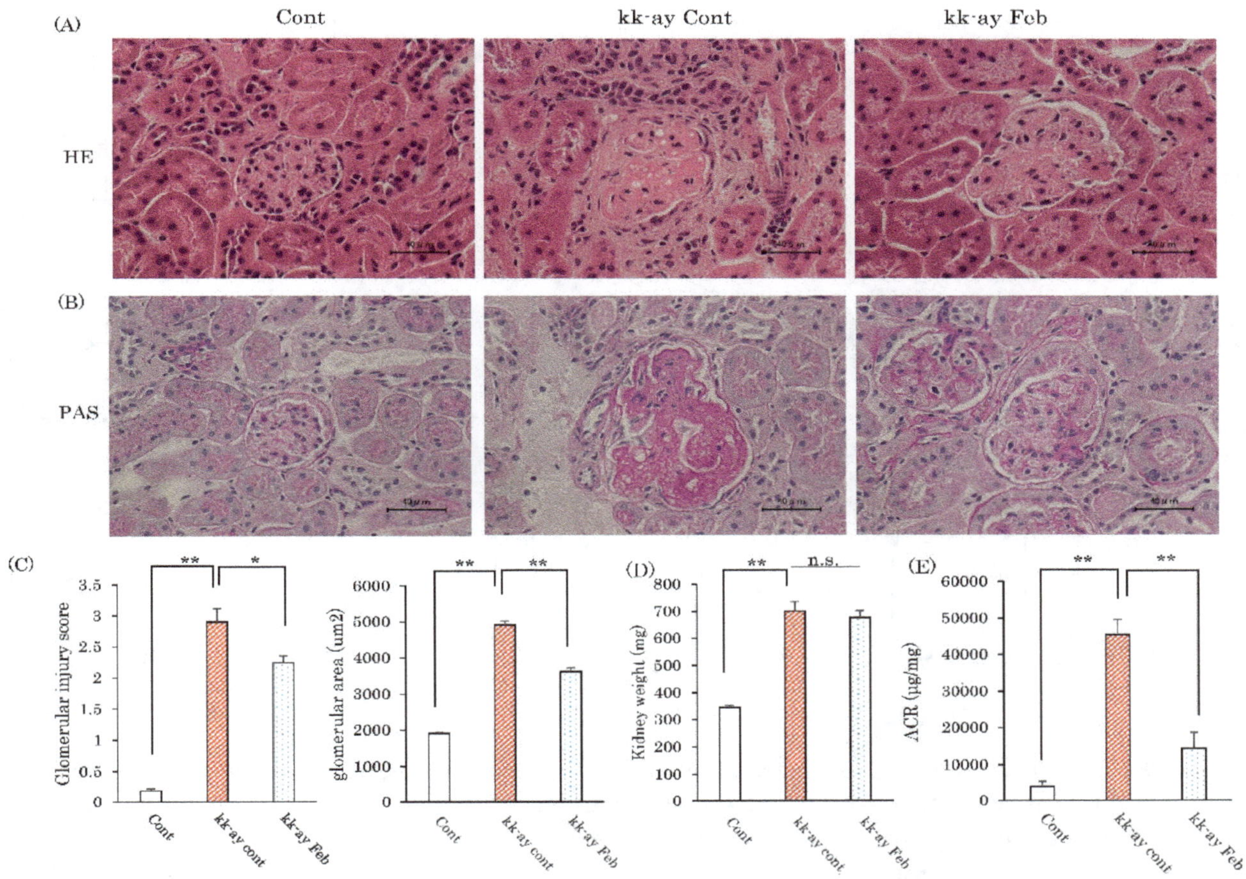

Figure 2. Febuxostat administered for prevention of glomerular sclerosis. (**A**) Hematoxylin–Eosin (HE) staining of kidney fractions. Scale bar = 40 μm. (**B**) Peroxide acid-Schiff (PAS) staining of kidney fractions. Scale bar = 40 μm. (**C**) Glomerular sclerosis score and glomerular area were calculated using image J. (**D**) Kidney weights and (**E**) the urinary albumin to creatinine ratio was measured at 20 weeks. Data are means ± SE. * $p < 0.05$, ** $p < 0.001$. n = 8 for control group, n = 10 for KK-Ay mice without febuxostat group and n = 8 for KK-Ay mice with febuxostat group.

2.3. Effects of Febuxostat on the Renal Expression Levels of Inflammatory Cytokines

Since elevated inflammation-related cytokine and chemokine expressions are reportedly involved in the pathogenesis in diabetic nephropathy, the effects of febuxostat on their mRNA levels were evaluated. In comparison with the normal mice, renal mRNA levels of IL-1β, IL-6, MCP-1, CXCL1, CXCL2, and CXCL5, but not those of the macrophage marker F4/80 and TNFα, were markedly elevated in the KK-Ay mice (Figure 3). Treatment with febuxostat essentially normalized the upregulated expressions of inflammatory cytokines (IL-1β, IL-6) without significantly affecting, though a tendency for reduction was observed, inflammatory chemokines (CKCL1, CXCL2, CXCL5) in KK-Ay mouse kidneys (Figure 3).

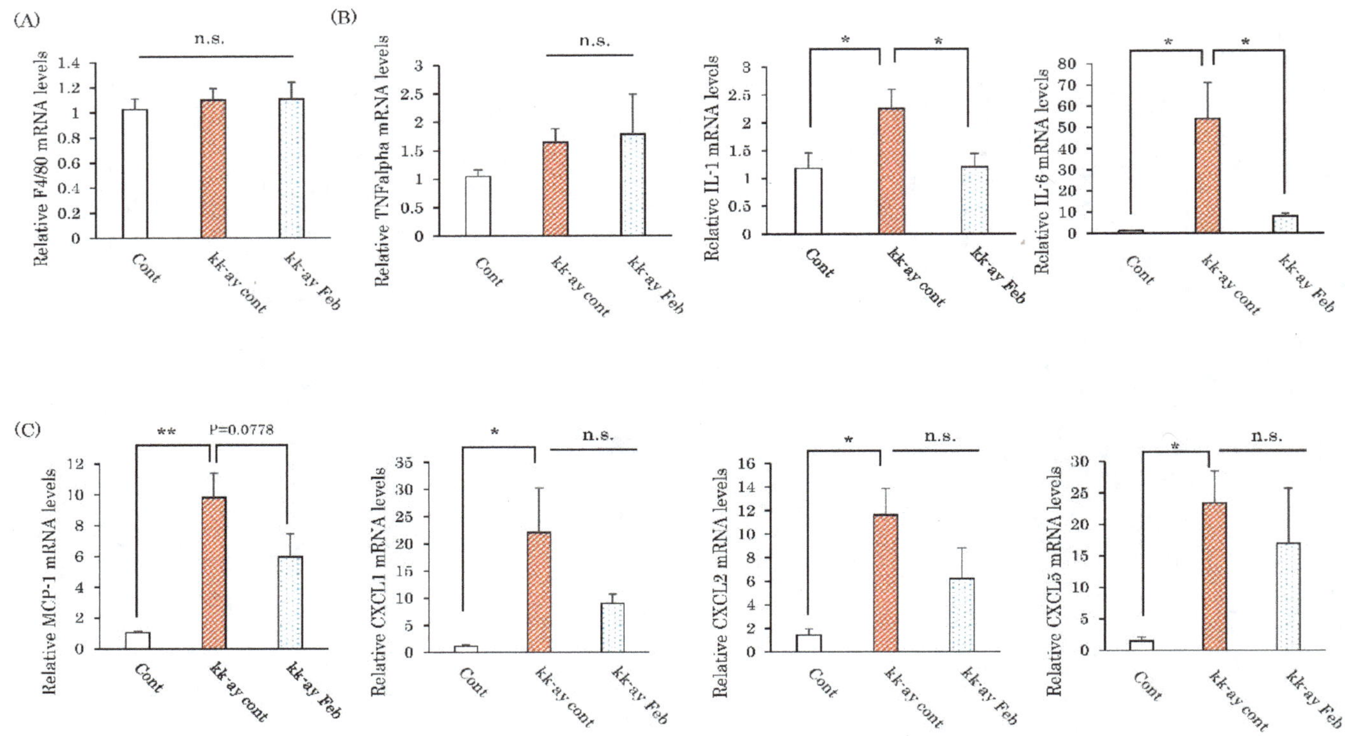

Figure 3. Febuxostat suppressed expressions of inflammatory cytokines in the kidneys of KK-Ay mice. (**A–C**) Relative mRNA levels of macrophage markers, cytokines, and chemokines in the kidneys were determined by employing real-time PCR. Data are means ± SE. * $p < 0.05$, ** $p < 0.001$. n = 8 for control group, n = 10 for KK-Ay mice without febuxostat group and n = 8 for KK-Ay mice with febuxostat group.

2.4. Effects of Febuxostat on Fibrosis-Related Collagen Gene Expressions

Azan staining was performed to evaluate the degree of fibrotic change, a change typical of the advanced stage of diabetic nephropathy. Imaging analysis of the fibrotic area based on Azan staining showed that the areas of increased fibrotic staining and fibrogenesis including glomerulosclerosis in the KK-Ay mice, as compared with control mice, were normalized by febuxostat treatment (Figure 4A). We next investigated the effects of febuxostat on the expression levels of the mRNA of genes related to the fibrotic process. The mRNA expression level of collagen 1a1 was increased in the kidneys of KK-Ay mice, but this elevation tended to be normalized by febuxostat treatment though the difference did not reach statistical significance (Figure 4B). On the other hand, mRNA expression levels of collagen 1a2, collagen 4a1, and collagen 4a2 did not show significant differences between KK-Ay and wild-type mice or between the presence and absence of febuxostat treatment (Figure 4B).

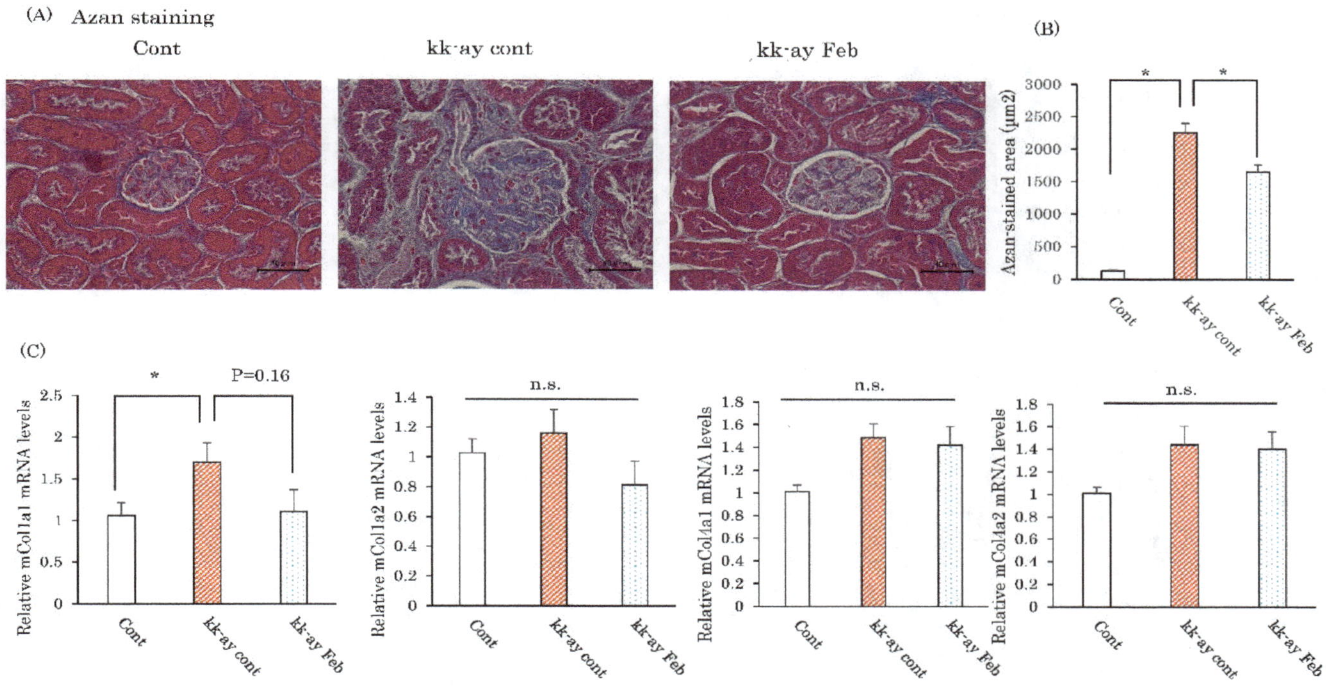

Figure 4. Febuxostat prevented progression of kidney fibrosis. (**A**) Azan staining of kidney fractions. Scale bar = 40 μm. (**B**) Relative mRNA levels of fibrotic markers in the kidneys. (**C**) The renal fibrotic area was assessed using Azan staining and then measured using image J. Data are means ± SE. * $p < 0.05$. n = 8 for control group, n = 10 for KK-Ay mice without febuxostat group and n = 8 for KK-Ay mice with febuxostat group.

2.5. *Effects of Febuxostat on Markers of Oxidative Stress and the Endoplasmic Reticulum*

Since febuxostat reportedly reduces the production of xanthine-induced oxidants, we measured oxidative stress in the kidneys of KK-Ay mice with and without febuxostat treatment and in wild-type mice. The amount of renal MDA, a product of lipid peroxidation, measured by the thiobarbituric acid reactive substances (TBARS) assay, showed no significant differences with wide variations among the three groups (Figure 5A). Expressions of endothelial damage markers (ICAM-1, VCAM-1) in the kidneys were elevated in KK-Ay mice as compared with wild-type mice, and febuxostat reduced these ICAM-1 elevations though not significantly (Figure 5B). Similarly, the mRNA levels of an endoplasmic reticulum stress marker (CHOP) were elevated in KK-Ay mice as compared to wild-type mice, with febuxostat reducing, though not significantly, these elevations (Figure 5C).

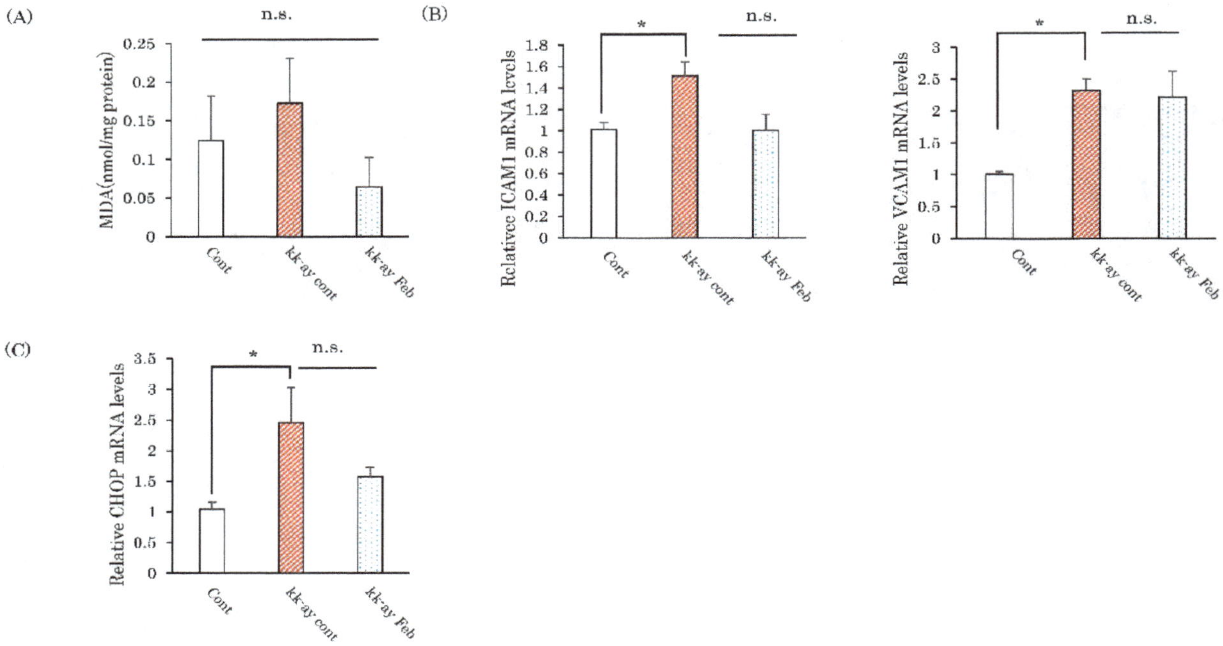

Figure 5. Febuxostat had no significant effect on either oxidative stress or endoplasmic reticulum stress. (**A**) Amounts of malondialdehyde were measured in renal tissues. (**B**) Relative mRNA levels of ICAM-1 and VCAM-1 in the kidneys. (**C**) Relative mRNA levels of CHOP in the kidney. Data are means ± SE. * $p < 0.05$, n = 8 in control group and KK-Ay mice with febuxostat, n = 10 in KK-Ay mice without febuxostat

3. Discussion

The relationship between hyperuricemia and the development of DKD is now widely recognized [18–20]. In the pathogenesis of DKD, inflammation appears to play essential roles via inflammatory mediators, adhesion molecules, and inflammatory signaling pathways directly or indirectly induced by hyperglycemia [1]. We previously demonstrated XO activity to promote inflammation in blood vessels [21] and the liver [22], while XO inhibitors suppress inflammation and oxidative stress [23] in macrophages. Thus, treatment with XO inhibitors prevented inflammatory and fibrotic changes in rodent models of atherosclerosis and non-alcoholic steatohepatitis. Another group also reported febuxostat to suppress angiotensin II-induced aortic fibrosis via XO inhibition in macrophages [24].

In this study, we showed febuxostat treatment to attenuate the development of proteinuria and to ameliorate mesangial structural changes in the kidneys of type 2 diabetic KK-Ay mice. A previous study using db/db mice also showed that allopurinol normalized hyperuricemia (to approximately 3 mg/dL) and reduced albuminuria with improvements in some of the features of diabetic nephropathy [15]. The authors insisted that high glucose accompanied by high uric acid (UA) is the causal mechanism of progressive renal function loss in db/db mice, based on a small increase in sICAM-1 detected by in vitro assay. In contrast, while KK/Ay mice showed slightly higher serum UA levels than control wild-type mice, these levels remained relatively low (around 1 mg/dL). The improved glucose tolerance and insulin tolerance test results by febuxostat obtained in this study might be consistent with the previous study using XO inhibitor [25]. However, it should be noted that the actual degree of hyperglycemia in KK/Ay mice, judging from blood sugar and glycated albumin levels, was not significantly altered by febuxostat administration. Furthermore, we recently reported treatment with febuxostat to provide significant protection from kidney failure, possibly via suppression of inflammation, in gddY mice [26], a model spontaneously developing IgA nephropathy [27] but showing no glucose metabolism defect. Taken together, these findings suggest that it would be inappropriate to interpret the mechanism underlying amelioration of renal dysfunction in KK/Ay mice as being via normalization of hyperuricemia and hyperglycemia.

The renal protective effects of febuxostat appear to be exerted through its potent anti-inflammatory actions. Despite macrophage infiltration, as indirectly evaluated by the F4/80 level, being unchanged by febuxostat treatment, renal injury was suppressed, and this was associated with reductions in inflammatory cytokines. XO inhibition was also reported to attenuate certain cellular migrations [28,29] and monocytic differentiations, such as those of foam cell formation and multinucleated giant cell formation [21,30]. Indeed, the renal protective effects of XO inhibition are consistent with previous reports showing the effects of febuxostat in mice with gddY IgA nephropathy [26] and in 5/6 nephrectomy rats, regardless of the coexisting hyperuricemia [31]. The suppressive effect on inflammation is a common feature of febuxostat treatment. Our present observations suggest febuxostat suppresses urinary albumin and glomerular injury at early stages of type 2 diabetic nephropathy, i.e., at the stage when inflammatory cytokines, such as IL-6 [32] and MCP-1, are secreted [33]. Repeated suppressions of ICAM-1 expression reportedly raised the possibility of preventing tissue injuries by administering XO inhibitors [15,34,35].

Collagenous proliferation evaluated by Azan as well as mesangial expansion, as evaluated by PAS staining, became more severe in KK/Ay mice and showed amelioration in response to febuxostat. In db/db, there are reportedly no changes in PAS staining with allopurinol treatment [15]. Febuxostat attenuated renal protein expression of TGF-β, CTGF, and collagen 4 in the kidneys of Zucker obese rats [14]. Studies using db/db mice [15] and our current experiments showed no reductions in collagen 4, though our data on collagen 1a1 and measurement of collagen 3 in db/db mice indicated both to be reduced by febuxostat administration. Despite variations in renal glomerular damage among animal models and/or species, it is reasonable to consider febuxostat to exert positive effects in terms of maintaining glomerular structure. Comparisons of the data from different sources imply that the effect of febuxostat might be more evident in KK/Ay than in db/db mice, although the mechanism underlying this difference is unclear.

Two mechanisms possibly underlying hyperuricemia-related DKD development have been suggested, elevation of the serum UA and increased superoxide free radical generation [36,37]. Oxidative stress indicators, such as the whole-kidney MDA level, and ER stress marker CHOP did not show a clearly significant difference and relatively large variance was noted. We speculate that the generation of oxidative stress would be limited to a highly localized area and that significant local changes might be difficult to detect at the whole-kidney level. Thus, we were not able to conclude that the effects of febuxostat are not due, even partially, to reduced free radical generation. Further studies are necessary to clarify this issue.

There are some limitations in this study. First, since febuxostat administration to kk-ay mice in this study showed significant changes in glomerular lesions and no obvious changes in the renal tubules or mesenchyme. Therefore, we focused on the histological glomerular change, however, the inflammation and/or fibrosis in tubulointerstitium should be evaluated in the future study. Finally, all the mRNA analysis is performed in whole kidney and not from the glomeruli, therefore the relationship between the gene expression and the effect of febuxostat on the glomerular protection might not be direct. Finally, the other xanthine oxidase inhibitors such as allopurinol, its metabolite oxypurinol, and topiroxostat should be evaluated in our model, to clarify the glomerular protective effect of febuxostat is class-effect.

In conclusion, we demonstrated that KK-Ay mice developed evident hyperglycemia and slight hyperuricemia, leading to diabetic nephropathy progression. XO inhibition by febuxostat ameliorated both proteinuria and glomerular damage, without affecting plasma glucose levels. Furthermore, the mechanism likely involves blocking intrarenal inflammation.

4. Materials and Methods

4.1. Animals

Male diabetic KK-Ay mice and age-matched C57BL/6 mice (8 weeks of age) were purchased from CLEA Japan (Tokyo, Japan). Febuxostat was obtained from Teijin Pharma Ltd., Tokyo, Japan. The mice were housed in temperature- and light-controlled rooms with free access to food (Oriental Yeast, Tokyo, Japan) and water. After the 12 weeks of treatment with or without drinking water containing febuxostat (15 μg/mL), which corresponds to approximately 1 mg/kg body weight per day, close to the clinical dose range of oral febuxostat, the mice were killed, and their kidneys and blood samples were collected. For uric acid (UA) measurement, 100 μL whole blood samples were collected with 100 μM allopurinol (Wako, Osaka, Japan). To measure the glucose concentration, blood samples were incubated on ice for 30 min and then centrifuged at 15,000 rpm for 30 min at 4 °C. All samples were preserved at −80 °C. All mice were handled in accordance with Guidelines for Care and Use of Experimental Animals published by Hiroshima University, and all protocols were approved by Hiroshima University (Approval #A17-178 Date 29 March 2018).

4.2. Metabolic Analysis

Mouse urine was collected for 24 h employing metabolic cages and preserved at −80 °C. Urine albumin and creatinine were quantified using a mouse albumin ELISA kit (FUJIFILM Wako Shibayagi, Gunma, Japan) and a mouse creatinine assay kit (Abcam, Cambridge, MA, USA), respectively. Serum UA concentrations were assayed with a UA assay kit (Cayman Chemical, Ann Arbor, UI, USA). All assays were conducted according to the manufacturers' protocols. The albumin-to-creatinine ratio (ACR) was calculated as urinary albumin/urinary creatinine.

4.3. Histological Study

Kidneys were fixed in 10% formalin, embedded in paraffin, and then cut into 2-μm sections. The sections were subjected to peroxide acid-Schiff (PAS) and Azan staining to identify glomerular sclerosis and fibrotic change, respectively [38].

Glomerular injury included mesangial matrix expansion and/or hyalinosis with focal adhesions, capillary dilation, and true glomerular tuft occlusion, and sclerosis. For the quantitative analysis of glomerular injury, the glomerular injury score (GIS) was determined on PAS-stained paraffin sections using a scale ranging from 0 to 4 for normal (0), with 1 = 25% sclerosis, 2 = 50% sclerosis, 3 = 75% sclerosis, and 4 = 100% sclerosis [39]. On average, 40 glomeruli were evaluated per mouse. GIS was calculated as [$\sum$ (each score × number of glomeruli)]/number of glomeruli. The glomerular area was measured in an average of 40 glomeruli per mouse employing image J (NIH, Bethesda, MD, USA). The renal fibrotic area was assessed using Azan staining, with an average of 10 glomeruli being measured per mouse using NIH Image J. All structural analyses were conducted in a blinded manner on unidentified sections.

4.4. Malondialdehyde (MDA) assay

Thiobarbituric acid reactive substances (TBARS) were measured using a TBARS assay kit (Cayman Chemical, Ann Arbor, UI, USA), according to the manufacturer's instructions, and absorbance was determined at 540 nm.

4.5. Quantitative Real-Time RT-PCR

Total RNA was extracted from mouse kidneys using Sepasol reagent (Nacalai Tesque, Kyoto, Japan). A 500 ng quantity of RNA was reverse transcribed using the Verso cDNA Synthesis kit (Thermo Scientific, Vilnius, Lithuania), which degrades double-stranded DNA. Quantitative real-time RT-PCR was performed using SYBR Green PCR master mix (Agilent Technologies, Santa Clara, CA, USA) on a CFX96 real-time PCR system (Bio-Rad, Hercules, CA, USA). Relative mRNA gene levels were normalized to the GAPDH mRNA level, and relative expressions were determined by the comparative Ct method. The designed primers used are shown previously [26].

4.6. Statistical Analysis

All results are expressed as means ± SE. Statistical analyses were conducted using ANOVA followed by Dunnett's test. A value of $p < 0.05$ was taken to indicate a statistically significant difference.

Author Contributions: Data curation, Y.N.; Formal analysis, T.Y., Y.N., T.K., M.T., and A.K.; Investigation, Y.M. (Yu Mizuno), T.Y., and K.U., Masa-ki Inoue, T.K., K.K., K.S., and A.K.; Methodology, K.K., K.S., T.M., and T.A.; Supervision, Y.M. (Yasuka Matsunaga), H.S., M.F., H.O., M.T., K.K., K.S., and T.M.; Validation, Y.M. (Yasuka Matsunaga); Writing—original draft, Y.M. (Yu Mizuno), T.A., and A.K.; Writing—review and editing, T.A. and A.K.

References

1. Matoba, K.; Takeda, Y.; Nagai, Y.; Kawanami, D.; Utsunomiya, K.; Nishimura, R. Unraveling the Role of Inflammation in the Pathogenesis of Diabetic Kidney Disease. *Int J. Mol. Sci.* **2019**. [CrossRef]
2. Vejakama, P.; Ingsathit, A.; McKay, G.J.; Maxwell, A.P.; McEvoy, M.; Attia, J.; Thakkinstian, A. Treatment effects of renin-angiotensin aldosterone system blockade on kidney failure and mortality in chronic kidney disease patients. *BMC Nephrol.* **2017**, *18*, 342. [CrossRef]
3. Riccio, E.; Di Nuzzi, A.; Pisani, A. Nutritional treatment in chronic kidney disease: The concept of nephroprotection. *Clin. Exp. Nephrol.* **2015**, *19*, 161–167. [CrossRef]
4. Tanaka, K.; Hara, S.; Hattori, M.; Sakai, K.; Onishi, Y.; Yoshida, Y.; Kawazu, S.; Kushiyama, A. Role of elevated serum uric acid levels at the onset of overt nephropathy in the risk for renal function decline in patients with type 2 diabetes. *J. Diabetes Investig.* **2015**, *6*, 98–104. [CrossRef]
5. Shichiri, M.; Iwamoto, H.; Marumo, F. Diabetic hypouricemia as an indicator of clinical nephropathy. *Am. J. Nephrol.* **1990**, *10*, 115–122. [CrossRef]
6. Ficociello, L.H.; Rosolowsky, E.T.; Niewczas, M.A.; Maselli, N.J.; Weinberg, J.M.; Aschengrau, A.; Eckfeldt, J.H.; Stanton, R.C.; Galecki, A.T.; Doria, A.; et al. High-normal serum uric acid increases risk of early progressive renal function loss in type 1 diabetes: Results of a 6-year follow-up. *Diabetes Care* **2010**, *33*, 1337–1343. [CrossRef]
7. Kushiyama, A.; Tanaka, K.; Hara, S.; Kawazu, S. Linking uric acid metabolism to diabetic complications. *World J. Diabetes* **2014**, *5*, 787–795. [CrossRef]
8. Pisano, A.; Cernaro, V.; Gembillo, G.; D'Arrigo, G.; Buemi, M.; Bolignano, D. Xanthine Oxidase Inhibitors for Improving Renal Function in Chronic Kidney Disease Patients: An Updated Systematic Review and Meta-Analysis. *Int. J. Mol. Sci.* **2017**. [CrossRef]
9. Siu, Y.P.; Leung, K.T.; Tong, M.K.; Kwan, T.H. Use of allopurinol in slowing the progression of renal disease through its ability to lower serum uric acid level. *Am. J. Kidney Dis.* **2006**, *47*, 51–59. [CrossRef]
10. Beddhu, S.; Filipowicz, R.; Wang, B.; Wei, G.; Chen, X.; Roy, A.C.; DuVall, S.L.; Farrukh, H.; Habib, A.N.; Bjordahl, T.; et al. A Randomized Controlled Trial of the Effects of Febuxostat Therapy on Adipokines and Markers of Kidney Fibrosis in Asymptomatic Hyperuricemic Patients With Diabetic Nephropathy. *Can. J. Kidney Health Dis.* **2016**, *3*, 2054358116675343. [CrossRef]
11. Mukri, M.N.A.; Kong, W.Y.; Mustafar, R.; Shaharir, S.S.; Shah, S.A.; Abdul Gafor, A.H.; Mohd, R.; Abdul Cader, R.; Kamaruzaman, L. Role of febuxostat in retarding progression of diabetic kidney disease with asymptomatic hyperuricemia: A 6-months open-label, randomized controlled trial. *Excli. J.* **2018**, *17*, 563–575.
12. Kojima, S.; Matsui, K.; Hiramitsu, S.; Hisatome, I.; Waki, M.; Uchiyama, K.; Yokota, N.; Tokutake, E.; Wakasa, Y.; Jinnouchi, H.; et al. Febuxostat for Cerebral and CaRdiorenovascular Events PrEvEntion StuDy. *Eur. Heart J.* **2019**, *40*, 1778–1786. [CrossRef]
13. Wang, C.; Pan, Y.; Zhang, Q.Y.; Wang, F.M.; Kong, L.D. Quercetin and allopurinol ameliorate kidney injury in STZ-treated rats with regulation of renal NLRP3 inflammasome activation and lipid accumulation. *PLoS ONE* **2012**, *7*, e38285. [CrossRef]

14. Komers, R.; Xu, B.; Schneider, J.; Oyama, T.T. Effects of xanthine oxidase inhibition with febuxostat on the development of nephropathy in experimental type 2 diabetes. *Br. J. Pharm.* **2016**, *173*, 2573–2588. [CrossRef]
15. Kosugi, T.; Nakayama, T.; Heinig, M.; Zhang, L.; Yuzawa, Y.; Sanchez-Lozada, L.G.; Roncal, C.; Johnson, R.J.; Nakagawa, T. Effect of lowering uric acid on renal disease in the type 2 diabetic db/db mice. *Am. J. Physiol. Ren. Physiol.* **2009**, *297*, F481–488. [CrossRef]
16. Iwatsuka, H.; Shino, A.; Suzuoki, Z. General survey of diabetic features of yellow KK mice. *Endocrinol Jpn.* **1970**, *17*, 23–35. [CrossRef]
17. Ruggenenti, P.; Remuzzi, G. Nephropathy of type-2 diabetes mellitus. *J. Am. Soc. Nephrol.* **1998**, *9*, 2157–2169.
18. Bo, S.; Cavallo-Perin, P.; Gentile, L.; Repetti, E.; Pagano, G. Hypouricemia and hyperuricemia in type 2 diabetes: Two different phenotypes. *Eur. J. Clin. Invest.* **2001**, *31*, 318–321. [CrossRef]
19. Rosolowsky, E.T.; Ficociello, L.H.; Maselli, N.J.; Niewczas, M.A.; Binns, A.L.; Roshan, B.; Warram, J.H.; Krolewski, A.S. High-normal serum uric acid is associated with impaired glomerular filtration rate in nonproteinuric patients with type 1 diabetes. *Clin. J. Am. Soc. Nephrol.* **2008**, *3*, 706–713. [CrossRef]
20. Tseng, C.H. Correlation of uric acid and urinary albumin excretion rate in patients with type 2 diabetes mellitus in Taiwan. *Kidney Int.* **2005**, *68*, 796–801. [CrossRef]
21. Kushiyama, A.; Okubo, H.; Sakoda, H.; Kikuchi, T.; Fujishiro, M.; Sato, H.; Kushiyama, S.; Iwashita, M.; Nishimura, F.; Fukushima, T.; et al. Xanthine oxidoreductase is involved in macrophage foam cell formation and atherosclerosis development. *Arter. Thromb. Vasc. Biol.* **2012**, *32*, 291–298. [CrossRef]
22. Nakatsu, Y.; Seno, Y.; Kushiyama, A.; Sakoda, H.; Fujishiro, M.; Katasako, A.; Mori, K.; Matsunaga, Y.; Fukushima, T.; Kanaoka, R.; et al. The xanthine oxidase inhibitor febuxostat suppresses development of nonalcoholic steatohepatitis in a rodent model. *Am. J. Physiol. Gastrointest. Liver Physiol.* **2015**, *309*, G42–51. [CrossRef]
23. Nomura, J.; Busso, N.; Ives, A.; Matsui, C.; Tsujimoto, S.; Shirakura, T.; Tamura, M.; Kobayashi, T.; So, A.; Yamanaka, Y. Xanthine oxidase inhibition by febuxostat attenuates experimental atherosclerosis in mice. *Sci. Rep.* **2014**, *4*, 4554. [CrossRef]
24. Kondo, M.; Imanishi, M.; Fukushima, K.; Ikuto, R.; Murai, Y.; Horinouchi, Y.; Izawa-Ishizawa, Y.; Goda, M.; Zamami, Y.; Takechi, K.; et al. Xanthine Oxidase Inhibition by Febuxostat in Macrophages Suppresses Angiotensin II-Induced Aortic Fibrosis. *Am. J. Hypertens* **2019**, *(3)*, 249–256. [CrossRef]
25. Yisireyili, M.; Hayashi, M.; Wu, H.; Uchida, Y.; Yamamoto, K.; Kikuchi, R.; Shoaib Hamrah, M.; Nakayama, T.; Wu Cheng, X.; Matsushita, T.; et al. Xanthine oxidase inhibition by febuxostat attenuates stress-induced hyperuricemia, glucose dysmetabolism, and prothrombotic state in mice. *Sci. Rep.* **2017**, *7*, 1266. [CrossRef]
26. Inoue, M.K.; Yamamotoya, T.; Nakatsu, Y.; Ueda, K.; Inoue, Y.; Matsunaga, Y.; Sakoda, H.; Fujishiro, M.; Ono, H.; Morii, K.; et al. The Xanthine Oxidase Inhibitor Febuxostat Suppresses the Progression of IgA Nephropathy, Possibly via Its Anti-Inflammatory and Anti-Fibrotic Effects in the gddY Mouse Model. *Int. J. Mol. Sci.* **2018**. [CrossRef]
27. Suzuki, H.; Suzuki, Y.; Novak, J.; Tomino, Y. Development of Animal Models of Human IgA Nephropathy. *Drug Discov. Today Dis. Models* **2014**, *11*, 5–11. [CrossRef]
28. Tsirmoula, S.; Lamprou, M.; Hatziapostolou, M.; Kieffer, N.; Papadimitriou, E. Pleiotrophin-induced endothelial cell migration is regulated by xanthine oxidase-mediated generation of reactive oxygen species. *Microvasc. Res.* **2015**, *98*, 74–81. [CrossRef]
29. Oh, S.H.; Choi, S.Y.; Choi, H.J.; Ryu, H.M.; Kim, Y.J.; Jung, H.Y.; Cho, J.H.; Kim, C.D.; Park, S.H.; Kwon, T.H.; et al. The emerging role of xanthine oxidase inhibition for suppression of breast cancer cell migration and metastasis associated with hypercholesterolemia. *FASEB J.* **2019**, *33*, 7301–7314. [CrossRef]
30. Mizuno, K.; Okamoto, H.; Horio, T. Inhibitory influences of xanthine oxidase inhibitor and angiotensin I-converting enzyme inhibitor on multinucleated giant cell formation from monocytes by downregulation of adhesion molecules and purinergic receptors. *Br. J. Derm.* **2004**, *150*, 205–210. [CrossRef]
31. Sanchez-Lozada, L.G.; Tapia, E.; Soto, V.; Avila-Casado, C.; Franco, M.; Wessale, J.L.; Zhao, L.; Johnson, R.J. Effect of febuxostat on the progression of renal disease in 5/6 nephrectomy rats with and without hyperuricemia. *Nephron Physiol.* **2008**, *108*, 69–78. [CrossRef]
32. Choudhary, N.; Ahlawat, R.S. Interleukin-6 and C-reactive protein in pathogenesis of diabetic nephropathy: New evidence linking inflammation, glycemic control, and microalbuminuria. *Iran. J. Kidney Dis.* **2008**, *2*, 72–79.
33. Morii, T.; Fujita, H.; Narita, T.; Shimotomai, T.; Fujishima, H.; Yoshioka, N.; Imai, H.; Kakei, M.; Ito, S. Association of monocyte chemoattractant protein-1 with renal tubular damage in diabetic nephropathy. *J.*

Diabetes Complicat. **2003**, *17*, 11–15. [CrossRef]

34. Eleftheriadis, T.; Pissas, G.; Antoniadi, G.; Liakopoulos, V.; Stefanidis, I. Allopurinol protects human glomerular endothelial cells from high glucose-induced reactive oxygen species generation, p53 overexpression and endothelial dysfunction. *Int. Urol. Nephrol.* **2018**, *50*, 179–186. [CrossRef]
35. Dong, G.; Ren, M.; Wang, X.; Jiang, H.; Yin, X.; Wang, S.; Wang, X.; Feng, H. Allopurinol reduces severity of delayed neurologic sequelae in experimental carbon monoxide toxicity in rats. *Neurotoxicology* **2015**, *48*, 171–179. [CrossRef]
36. Yang, C.C.; Ma, M.C.; Chien, C.T.; Wu, M.S.; Sun, W.K.; Chen, C.F. Hypoxic preconditioning attenuates lipopolysaccharide-induced oxidative stress in rat kidneys. *J. Physiol.* **2007**, *582*, 407–419. [CrossRef]
37. Szalay, C.I.; Erdelyi, K.; Kokeny, G.; Lajtar, E.; Godo, M.; Revesz, C.; Kaucsar, T.; Kiss, N.; Sarkozy, M.; Csont, T.; et al. Oxidative/Nitrative Stress and Inflammation Drive Progression of Doxorubicin-Induced Renal Fibrosis in Rats as Revealed by Comparing a Normal and a Fibrosis-Resistant Rat Strain. *PLoS ONE* **2015**, *10*, e0127090. [CrossRef]
38. Afroz, T.; Sagar, R.; Reddy, S.; Gandhe, S.; Rajaram, K.G. Clinical and histological correlation of diabetic nephropathy. *Saudi J. Kidney Dis. Transpl.* **2017**, *28*, 836–841.
39. Lassila, M.; Seah, K.K.; Allen, T.J.; Thallas, V.; Thomas, M.C.; Candido, R.; Burns, W.C.; Forbes, J.M.; Calkin, A.C.; Cooper, M.E.; et al. Accelerated nephropathy in diabetic apolipoprotein e-knockout mouse: Role of advanced glycation end products. *J. Am. Soc. Nephrol.* **2004**, *15*, 2125–2138. [CrossRef]

8

Efficacy of Polyunsaturated Fatty Acids on Inflammatory Markers in Patients Undergoing Dialysis

Po-Kuan Wu [1], Shu-Ching Yeh [2], Shan-Jen Li [3,*] and Yi-No Kang [4,*]

1 School of Medicine, College of Medicine, Taipei Medical University, Taipei 11042, Taiwan
2 Division of Nephrology, Department of Internal Medicine, Taipei Medical University Hospital, Taipei 11042, Taiwan
3 Department of Emergency Medicine, Taipei Medical University Hospital, Taipei 11042, Taiwan
4 Evidence-Based Medicine Center, Wan Fang Hospital, Taipei Medical University, Taipei 11696, Taiwan
* Correspondence: b8401121@gmail.com (S.-J.L.); academicnono@gmail.com (Y.-N.K.)

Abstract: The effects of polyunsaturated fatty acids (PUFAs) on inflammatory markers among patients receiving dialysis have been discussed for a long time, but previous syntheses made controversial conclusion because of highly conceptual heterogeneity in their synthesis. Thus, to further understanding of this topic, we comprehensively gathered relevant randomized clinical trials (RCTs) before April 2019, and two authors independently extracted data of C-reactive protein (CRP), high-sensitivity C-reactive protein (hs-CRP), and interleukin-6 (IL-6) for conducting network meta-analysis. Eighteen eligible RCTs with 962 patients undergoing dialysis were included in our study. The result showed that with placebo as the reference, PUFAs was the only treatment showing significantly lower CRP (weighted mean difference (WMD): −0.37, 95% confidence interval (CI): −0.07 to −0.68), but the CRP in PUFAs group was not significantly lower than vitamin E, PUFAs plus vitamin E, or medium-chain triglyceride. Although no significant changes were noted for hs-CRP and IL-6 levels, PUFAs showed the best ranking among treatments according to surface under the cumulative ranking. Therefore, PUFAs could be a protective option for patients receiving dialysis in clinical practice.

Keywords: polyunsaturated fatty acids; omega-3 fatty acid; inflammatory maker; C-reactive protein; interleukin-6

---

1. Introduction

Patients with end-stage renal disease around the world suffer from chronic inflammation caused by dialysis, especially hemodialysis. For instance, vascular access of hemodialysis [1], filter membrane of hemodialysis machine [2], and endotoxin from the dialysate [3] all cause chronic inflammation. Chronic inflammation not only reduces the quality-of-life among patients with chronic kidney disease, but also increases the mortality rate of these populations [4,5]. Previous reports have noted about 30% to 50% of patients undergoing hemodialysis have activated inflammatory response [6]. Chronic inflammation is related to pathogenesis of atherosclerosis [7], and cardiovascular disease accounts for the largest proportion of mortality in patients with chronic kidney disease [8]. As a result, detecting Interleukin-6 (IL-6), C-reactive protein (CRP), and high-sensitivity C-reactive protein (hs-CRP) are imperative for understanding and managing inflammatory conditions among these patients [4,5]. The association between IL-6, CRP, and cardiovascular disease is well known. Also, hs-CRP is another important marker manifesting inflammation and endothelial damage; it is also an indicator of defective coronary artery blood flow [9].

To improve the outcomes among patients with hemodialysis, controlling their inflammatory status is an important aspect in clinical practice. In the past decade, many trials have tried to control these inflammations among this group of patients through nutrient supplements [10–30]. Commonly-used nutrient supplements such as polyunsaturated fatty acids (PUFAs), vitamin D, antioxidants, polyphenol-rich foods, fibers, and probiotics to modulate patient's immune response are becoming more and more popular [31]. Unlike consuming drugs, nutrient supplements are usually free from increment of patients' physical stress. PUFAs are the top two popular nutrient supplements with many trials and Omega-3 fatty acids are the main nutrients as trials used PUFAs for reducing inflammatory among patients with chronic kidney disease [31]. The association of PUFA and inflammatory processes has been widely discussed in the past decade [32–40]. With regard to Omega-3 fatty acids, it commonly involves eicosapentaenoic acid, docosahexaenoic acid, and alpha-linolenic acid. Eicosapentaenoic acid and docosahexaenoic acid upregulate peroxisome proliferators' active receptors, and decrease CRP and IL-6. The peroxisome proliferators' active receptors also decrease CRP and IL-6 through downregulation of nuclear factor kappa B (NF-κB) [41,42].

A good synthesis for the topic of nutrients on inflammatory markers among patients with hemodialysis in 2018, yet there is a very high heterogeneity (I-square = 84.3%) existing in the result of CRP mean changes after Omega-3 fatty acids supplementation [31]. Therefore, this topic needs further analysis to provide a clearer picture for the effects of PUFAs on inflammatory markers among patients undergoing hemodialysis. Moreover, there is another meta-analysis in 2018 showing that alpha-linolenic acid cannot affect relevant inflammatory markers [43]. Therefore, our study aimed to clarify whether using PUFAs can reduce inflammatory cytokines (CRP, IL-6, hs-CRP) among patients undergoing dialysis through systematic review and meta-analysis of randomized clinical trials.

2. Results

Through comprehensive search, this systematic review identified 1485 references from the EMBASE (n = 656), PubMed (n = 388), and Web of Science (n = 441). Three records were found from hand search of reference lists. After the exclusion of 437 duplications, 1051 references were reviewed for eligibility. Then, two systematic reviews and 25 randomized clinical trials without relevant outcomes were excluded [31,44–69]. There were 21 references from 18 RCTs meeting the eligibility criteria (Figure 1) [10–30].

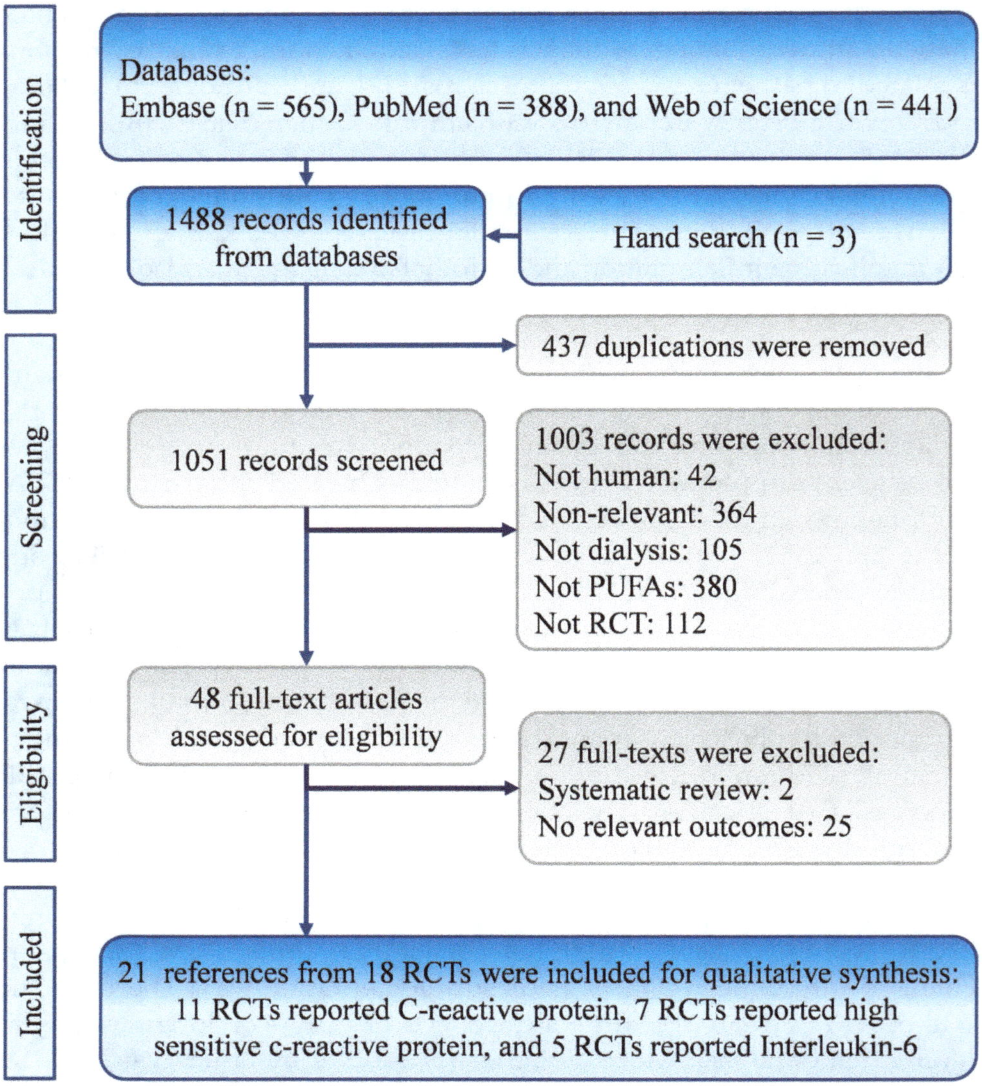

Figure 1. Flowchart of the systematic review and meta-analysis according to PRISMA guidelines.

2.1. Characteristics and Quality of Included Studies

The 18 trials recruited 962 patient undergoing dialysis from Brazil [24], Denmark [13,18], Greece [27], Egypt [30], Iran [10,14,21,22,25,26], Korea [23], United States [11,12,19,20,29], and Sweden [28]. The treatments in the 18 trials could be categorized into five treating strategies including placebo, PUFAs, vitamin E, medium chain triglyceride (MCT), and PUFAs plus vitamin E. The available data in each study showed mean ages from 46.4 to 68 years old, and a total of 598 (62.2%) men were included in the studies. Other information about trial location, inclusion years, treatments, number of patients, and dialysis period are shown in Table 1. Overall, the quality of the studies is presented in Table 2.

Table 1. Characteristics of the included randomized clinical trials.

Author	Location	Inclusion Year	Treatments	Patients	Mean Age	Sex (M/F)	Dialysis Period
Asemi [10]	Iran	2014	1. ω-3	30	55.2	20/10	3.6
			2. αT	30	61.2	20/10	3.5
			3. ω-3 + αT	30	54.9	20/10	3.4
			4. Placebo	30	59.9	20/10	3.4
Bowden [11]	USA	NR	1. ω-3	18	57.2	11/7	1.5
			2. corn oil	15	64.3	8/7	2.8
Daud [12]	USA	NR	1. ω-3	28	59	20/11	3.6
			2. placebo	27	58	12/20	3.3
Ewers [13]	Denmark	2007	1. ω-3	14	64.6	30/10	NR
			2. No supplement	14	64.6	30/10	NR
Gharekhani [14–17]	Iran	NR	1. ω-3	25	56.8	12/13	5
			2. paraffin (placebo)	20	57.2	8/12	6
Harving [18]	Denmark	NR	1. ω-3	83	65.5	55/28	4
			2. Olive oil	79	68	51/28	3.6
Himmelifarb [19]	USA	2008 to 2011	1. ω-3	31	58	23/8	2.1
			2. placebo	32	61.2	17/15	2.6
Hung [20]	USA	2008 to 2011	1. ω-3	17	50	14/3	4.2
			2. placebo	17	53	13/4	3.6
Khalatbari Soltani [21]	Iran	NR	1. ground flaxseed	15	54	10/5	2.6
			2. Usual diet	15	54.5	6/9	2.8
Kooshki [22]	Iran	NR	1. ω-3	17	50	10/7	1.75
			2. placebo	17	50	11/6	2.3
Lemos [24]	Brazil	NR	1. flaxseed oil + αT	70	55.7	39/31	2.4
			2. mineral oil + αT	75	58.3	46/29	2.9
Lee [23]	Korea	2012	1. ω-3	8	60	2/6	NR
			2. Olive oil	7	64	3/4	NR
Mirfatahi [25]	Iran	NR	1. flaxseed oil	17	68	12/5	4.4
			2. medium-chain triglycerides oil	17	59	10/7	4.6
Naini [26]	Iran	NR	1. ω-3	20	57.7	11/9	NR
			2. placebo	20	59.3	12/8	NR
Poulia [27]	Greece	NR	1. ω-3 + αT	22	51	16/9	9.4
			2. αT	23	51	16/9	
Rodhe [28]	Sweden	NR	1. sea buckthorn + vit-E	24	62	29/16	NR
			2. Coconut oil	21	62	29/16	NR
Saifullah [29]	USA	NR	1. ω-3	15	58	11/4	NR
			2. placebo	8	57	7/1	NR
Zakaria [30]	Egypt	NR	1. ω-3 + vit-E	20	50.2	12/8	4
			2. Placebo	20	46.4	11/9	4.5

CRP, C-reactive protein; hs-CRP, high-sensitivity C-reactive protein; IL-6, interleukin-6; NR, no report; vit-E, vitamin E; αT, alpha-tocopherol; ω-3, omega-3 fatty acids.

Table 2. Quality of the included randomized clinical trials.

Study	Randomization	Concealment	Blinding	Follow-Up Duration	Loss Follow-Up	Type of Analysis	Relevant Outcomes	Quality Judgement
Asemi	Computer generated	Yes	Double-blind	12 weeks	0	ITT	hs-CRP	Low risk
Bowden	4-block permuted randomization	No	Double-blind	26 weeks	7	PP	hs-CRP	High risk
Daud	NR	NR	Triple-blind	26 weeks	2	ITT	CRP	Moderate
Ewers	Computer generated	NR	Single-blind	6 weeks	10	PP	CRP	High risk
Gharekhani	Blocked randomization	NR	Single-blind	16 weeks	9	PP	CRP, IL-6	High risk
Harving	NR	NR	NR	12 weeks	44	PP	hs-CRP	High risk
Himmelifarb	4-block permuted randomization	NR	Double-blind	8 weeks	0	ITT	CRP, IL-6	Moderate
Hung	Randomized in 1:1 ratio	NR	Double-blind	12 weeks	4	PP	hs-CRP, IL-6	Moderate
KhalatbariSoltani	NR	NR	Unblind	8 weeks	8	PP	CRP	High risk
Kooshki	Blocked randomization	Yes	Double-blind	10 weeks	0	ITT	CRP, IL-6	Low risk
Lee	Random number table	NR	Double-blind	12 weeks	0	PP	CRP	Moderate
Lemos	NR	Yes	Double-blind	7 weeks	22	ITT	CRP	High risk
Mirfatahi	Blocked randomization	NR	Double-blind	8 weeks	0	PP	hs-CRP	Moderate
Naini	NR	Yes	Double-blind	8 weeks	0	ITT	CRP, IL-6	Moderate
Poulia	Flip coin	NR	Single-blind	4 weeks	8	PP	CRP	High risk
Rodhe	NR	Yes	Double-blind	8 weeks	21	PP	hs-CRP	High risk
Saifullah	Computer generated	Yes	Double-blind	12 weeks	3	PP	CRP	Moderate
Zakaria	Flip coin	NR	Double-blind	16 weeks	0	PP	hs-CRP	Moderate

CRP, C-reactive protein; hs-CRP, high-sensitivity C-reactive protein; IL-6, interleukin-6; ITT, intention to treat; NR, no report; PP, per protocol.

2.2. *C-Reactive Protein*

A total of 11 RCTs with 632 cases in five treatments were included in the network meta-analysis of CRP (Figure 2A) [12–14,18,21–24,26,27,29]. The result showed that with placebo as the reference, PUFAs was the only one treatment showing significantly lower CRP (WMD: −0.37, 95% CI: −0.07 to −0.68), but the CRP in PUFAs group was not significantly lower than vitamin E, PUFAs plus vitamin E, and MCT (Figure 3A; Supplementary File 1). Similarly, in SUCRA, PUFAs also had the highest value (Mean rank = 2.1; SUCRA = 72.7) and placebo had the lowest value (Mean rank = 4.3; SUCRA = 16.3; Supplementary File 2). Because placebo, PUFA, vitamin E, PUFAs plus vitamin E, and MCT did not form any loop in the network meta-analysis of CRP, it is not required to test inconsistency in this consistency model. Moreover, no evidence detected serious small study effects (t = 0.49, 95% CI: −1.27 to 1.98; Supplementary File 3).

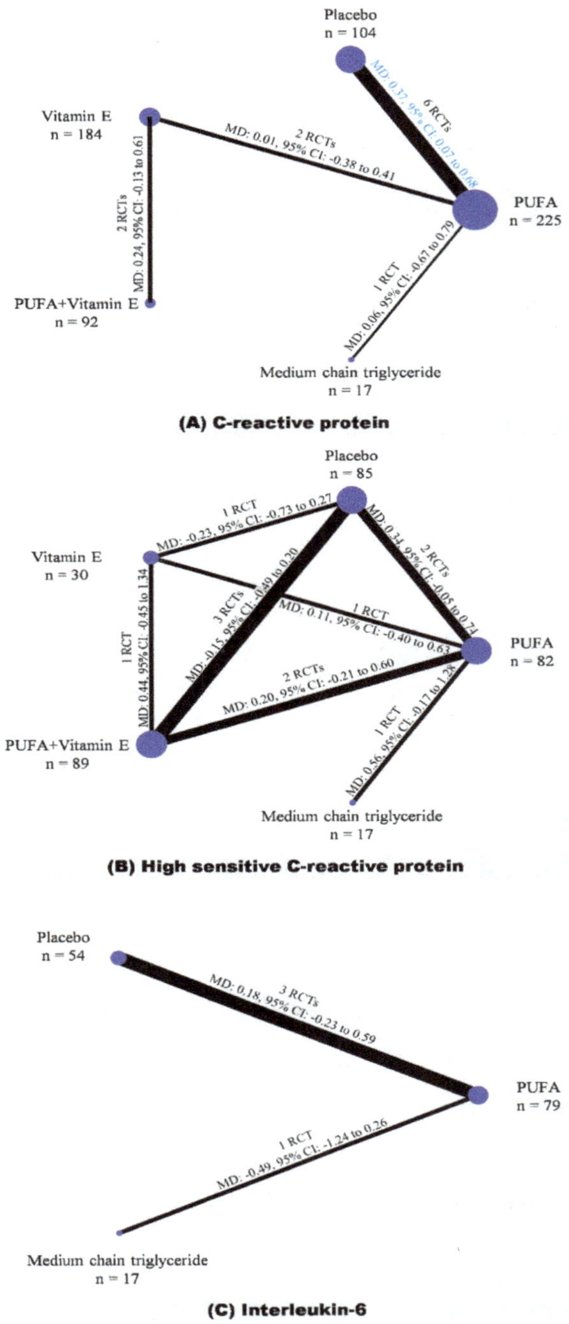

Figure 2. Network plots of (**A**) CRP, (**B**) high sensitivity CRP, and (**C**) IL-6.

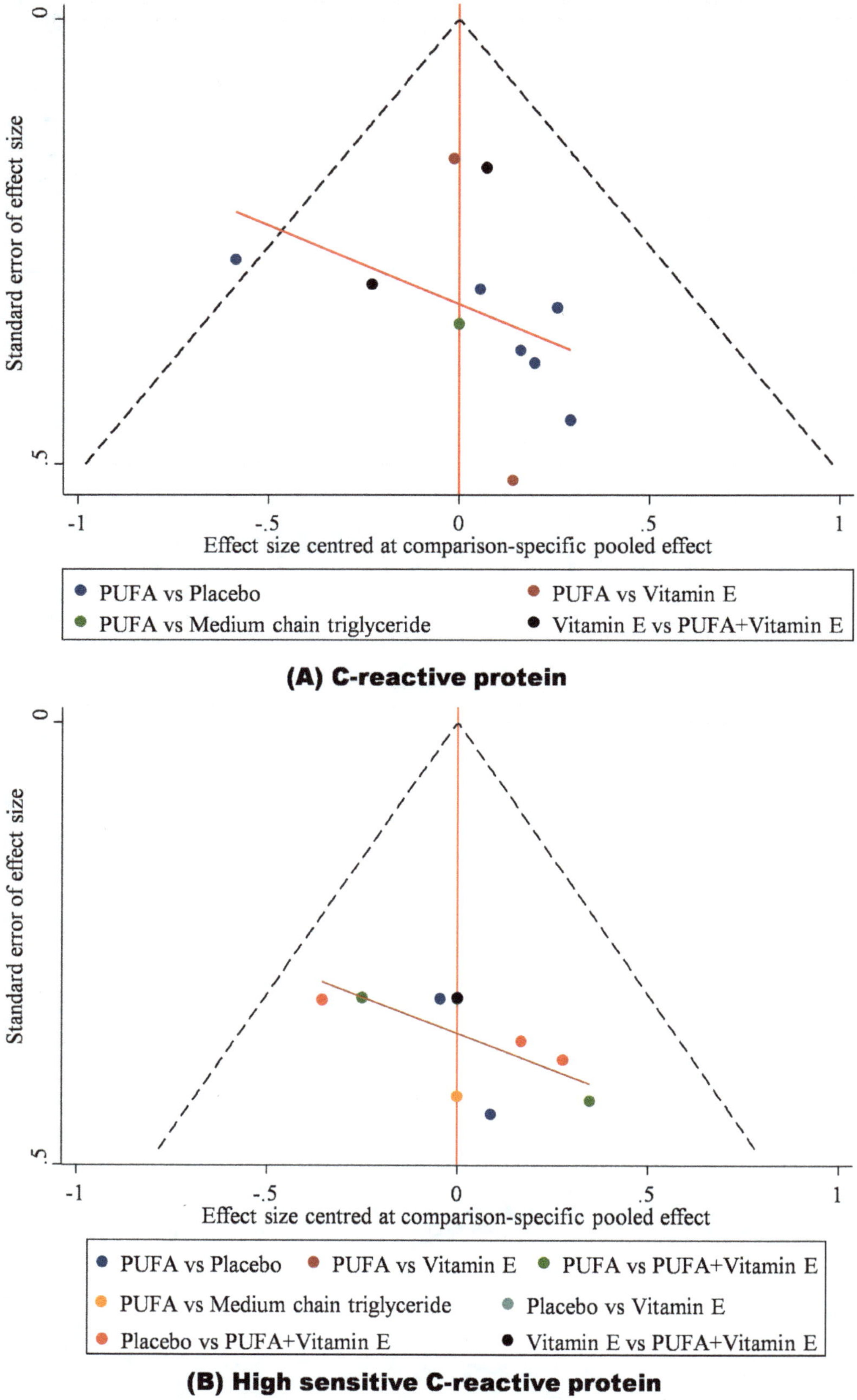

Figure 3. Funnel plots of (**A**) CRP and (**B**) high sensitivity CRP.

2.3. *High-Sensitivity C-Reactive Protein*

Six trials provided data on hs-CRP among the five treatments (n = 303) (Figure 2B) [10,11,20,25,28,30]. According to the available data, our network meta-analysis of hs-CRP showed no significant differences among placebo, PUFA, vitamin E, PUFAs plus vitamin E, and MCT (Supplementary File 4). There were some hints from ranking the best hs-CRP probability showing that PUFAs (54.7%) was the best choice, whereas placebo (1.2%) should be avoided. Similarly, in SUCRA, PUFAs had the highest value (Mean rank = 1.6; SUCRA = 84.6), whereas placebo (Mean rank = 3.9; SUCRA = 28.2) and MCT (Mean rank = 4.3; SUCRA = 18.4; Supplementary File 5) were the two treatments with lowest values. The loop inconsistency test for the network meta-analysis of hs-CRP showed insignificance (chi-square = 2.25, $p < 0.13$; Supplementary File 6), yet the Egger's test detected small study effects ($t = 2.34$, 95% CI: 0.10 to 6.06, $p = 0.04$; Supplementary File 7).

2.4. *Interleukin-6*

Four of the included trials provided data on IL-6 among placebo, PUFA, and MCT (n = 140) (Figure 2A) [14,20,22,26]. The network meta-analysis of IL-6 also showed no significant differences among placebo, PUFA, and MCT (Supplementary File 8). Interestingly, ranking the best IL-6 probability showing that MCT (88.8%) had the highest probability, whereas placebo (3.2%) and PUFAs (8.0%) were the two treatments with lowest probabilities. SUCRA also depicted similar phenomenon showing that MCT had the highest value (Mean rank = 1.2; SUCRA = 92.0), whereas placebo (Mean rank = 2.7; SUCRA = 12.7) and MCT (Mean rank = 2.1; SUCRA = 45.2) were the two treatments with lowest values. The loop inconsistency test for the network meta-analysis of hs-CRP showed no significance (chi-square = 1.64, $p < 0.20$; Supplementary File 9), and the Egger's test also detected no small study effects ($t = 1.44$, 95% CI: −14.26 to 28.63, $p = 0.29$; Supplementary File 10).

2.5. *Further Analysis*

We further examined albumin, a minor parameter of inflammatory, based on the included evidence, and we also detected the influences from regions because of lifestyle and dietary style. For albumin, A total of nine trials formed network for placebo, PUFA, vitamin E, and PUFAs plus vitamin E with 407 cases [10,12,13,15,20,23,27–29]. The pooled result also showed insignificant differences among those four treatments (Supplementary File 11). Yet, SUCRA indicated that PUFA had the highest value (Mean rank = 1.4, SUCRA = 86.9; Supplementary File 12). We did not observe significant inconsistency (chi-square = 5.38, $p < 0.06$; Supplementary File 13) and small study effects ($t = 1.02$, 95% CI: −1.69 to 4.65, $p = 0.33$; Supplementary File 14).

Moreover, we only found available and appropriate information for detecting region effects on the pooled results of CRP and hs-CRP. Then, the meta-regression did not show any significant findings. Current evidence is insufficient to prove that region plays an important role in the effects of PUFA on CRP (Supplementary File 15) and hs-CRP (Supplementary File 16).

A cluster plot for CRP and hs-CRP scores demonstrated that the best balance was achieved by PUFAs (Cophenetic Correlation Coefficient = 0.86; Supplementary File 17). Therefore, PUFAs may be recommended for treating patients undergoing dialysis. By contrast, placebo exhibited poor performance in the cluster plot.

3. Discussion

In our systematic review, we successfully identified 18 randomized clinical trials (n = 962) investigating the effect of PUFAs on inflammatory markers among patients undergoing dialysis. In our network meta-analysis, we depicted an overview of comparisons among placebo, PUFA, vitamin E, PUFAs plus vitamin E, and MCT. Then, the results showed that the current evidence only supports PUFAs group having significant lower CRP than placebo. Yet, other active treatments did not reach the statistical significance when they were compared to placebo. The results of hs-CRP and IL-6 failed to support PUFAs having more benefits than other treatment, even no significant benefit as it was compared to placebo. These results about limited anti-inflammatory effects from PUFAs are similar to a previous synthesis indicating that alpha-linolenic acid has no effects on blood inflammatory markers [43].

These insignificant results may relate to the complex comparators among trials. Some of the trials treated control group with vitamin E, and some of them used combined supplements of PUFAs and vitamin E. Apart from PUFA, antioxidants such as vitamin E can also reduce the inflammatory responses by decreasing reactive oxygen species and NF-κB [70]. Besides, combination of PUFAs and antioxidants can reduce the oxidative stress caused by PUFAs [1]. Thus, our synthesis separated PUFAs alone and combined supplements of PUFAs and vitamin E. Then, we found PUFAs alone having a significantly higher CRP level than placebo, whereas no significant difference in CRP level between combined supplements of PUFAs and vitamin E and placebo. The pooled result also did not support that combined supplements of PUFAs and vitamin E having significant benefits on hs-CRP.

We agree that Omega-3 fatty acids play some roles in anti-inflammatory among patients undergoing dialysis because eicosapentaenoic acid and docosahexaenoic acid have been well-known in anti-inflammatory action through regulating gene expression, lowering membrane content of arachidonic acid, inhibiting arachidonic acid metabolism, and competing with arachidonic acid [41,71]. To be more specific, eicosapentaenoic acid and docosahexaenoic acid affect cyclooxygenase and lipoxygenase pathway through being substrates for the key enzymes. The patients of chronic kidney disease have much higher systemic concentration of inflammatory cytokine because of the decrease renal clearance and the insufficiency of nutrient [72,73]. This situation will cause the destruction of endothelial cell and eventually lead to cardiovascular disease [72,74]. To control the chronic inflammation of these patients, dietary fat supplement has important biological effect. PUFA can clean up the reactive oxygen species and inhibit activation of NF-κB, which plays a significant role in regulating inflammatory response [31]. Furthermore, PUFA will compete with arachidonic acid for the substance in the cyclooxygenase pathway to produce less pro-inflammatory cytokine [41]. Collectively, PUFA can decrease the systemic inflammation and the cardiovascular disease mortality among patients with chronic kidney disease. Although our evidence did not show the significant benefit of Omega-3 fatty acids on hs-CRP among patients receiving dialysis, the pooled hs-CRP had similar trends with the pooled results of CRP. A potential reason for the insignificant difference in hs-CRP may be smaller sample size (n = 303). In addition, another important potential factor causing the insignificant finding is that hs-CRP detects inflammatory with better sensitivity than CRP, especially for those patients with cardiovascular problems. It is well-published that cardiovascular problems are common comorbidities of chronic kidney disease. Thus, the difference between hs-CRP and traditional CRP may be more obvious for patients undergoing dialysis than for healthy people.

3.1. *Comparing to the Previous Syntheses*

Besides the good systematic review and meta-analysis in 2018 we mentioned above [31], there is another important synthesis in 2016 on this topic [69]. These two systematic reviews concluded similarly by declaring that Omega-3 fatty acids are effective supplements for reducing CRP levels among patients undergoing dialysis. However, their meta-analyses of CRP reflected very high heterogeneities. They did not successfully explain the source of heterogeneities though the systematic review by Khor et al. in 2018 separated alpha-linolenic acid (I-square = 93.4%) from eicosapentaenoic acid and docosahexaenoic acid. As we know, the anti-inflammatory effects of alpha-linolenic acid share similar pathway with eicosapentaenoic acid and docosahexaenoic acid [31]. Thus, subgroup analysis for alpha-linolenic acid may be not the best way to explore the heterogeneity in the pooled result of CRP mean change.

To face the challenge of high heterogeneity in the pooled CRP reported by the previous syntheses, in our study, we carefully clarified comparators by mainly relevant nutrients and outcomes for giving fewer biased results because of conceptual heterogeneity according to methodological guidance [75]. These two conceptual heterogeneities may result in the statistical heterogeneity in the pooled CRP level. Our study not only distinguished placebo, PUFA, vitamin E, PUFAs plus vitamin E, and MCT for comparators, but also separated hs-CRP from CRP for outcome synthesis. For instance, four trials included in the previous synthesis used hs-CRP [10,11,20,25], and we pooled these four trials with the other two trials that were not included in the previous synthesis for hs-CRP [28,30]. As a result of reduction of conceptual heterogeneity, we successfully gave this topic reasonable results without inconsistency and highly statistical heterogeneity.

3.2. Limitations

Although our synthesis overcame some limitations in previous syntheses and clarified the effects of PUFAs on inflammatory markers among patients receiving dialysis, the present synthesis still has three limitations. Firstly, the use of PUFAs is not clear, though our study separated combined supplements of PUFAs and vitamin E from PUFAs alone. The separation resulted in lower heterogeneity than previous syntheses, but our study cannot make a practical suggestion with a specific dosage for the use of PUFAs. Secondly, interaction of PUFAs and vitamin E on the anti-inflammatory effects remains unclear. Our synthesis did not find better results as the trials treating patients with combined supplements of PUFAs and vitamin E. Thirdly, our synthesis showed some trends about the benefits of PUFAs on hs-CRP and IL-6, but the results may be under power because of small sample size. We suggest that future studies should use hs-CRP measurement to confirm whether using PUFAs can reduce inflammatory responses, especially among those patients undergoing dialysis.

4. Materials and Methods

This comprehensive review team consisting of nephrologists and an experienced researcher conducted this study according to the Cochrane handbook, and reported the systematic review and meta-analysis according to the PRISMA guidelines [76]. The experienced researcher previously participated in some studies about nutrient, internal medicine, and chronic kidney disease [77–80]. The researcher also has some experience in conducting network meta-analysis [81,82]. Because this meta-analysis uses published data, it was exempted from institutional review board approval.

4.1. Study Selection Criteria

According to our study purpose, this comprehensive review selected evidence if (1) the study recruited patients undergoing dialysis, (2) the intervention was PUFA, and (3) the study prospectively randomized patients into two or more groups. However, this comprehensive review removed studies when they met following exclusion criteria: (1) the reference was gray literature without detailed information or data, (2) the study did not separate outcome reporting as it concurrently recruited patients with and without dialysis, and (3) the article did not report any relevant outcomes (CRP, hs-CRP, and IL-6).

4.2. Search Strategy and Study Selection

Data sources were three important online databases including EMBASE, PubMed, and the Web of Science. PubMed was the platform for building search strategy with relevant terms of dialysis and PUFA, and the search strategy was adapted to the other two databases. The relevant terms involved free-text and medical subject heading. Boolean operator "OR" combined the relevant terms of dialysis, and we also used "OR" for combining relevant terms of PUFA. Then, Boolean operator "AND" connected both dialysis part and PUFAs part. This search strategy did not restrict language and publication date from database inception until April 2019. Supplemental Material 18 showed the detail of the searching strategy.

After relevant references were identified from online databases, two investigators excluded ineligible references according to criteria in two phases. The first phase was title and abstract screening, and the second phase was full-text review. Any references meeting exclusion criteria were removed.

4.3. *Quality Assessment and Data Extraction*

The two investigators independently identified relevant information, and extracted outcome data. They identified the data about the details of trial design, location, inclusion year, treatments, sample size, mean age, sex, and dialysis period. The outcome data included three inflammatory markers, namely CRP, hs-CRP, IL-6, and albumin at the end of treatment. Because these data were continuous, the investigators extracted them in mean and standard deviation (SD). This network meta-analysis estimated SD from standard error (SE) according to the formula $SE = SD/\sqrt{N}$ when the trial only provided SE. When the trial only presented interquartile range (IQR), this study estimated SD using formula IQR/1.35. Moreover, the network meta-analysis estimated SD from maximum and minimum according to Hozo's method [83].

Based on the identified information, the investigators completed the risk of bias in each trial. The assessment involved randomization, concealment, blinding, follow-up duration, loss follow-up, and analysis type. These items reflected selection bias, performance bias, detection bias, and attrition bias. In case of any disagreements on risk of bias between the two investigators, a third reviewer participated into discussion to resolve the disagreement.

4.4. *Evidence Synthesis and Statistical Analysis*

Evidence synthesis consisted of qualitative and quantitative parts. The quantitative synthesis was contrast-based network meta-analysis. Because of conceptual heterogeneity among trial design, the network meta-analysis should be in random-effects model. The main outcomes were CRP, hs-CRP, and IL-6 at the end of treatment. Thus, the analysis performed weighted mean difference (WMD) and 95% confidence interval (CI). Standardized mean difference was the solution for units of measurement including mg/L, mg/dL, ng/L, ng/mL, and pg/mL. To clarify the effects among active treatments, the quantitative synthesis also showed surface under the cumulative ranking (SUCRA). This statistical technique estimated the probability of each treatment among the most effective treatments, and formed a hierarchy through the treatment ranking of probability. We would like to foster the understanding on this topic, and therefore we further analyzed albumin and the influence from region. The influence from region was detected by using meta-regression in network meta-analysis model. For conducting meta-regression, we applied dummy variables for America, Asia, and Europe. To confirm the quality of the quantitative synthesis, the network meta-analysis detected both the small-study effect and inconsistency. The small-study effect in a network meta-analysis can be assessed by an adjusted funnel plot and Egger's regression intercept. Concerning inconsistency, the meta-analysis implemented Lu–Ades' loop inconsistency test. The analyses mentioned above were completed using STATA version 14 for Microsoft Windows. In all analysis, $p < 0.05$ was considered as statistically significant.

5. Conclusions

Based on available evidence, the very first network meta-analysis on this topic, PUFAs could be an option for controlling inflammatory to patients undergoing dialysis. However, the evidence is not strong enough, especially with regards to the results of hs-CRP and IL-6. For practical recommendation, we anticipate further studies investigating in this topic to further elucidate how PUFAs reduce inflammatory among patients receiving dialysis.

Author Contributions: P.-K.W.: Conception of the study, data acquisition, manuscript drafting, and final approval of the version to be published. S.-C.Y.: Critical revision of the draft for enhancing crucial intellectual content, and final approval of the version to be published. S.-J.L.: Interpretation of data, supervision of the study, critical revision of the draft for enhancing crucial intellectual content, and final approval of the version to be published. Y.-N.K.: Design of the study, formal analysis and interpretation of data, manuscript drafting, and final approval of the version to be published.

Abbreviations

CI	confidence interval
CRP	C-reactive protein
hs-CRP	high-sensitivity C-reactive protein
IQR	interquartile range
IL-6	interleukin-6
MCT	medium chain triglyceride
NF-κB	nuclear factor kappa B
PUFA	polyunsaturated fatty acids
RCT	randomized clinical trial
SD	standard deviation.
SE	standard error
SUCRA	surface under the cumulative ranking curve
WMD	weighted mean difference

References

1. Sachdeva, M.; Hung, A.; Kovalchuk, O.; Bitzer, M.; Mokrzycki, M.H. The initial vascular access type contributes to inflammation in incident hemodialysis patients. *Int. J. Nephrol.* **2012**, *2012*, 917465. [CrossRef] [PubMed]
2. Caglar, K.; Peng, Y.; Pupim, L.B.; Flakoll, P.J.; Levenhagen, D.; Hakim, R.M.; Ikizler, T.A. Inflammatory signals associated with hemodialysis. *Kidney Int.* **2002**, *62*, 1408–1416. [CrossRef] [PubMed]
3. Carrero, J.J.; Stenvinkel, P. Inflammation in end-stage renal disease—What have we learned in 10 years? *Semin. Dial.* **2010**, *23*, 498–509. [CrossRef] [PubMed]
4. Bazeley, J.; Bieber, B.; Li, Y.; Morgenstern, H.; de Sequera, P.; Combe, C.; Yamamoto, H.; Gallagher, M.; Port, F.K.; Robinson, B.M. C-reactive protein and prediction of 1-year mortality in prevalent hemodialysis patients. *Clin. J. Am. Soc. Nephrol. CJASN* **2011**, *6*, 2452–2461. [CrossRef] [PubMed]
5. Panichi, V.; Maggiore, U.; Taccola, D.; Migliori, M.; Rizza, G.M.; Consani, C.; Bertini, A.; Sposini, S.; Perez-Garcia, R.; Rindi, P.; et al. Interleukin-6 is a stronger predictor of total and cardiovascular mortality than c-reactive protein in haemodialysis patients. *Nephrol. Dial. Transplant. Off. Publ. Eur. Dial. Transplant. Assoc. Eur. Ren. Assoc.* **2004**, *19*, 1154–1160. [CrossRef] [PubMed]
6. Stenvinkel, P. Inflammation in end-stage renal failure: Could it be treated? *Nephrol. Dial. Transplant. Off. Publ. Eur. Dial. Transplant. Assoc. Eur. Ren. Assoc.* **2002**, *17* (Suppl. 8), 33–38. [CrossRef] [PubMed]
7. Stenvinkel, P.; Alvestrand, A. Inflammation in end-stage renal disease: Sources, consequences, and therapy. *Semin. Dial.* **2002**, *15*, 329–337. [CrossRef]
8. Machowska, A.; Carrero, J.J.; Lindholm, B.; Stenvinkel, P. Therapeutics targeting persistent inflammation in chronic kidney disease. *Transl. Res. J. Lab. Clin. Med.* **2016**, *167*, 204–213. [CrossRef]
9. Barutcu, I.; Sezgin, A.T.; Sezgin, N.; Gullu, H.; Esen, A.M.; Topal, E.; Ozdemir, R.; Kosar, F.; Cehreli, S. Increased high sensitive crp level and its significance in pathogenesis of slow coronary flow. *Angiology* **2007**, *58*, 401–407. [CrossRef]
10. Asemi, Z.; Soleimani, A.; Shakeri, H.; Mazroii, N.; Esmaillzadeh, A. Effects of omega-3 fatty acid plus alpha-tocopherol supplementation on malnutrition-inflammation score, biomarkers of inflammation and oxidative stress in chronic hemodialysis patients. *Int. Urol. Nephrol.* **2016**, *48*, 1887–1895. [CrossRef]
11. Bowden, R.G.; Wilson, R.L.; Deike, E.; Gentile, M. Fish oil supplementation lowers c-reactive protein levels independent of triglyceride reduction in patients with end-stage renal disease. *Nutr. Clin. Pract.* **2009**, *24*, 508–512. [CrossRef] [PubMed]
12. Daud, Z.A.; Tubie, B.; Adams, J.; Quainton, T.; Osia, R.; Tubie, S.; Kaur, D.; Khosla, P.; Sheyman, M. Effects of protein and omega-3 supplementation, provided during regular dialysis sessions, on nutritional and inflammatory indices in hemodialysis patients. *Vasc. Health Risk Manag.* **2012**, *8*, 187–195. [PubMed]
13. Ewers, B.; Riserus, U.; Marckmann, P. Effects of unsaturated fat dietary supplements on blood lipids, and on markers of malnutrition and inflammation in hemodialysis patients. *J. Ren. Nutr.* **2009**, *19*, 401–411. [CrossRef] [PubMed]
14. Gharekhani, A.; Dashti-Khavidaki, S.; Lessan-Pezeshki, M.; Khatami, M.R. Potential effects of omega-3

fatty acids on insulin resistance and lipid profile in maintenance hemodialysis patients a randomized placebo-controlled trial. *Iran. J. Kidney Dis.* **2016**, *10*, 310–318. [PubMed]
15. Gharekhani, A.; Khatami, M.R.; Dashti-Khavidaki, S.; Razeghi, E.; Abdollahi, A.; Hashemi-Nazari, S.S.; Mansournia, M.A. Effects of oral supplementation with omega-3 fatty acids on nutritional state and inflammatory markers in maintenance hemodialysis patients. *J. Ren. Nutr.* **2014**, *24*, 177–185. [CrossRef] [PubMed]
16. Gharekhani, A.; Khatami, M.R.; Dashti-Khavidaki, S.; Razeghi, E.; Abdollahi, A.; Hashemi-Nazari, S.S.; Mansournia, M.A. Potential effects of omega-3 fatty acids on anemia and inflammatory markers in maintenance hemodialysis patients. *DARU* **2014**, *22*, 11. [CrossRef] [PubMed]
17. Gharekhani, A.; Khatami, M.R.; Dashti-Khavidaki, S.; Razeghi, E.; Noorbala, A.A.; Hashemi-Nazari, S.S.; Mansournia, M.A. The effect of omega-3 fatty acids on depressive symptoms and inflammatory markers in maintenance hemodialysis patients: A randomized, placebo-controlled clinical trial. *Eur. J. Clin. Pharmacol.* **2014**, *70*, 655–665. [CrossRef]
18. Harving, F.; Svensson, M.; Flyvbjerg, A.; Schmidt, E.B.; Jorgensen, K.A.; Eriksen, H.H.; Christensen, J.H. N-3 polyunsaturated fatty acids and adiponectin in patients with end-stage renal disease. *Clin. Nephrol.* **2015**, *83*, 279–285. [CrossRef]
19. Himmelifarb, J.; Phinney, S.; Ikizler, T.A.; Kane, J.; McMonagle, E.; Miller, G. Gamma-tocopherol and docosahexaenoic acid decrease inflammation in dialysis patients. *J. Ren. Nutr.* **2007**, *17*, 296–304. [CrossRef]
20. Hung, A.M.; Booker, C.; Ellis, C.D.; Siew, E.D.; Graves, A.J.; Shintani, A.; Abumrad, N.N.; Himmelfarb, J.; Ikizler, T.A. Omega-3 fatty acids inhibit the up-regulation of endothelial chemokines in maintenance hemodialysis patients. *Nephrol. Dial. Transplant.* **2015**, *30*, 266–274. [CrossRef]
21. Khalatbari Soltani, S.; Jamaluddin, R.; Tabibi, H.; Mohd Yusof, B.N.; Atabak, S.; Loh, S.P.; Rahmani, L. Effects of flaxseed consumption on systemic inflammation and serum lipid profile in hemodialysis patients with lipid abnormalities. *Hemodial. Int.* **2013**, *17*, 275–281. [CrossRef] [PubMed]
22. Kooshki, A.; Taleban, F.A.; Tabibi, H.; Hedayati, M. Effects of marine omega-3 fatty acids on serum systemic and vascular inflammation markers and oxidative stress in hemodialysis patients. *Ann. Nutr. Metab.* **2011**, *58*, 197–202. [CrossRef] [PubMed]
23. Lee, S.M.; Son, Y.K.; Kim, S.E.; An, W.S. The effects of omega-3 fatty acid on vitamin d activation in hemodialysis patients: A pilot study. *Mar. Drugs* **2015**, *13*, 741–755. [CrossRef] [PubMed]
24. Lemos, J.R.N.; de Alencastro, M.G.; Konrath, A.V.; Cargnin, M.; Manfro, R.C. Flaxseed oil supplementation decreases c-reactive protein levels in chronic hemodialysis patients. *Nutr. Res.* **2012**, *32*, 921–927. [CrossRef] [PubMed]
25. Mirfatahi, M.; Tabibi, H.; Nasrollahi, A.; Hedayati, M.; Taghizadeh, M. Effect of flaxseed oil on serum systemic and vascular inflammation markers and oxidative stress in hemodialysis patients: A randomized controlled trial. *Int. Urol. Nephrol.* **2016**, *48*, 1335–1341. [CrossRef]
26. Naini, A.E.; Asiabi, R.E.; Keivandarian, N.; Moeinzadeh, F. Effect of omega-3 supplementation on inflammatory parameters in patients on chronic ambulatory peritoneal dialysis. *Adv. Biomed. Res.* **2015**, *4*, 167. [PubMed]
27. Poulia, K.A.; Panagiotakos, D.B.; Tourlede, E.; Rezou, A.; Stamatiadis, D.; Boletis, J.; Zampelas, A. Omega-3 fatty acids supplementation does not affect serum lipids in chronic hemodialysis patients. *J. Ren. Nutr.* **2011**, *21*, 479–484. [CrossRef]
28. Rodhe, Y.; Woodhill, T.; Thorman, R.; Moller, L.; Hylander, B. The effect of sea buckthorn supplement on oral health, inflammation, and DNA damage in hemodialysis patients: A double-blinded, randomized crossover study. *J. Ren. Nutr.* **2013**, *23*, 172–179. [CrossRef]
29. Saifullah, A.; Watkins, B.A.; Saha, C.; Li, Y.; Moe, S.M.; Friedman, A.N. Oral fish oil supplementation raises blood omega-3 levels and lowers c-reactive protein in haemodialysis patients—A pilot study. *Nephrol. Dial. Transplant.* **2007**, *22*, 3561–3567. [CrossRef]
30. Zakaria, H.; Mostafa, T.M.; El-Azab, G.A.; Abd El Wahab, A.M.; Elshahawy, H.; Sayed-Ahmed, N.A.H. The impact of fish oil and wheat germ oil combination on mineral-bone and inflammatory markers in maintenance hemodialysis patients: A randomized, double-blind, placebo-controlled clinical trial. *Int. Urol. Nephrol.* **2017**, *49*, 1851–1858. [CrossRef]
31. Khor, B.H.; Narayanan, S.S.; Sahathevan, S.; Gafor, A.H.A.; Daud, Z.A.M.; Khosla, P.; Sabatino, A.; Fiaccadori, E.; Chinna, K.; Karupaiah, T. Efficacy of nutritional interventions on inflammatory markers in haemodialysis patients: A systematic review and limited meta-analysis. *Nutrients* **2018**, *10*, 397. [CrossRef] [PubMed]

32. Bersch-Ferreira, A.C.; Sampaio, G.R.; Gehringer, M.O.; Ross-Fernandes, M.B.; Kovacs, C.; Alves, R.; Pereira, J.L.; Magnoni, C.D.; Weber, B.; Rogero, M.M. Association between polyunsaturated fatty acids and inflammatory markers in patients in secondary prevention of cardiovascular disease. *Nutr.* **2017**, *37*, 30–36. [CrossRef] [PubMed]
33. Calder, P.C. N-3 polyunsaturated fatty acids, inflammation, and inflammatory diseases. *Am. J. Clin. Nutr.* **2006**, *83*, 1505s–1519s. [CrossRef] [PubMed]
34. Calder, P.C. Omega-3 polyunsaturated fatty acids and inflammatory processes: Nutrition or pharmacology? *Br. J. Clin. Pharmacol.* **2013**, *75*, 645–662. [CrossRef] [PubMed]
35. Calder, P.C. Omega-3 fatty acids and inflammatory processes: From molecules to man. *Biochem. Soc. Trans.* **2017**, *45*, 1105–1115. [CrossRef] [PubMed]
36. Laye, S.; Nadjar, A.; Joffre, C.; Bazinet, R.P. Anti-inflammatory effects of omega-3 fatty acids in the brain: Physiological mechanisms and relevance to pharmacology. *Pharmacol. Rev.* **2018**, *70*, 12–38. [CrossRef] [PubMed]
37. Scaioli, E.; Liverani, E.; Belluzzi, A. The imbalance between n-6/n-3 polyunsaturated fatty acids and inflammatory bowel disease: A comprehensive review and future therapeutic perspectives. *Int. J. Mol. Sci.* **2017**, *18*, 2619. [CrossRef]
38. Thomas, J.; Thomas, C.J.; Radcliffe, J.; Itsiopoulos, C. Omega-3 fatty acids in early prevention of inflammatory neurodegenerative disease: A focus on alzheimer's disease. *Biomed. Res. Int* **2015**, *2015*, 172801. [CrossRef]
39. Tortosa-Caparros, E.; Navas-Carrillo, D.; Marin, F.; Orenes-Pinero, E. Anti-inflammatory effects of omega 3 and omega 6 polyunsaturated fatty acids in cardiovascular disease and metabolic syndrome. *Crit. Rev. Food Sci. Nutr.* **2017**, *57*, 3421–3429. [CrossRef]
40. Yates, C.M.; Calder, P.C.; Ed Rainger, G. Pharmacology and therapeutics of omega-3 polyunsaturated fatty acids in chronic inflammatory disease. *Pharmacol. Ther.* **2014**, *141*, 272–282. [CrossRef]
41. Calder, P.C. Mechanisms of action of (n-3) fatty acids. *J. Nutr.* **2012**, *142*, 592s–599s. [CrossRef] [PubMed]
42. Reiter, E.; Jiang, Q.; Christen, S. Anti-inflammatory properties of alpha- and gamma-tocopherol. *Mol. Asp. Med.* **2007**, *28*, 668–691. [CrossRef] [PubMed]
43. Su, H.; Liu, R.J.; Chang, M.; Huang, J.H.; Jin, Q.Z.; Wang, X.G. Effect of dietary alpha-linolenic acid on blood inflammatory markers: A systematic review and meta-analysis of randomized controlled trials. *Eur. J. Nutr.* **2018**, *57*, 877–891. [CrossRef] [PubMed]
44. Yoshimoto-Furuie, K.; Yoshimoto, K.; Tanaka, T.; Saima, S.; Kikuchi, Y.; Shay, J.; Horrobin, D.F.; Echizen, H. Effects of oral supplementation with evening primrose oil for six weeks on plasma essential fatty acids and uremic skin symptoms in hemodialysis patients. *Nephron* **1999**, *81*, 151–159. [CrossRef] [PubMed]
45. Taziki, O.; Lessan-Pezeshki, M.; Akha, O.; Vasheghani, F. The effect of low dose omega-3 on plasma lipids in hemodialysis patients. *Saudi J. Kidney Dis. Transplant. Off. Publ. Saudi Cent. Organ. Transplant. Saudi Arab.* **2007**, *18*, 571–576.
46. Tabibi, H.; Mirfatahi, M.; Hedayati, M.; Nasrollahi, A. Effects of flaxseed oil on blood hepcidin and hematologic factors in hemodialysis patients. *Hemodial. Int.* **2017**, *21*, 549–556. [CrossRef] [PubMed]
47. Svensson, M.; Schrnidt, E.B.; Jorgense, K.A.; Christensen, J.H. The effect of n-3 fatty acids on lipids and lipoproteins in patients treated with chronic haemodialysis: A randomized placebo-controlled intervention study. *Nephrol. Dial. Transplant.* **2008**, *23*, 2918–2924. [CrossRef]
48. Svensson, M.; Schmidt, E.B.; Jorgensen, K.A.; Christensen, J.H. The effect of n-3 fatty acids on heart rate variability in patients treated with chronic hemodialysis. *J. Ren. Nutr.* **2007**, *17*, 243–249. [CrossRef]
49. Sorensen, G.V.B.; Svensson, M.; Strandhave, C.; Schmidt, E.B.; Jorgensen, K.A.; Christensen, J.H. The effect of n-3 fatty acids on small dense low-density lipoproteins in patients with end-stage renal disease: A randomized placebo-controlled intervention study. *J. Ren. Nutr.* **2015**, *25*, 376–380. [CrossRef]
50. Schmitz, P.G.; McCloud, L.K.; Reikes, S.T.; Leonard, C.L.; Gellens, M.E. Prophylaxis of hemodialysis graft thrombosis with fish oil: Double-blind, randomized, prospective trial. *J. Am. Soc. Nephrol.* **2002**, *13*, 184–190.
51. Rantanen, J.M.; Riahi, S.; Johansen, M.B.; Schmidt, E.B.; Christensen, J.H. Effects of marine n-3 polyunsaturated fatty acids on heart rate variability and heart rate in patients on chronic dialysis: A randomized controlled trial. *Nutrients* **2018**, *10*, 1313. [CrossRef] [PubMed]
52. Omrani, H.R.; Pasdar, Y.; Raisi, D.; Najafi, F.; Esfandiari, A. The effect of omega-3 on serum lipid profile in hemodialysis patients. *J. Ren. Inj. Prev.* **2015**, *4*, 68–72. [PubMed]
53. Madsen, T.; Hagstrup Christensen, J.; Toft, E.; Aardestrup, I.; Lundbye-Christensen, S.; Schmidt, E.B. Effect of intravenous ω-3 fatty acid infusion and hemodialysis on fatty acid composition of free fatty acids and

phospholipids in patients with end-stage renal disease. *J. Parenter. Enter. Nutr.* **2011**, *35*, 97–106. [CrossRef] [PubMed]

54. Lok, C.E.; Moist, L.; Hemmelgarn, B.R.; Tonelli, M.; Vazquez, M.A.; Dorval, M.; Oliver, M.; Donnelly, S.; Allon, M.; Stanley, K. Effect of fish oil supplementation on graft patency and cardiovascular events among patients with new synthetic arteriovenous hemodialysis grafts a randomized controlled trial. *JAMA J. Am. Med. Assoc.* **2012**, *307*, 1809–1816. [CrossRef] [PubMed]
55. Khosroshahi, H.T.; Dehgan, R.; Asl, B.H.; Safaian, A.; Panahi, F.; Estakhri, R.; Purasgar, B. Effect of omega-3 supplementation on serum level of homocysteine in hemodialysis patients. *Iran. J. Kidney Dis.* **2013**, *7*, 479–484.
56. Khajehdehi, P. Lipid-lowering effect of polyunsaturated fatty acids in hemodialysis patients. *J. Ren. Nutr. Off. J. Counc. Ren. Nutr. Natl. Kidney Found.* **2000**, *10*, 191–195. [CrossRef]
57. Kajbaf, M.H.; Khorvash, F.; Mortazavi, M.; Shahidi, S.; Moeinzadeh, F.; Farajzadegan, Z.; Tirani, S.A. Does omega-3 supplementation decrease carotid intima-media thickening in hemodialysis patients? *J. Res. Pharm. Pract.* **2016**, *5*, 252–256.
58. Jabbari, M.; Khoshnevis, T.; Jenabi, A.; Yousefi, F. The effect of omega-3 supplement on serum lipid profile in patients undergoing hemodialysis: A randomized clinical trial. *Rom. J. Intern. Med. Rev. Roum. Med. Interne* **2016**, *54*, 222–227. [CrossRef]
59. Irish, A.B.; Viecelli, A.K.; Hawley, C.M.; Hooi, L.S.; Pascoe, E.M.; Paul-Brent, P.A.; Badve, S.V.; Mori, T.A.; Cass, A.; Kerr, P.G.; et al. Effect of fish oil supplementation and aspirin use on arteriovenous fistula failure in patients requiring hemodialysis a randomized clinical trial. *JAMA Intern. Med.* **2017**, *177*, 184–193. [CrossRef]
60. Ghanei, E.; Zeinali, J.; Borghei, M.; Homayouni, M. Efficacy of omega-3 fatty acids supplementation in treatment of uremic pruritus in hemodialysis patients: A double-blind randomized controlled trial. *Iran. Red Crescent Med. J.* **2012**, *14*, 515–522.
61. Deger, S.M.; Hung, A.M.; Ellis, C.D.; Booker, C.; Bian, A.H.; Chen, G.H.; Abumrad, N.N.; Ikizler, T.A. High dose omega-3 fatty acid administration and skeletal muscle protein turnover in maintenance hemodialysis patients. *Clin. J. Am. Soc. Nephrol.* **2016**, *11*, 1227–1235. [CrossRef] [PubMed]
62. De Mattos, A.M.; da Costa, J.A.C.; Jordao, A.A.; Chiarello, P.G. Omega-3 fatty acid supplementation is associated with oxidative stress and dyslipidemia, but does not contribute to better lipid and oxidative status on hemodialysis patients. *J. Ren. Nutr.* **2017**, *27*, 333–339. [CrossRef] [PubMed]
63. Dashti-Khavidaki, S.; Gharekhani, A.; Khatami, M.R.; Miri, E.S.; Khalili, H.; Razeghi, E.; Hashemi-Nazari, S.S.; Mansournia, M.A. Effects of omega-3 fatty acids on depression and quality of life in maintenance hemodialysis patients. *Am. J. Ther.* **2014**, *21*, 275–287. [CrossRef] [PubMed]
64. Begum, R.; Belury, M.A.; Burgess, J.R.; Peck, L.W. Supplementation with n-3 and n-6 polyunsaturated fatty acids: Effects on lipoxygenase activity and clinical symptoms of pruritus in hemodialysis patients. *J. Ren. Nutr.* **2004**, *14*, 233–241. [CrossRef]
65. Beavers, K.M.; Beavers, D.P.; Bowden, R.G.; Wilson, R.L.; Gentile, M. Effect of over-the-counter fish-oil administration on plasma lp(a) levels in an end-stage renal disease population. *J. Ren. Nutr.* **2009**, *19*, 443–449. [CrossRef] [PubMed]
66. Beavers, K.M.; Beavers, D.P.; Bowden, R.G.; Wilson, R.L.; Gentile, M. Omega-3 fatty acid supplementation and total homocysteine levels in end-stage renal disease patients. *Nephrology* **2008**, *13*, 284–288. [CrossRef]
67. Ateya, A.M.; Sabri, N.A.; El Hakim, I.; Shaheen, S.M. Effect of omega-3 fatty acids on serum lipid profile and oxidative stress in pediatric patients on regular hemodialysis: A randomized placebo-controlled study. *J. Ren. Nutr.* **2017**, *27*, 169–174. [CrossRef] [PubMed]
68. Allawi, A.A.D.; Wahab Alwardi, M.A.; Altemimi, H.M. Effects of omega-3 on vitamin d activation in iraqi patients with chronic kidney disease treated by maintenance hemodialysis. *J. Pharm. Sci. Res.* **2017**, *9*, 1812–1816.
69. Xu, T.H.; Sun, Y.T.; Sun, W.; Yao, L.; Sun, L.; Liu, L.L.; Ma, J.F.; Wang, L.N. Effect of omega-3 fatty acid supplementation on serum lipids and vascular inflammation in patients with end-stage renal disease: A meta-analysis. *Sci Rep.* **2016**, *6*, 39346. [CrossRef]
70. Khan, A.Q.; Khan, R.; Rehman, M.U.; Lateef, A.; Tahir, M.; Ali, F.; Sultana, S. Soy isoflavones (daidzein & genistein) inhibit 12-o-tetradecanoylphorbol-13-acetate (tpa)-induced cutaneous inflammation via modulation of cox-2 and nf-kappab in swiss albino mice. *Toxicology* **2012**, *302*, 266–274.
71. Mori, T.A.; Beilin, L.J. Omega-3 fatty acids and inflammation. *Curr. Atheroscler. Rep.* **2004**, *6*, 461–467. [CrossRef] [PubMed]

72. Carrero, J.J.; Stenvinkel, P. Persistent inflammation as a catalyst for other risk factors in chronic kidney disease: A hypothesis proposal. *Clin. J. Am. Soc. Nephrol. CJASN* **2009**, *4* (Suppl. 1), S49–S55. [CrossRef] [PubMed]
73. Huang, X.; Stenvinkel, P.; Qureshi, A.R.; Riserus, U.; Cederholm, T.; Barany, P.; Heimburger, O.; Lindholm, B.; Carrero, J.J. Essential polyunsaturated fatty acids, inflammation and mortality in dialysis patients. *Nephrol. Dial. Transplant. Off. Publ. Eur. Dial. Transplant. Assoc. Eur. Ren. Assoc.* **2012**, *27*, 3615–3620. [CrossRef]
74. Foley, R.N.; Parfrey, P.S.; Sarnak, M.J. Clinical epidemiology of cardiovascular disease in chronic renal disease. *Am. J. Kidney Dis. Off. J. Natl. Kidney Found.* **1998**, *32*, S112–S119. [CrossRef]
75. Mills, E.J.; Thorlund, K.; Ioannidis, J.P. Demystifying trial networks and network meta-analysis. *BMJ (Clin. Res. Ed.)* **2013**, *346*, f2914. [CrossRef] [PubMed]
76. Hutton, B.; Salanti, G.; Caldwell, D.M.; Chaimani, A.; Schmid, C.H.; Cameron, C.; Ioannidis, J.P.; Straus, S.; Thorlund, K.; Jansen, J.P.; et al. The prisma extension statement for reporting of systematic reviews incorporating network meta-analyses of health care interventions: Checklist and explanations. *Ann. Intern. Med.* **2015**, *162*, 777–784. [CrossRef] [PubMed]
77. Chi, S.C.; Tuan, H.I.; Kang, Y.N. Effects of polyunsaturated fatty acids on nonspecific typical dry eye disease: A systematic review and meta-analysis of randomized clinical trials. *Nutrients* **2019**, *11*, 942. [CrossRef] [PubMed]
78. Kang, Y.N.; Chi, S.C.; Wu, M.H.; Chiu, H.H. The effects of losartan versus beta-blockers on cardiovascular protection in marfan syndrome: A systematic review and meta-analysis. *J. Formos. Med Assoc. Taiwan Yi Zhi* **2019**, in press. [CrossRef]
79. Lin, T.M.; Chi, J.E.; Chang, C.C.; Kang, Y.N. Do etoricoxib and indometacin have similar effects and safety for gouty arthritis? A meta-analysis of randomized controlled trials. *J. Pain Res.* **2019**, *12*, 83–91. [CrossRef]
80. Lin, Y.C.; Lin, J.W.; Wu, M.S.; Chen, K.C.; Peng, C.C.; Kang, Y.N. Effects of calcium channel blockers comparing to angiotensin-converting enzyme inhibitors and angiotensin receptor blockers in patients with hypertension and chronic kidney disease stage 3 to 5 and dialysis: A systematic review and meta-analysis. *PLoS ONE* **2017**, *12*, e0188975. [CrossRef]
81. Kao, C.C.; Lin, Y.S.; Chu, H.C.; Fang, T.C.; Wu, M.S.; Kang, Y.N. Association of renal function and direct-acting antiviral agents for hcv: A network meta-analysis. *J. Clin. Med.* **2018**, *7*, 341. [CrossRef] [PubMed]
82. Lin, E.Y.; Kuo, Y.K.; Kang, Y.N. Effects of three common lumbar interbody fusion procedures for degenerative disc disease: A network meta-analysis of prospective studies. *Int. J. Surg.* **2018**, *60*, 224–230. [CrossRef] [PubMed]
83. Hozo, S.P.; Djulbegovic, B.; Hozo, I. Estimating the mean and variance from the median, range, and the size of a sample. *BMC Med Res. Methodol.* **2005**, *5*, 13. [CrossRef] [PubMed]

9

Non-Coding RNAs as New Therapeutic Targets in the Context of Renal Fibrosis

Cynthia Van der Hauwaert [1,2], François Glowacki [1,3], Nicolas Pottier [1,4] and Christelle Cauffiez [1,*]

1 EA 4483-IMPECS-IMPact of Environmental ChemicalS on Human Health, Univ. Lille, 59045 Lille CEDEX, France; cynthia.vanderhauwaert@gmail.com (C.V.d.H.); francois.glowacki@chru-lille.fr (F.G.); nicolas.pottier@univ-lille.fr (N.P.)

2 Département de la Recherche en Santé, CHU Lille, 59037 Lille, France

3 Service de Néphrologie, CHU Lille, 59037 Lille, France

4 Service de Toxicologie et Génopathies, CHU Lille, 59037 Lille, France

* Correspondence: christelle.cauffiez@univ-lille2.fr

Abstract: Fibrosis, or tissue scarring, is defined as the excessive, persistent and destructive accumulation of extracellular matrix components in response to chronic tissue injury. Renal fibrosis represents the final stage of most chronic kidney diseases and contributes to the progressive and irreversible decline in kidney function. Limited therapeutic options are available and the molecular mechanisms governing the renal fibrosis process are complex and remain poorly understood. Recently, the role of non-coding RNAs, and in particular microRNAs (miRNAs), has been described in kidney fibrosis. Seminal studies have highlighted their potential importance as new therapeutic targets and innovative diagnostic and/or prognostic biomarkers. This review will summarize recent scientific advances and will discuss potential clinical applications as well as future research directions.

Keywords: non-coding RNAs; microRNAs; long non-coding RNAs; renal fibrosis; biomarkers; therapeutics targets

---

1. Introduction

Chronic kidney disease (CKD) is increasingly recognized as a major public health concern. CKD prevalence has been estimated to be 8–16% worldwide [1]. In particular, CKD has been evaluated to affect more than 10% of the western population [2]. The common feature of CKD is renal fibrosis, which contributes to the progressive and irreversible decline in renal function and is associated with high morbidity and mortality.

Renal fibrosis, defined as an aberrant wound healing process in response to chronic injury, is characterized by the progressive and persistent accumulation of extracellular matrix components (ECM) in the kidney, ultimately leading to renal failure. As tissue scarring affects all compartments of the kidney, renal fibrosis is typically associated with glomerulosclerosis, arteriosclerosis and tubulointerstitial fibrosis [2]. Disruption of the epithelium and/or endothelium integrity during injury results in the activation of a complex cascade of molecular and cellular events. First, an inflammatory response initiates the release of profibrotic cytokines, chemokines and growth factors, which in turn promotes the proliferative phase of the scarring process characterized in particular by the recruitment and activation of fibroblasts into ECM-secreting myofibroblasts [3,4]. Finally, ECM accumulation results in the formation of a permanent fibrotic scar associated with renal tissue remodeling [5]. Once deposited, ECM components are further cross-linked and acquire resistance properties to degradation, precluding fibrosis resolution [6].

Although histological analysis of renal biopsies represents the gold standard to evaluate fibrosis, indirect biological parameters such as evolution of estimated Glomerular Filtration Rate are widely used in clinical practice for monitoring the progression of fibrotic lesions [7,8]. Furthermore, no specific treatment directly targeting fibrosis is currently approved [2]. Therefore, identifying new therapeutic targets and innovative diagnostic and/or prognostic biomarkers remains critical.

Recently, among the various mechanisms triggering fibrogenesis, non-coding RNAs (ncRNAs) have emerged as important regulators of this deleterious process [9–13].

In this review, we summarize the implication of ncRNAs in renal fibrosis and their potential value as either biomarkers or therapeutic targets, with an emphasis on microRNAs (miRNAs) and long non-coding RNAs (lncRNAs).

2. Non-Coding RNAs

New high-throughput technologies have revolutionized our understanding of the genome. Indeed, transcriptome of higher eukaryotic organism is far more complex than anticipated and contains large amounts of RNA molecules without coding potential (only 2% mRNAs in humans). Besides transfer and ribosomal RNAs that have been known since the 1950s, non-coding RNAs (ncRNAs) form a large and heterogenous class of RNA species involved in the regulation of gene expression. Non-coding RNAs are classified according to their length, localization and/or function into long non-coding RNAs (lncRNAs), microRNAs (miRNAs), small interfering RNAs (siRNAs), small nucleolar RNAs (snoRNAs), small nuclear RNAs (snRNAs) and PIWI-interacting RNAs (piRNAs) (Figure 1) [14–17]. Given that the role of some classes of ncRNAs (including siRNAs, snoRNAs or piRNAs) in kidney fibrosis remains largely unknown, this review will be restricted to miRNAs and lncRNAs.

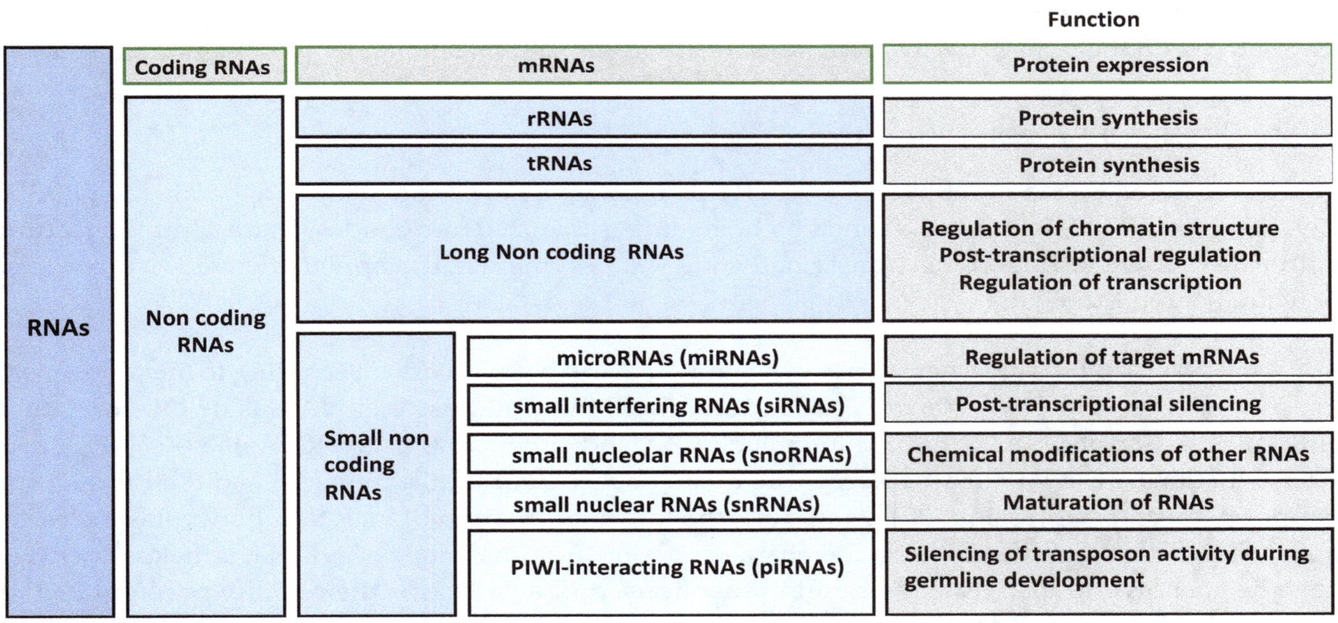

Figure 1. Classification and function of non-coding RNAs (ncRNAs).

2.1. *microRNAs (miRNAs)*

miRNAs are ncRNAs of about 22 nucleotides usually conserved between species and involved in post-transcriptional regulation of gene expression. Currently, about 2700 mature miRNAs have been identified in humans, regulating at least 60% of mRNAs (miRbase v.22.1, October 2018 [18]). As miRNAs are involved in a vast array of physiological processes, such as embryogenesis, cellular homeostasis and differentiation [19]. Their aberrant expression plays a causative role in most complex disorders such as cancer, cardio-vascular diseases and fibro-proliferative disorders [20–23].

About 60% of miRNAs are localized in intergenic regions and possess their own transcriptional unit [24]. Other miRNAs are localized in intron of coding genes and are either co-transcribed with their host genes or under the control of a specific promoter [25,26]. miRNAs are usually transcribed by RNA polymerase II into a primary transcript, termed pri-miRNA. This pri-miRNA is then processed into a pre-miRNA of about 70 nucleotides by a multiproteic complex, called microprocessor and composed of two subunits: The RNAse III endonuclease DROSHA and the RNA binding protein DGCR8 (DiGiorge Critical Region 8). The pre-miRNA is recognized by EXP5 (Exportin 5)-Ran-GTP and exported to the cytoplasm. The last step of maturation is catalyzed by the RNAse III DICER associated with TRBP (TAR RNA binding protein). The PAZ domain (PIWI-AGOZWILLE) of the complex allows the recognition and positioning of DICER, then the RNAse III domain cleaves the pre-miRNA loop, generating a 22-nucleotide miRNA duplex [27]. The association with an Argonaute protein into the RISC (RNA-induced silencing complex) allows the dissociation of the duplex [28]. The passenger strand (termed miRNA*) is then cleaved and released into the cytoplasm for degradation [29] whereas the guide strand, or mature miRNA, persists within RISC [30]. When both strands lead to a mature miRNA, they are identified by the suffix -3p or -5p depending on whether they come from the 3′ or 5′ end of their precursor.

By preferentially binding on specific sequences, called "seed" sequences, which are mainly localized in the mRNA 3′-UTR (UnTranslated Region), mature miRNAs induce the degradation of the target mRNAs if miRNA-mRNA complementarity is perfect. However, this mechanism is minor in animals. Indeed, in the majority of cases, miRNAs regulate the expression levels of their target mRNAs by the recruitment of protein partners responsible for the activation of de-adenylation and de-capping associated with the 5′-to-3′ decay of mRNAs and possibly to translational repression mechanisms [30].

2.2. Long Non-Coding RNAs (lncRNAs)

In the human genome, about 30,000 lncRNA transcripts have been identified to date (GENCODE v29, [31]). LncRNAs, which are defined by being larger than 200 nucleotides, share common features with mRNAs, including being transcribed by RNA polymerase II, capped, cleaved, spliced, and polyadenylated [32,33].

LncRNA members are a heterogeneous family that can be subdivided according to their biogenesis loci into intergenic lncRNAs (lincRNAs), intronic lncRNAs, antisense lncRNAs (aslncRNA or natural antisense transcripts, NATs), bidirectional lncRNAs, and enhancer RNAs (eRNAs) [34–37] (Figure 2). Their functions are still poorly explored due to their subcellular localization [34] and their tissue- and temporal-specific expression [38]. Moreover, the low conservation of lncRNAs between species is a major obstacle to their identification and characterization in animal models [39]. Nevertheless, lncRNAs have been shown to display wide-ranging functions, probably due to their ability to bind to either DNA, RNA or protein. In particular, seminal functional studies have demonstrated their important role in the modulation of gene expression or DNA remodeling in physiological and pathological processes [32].

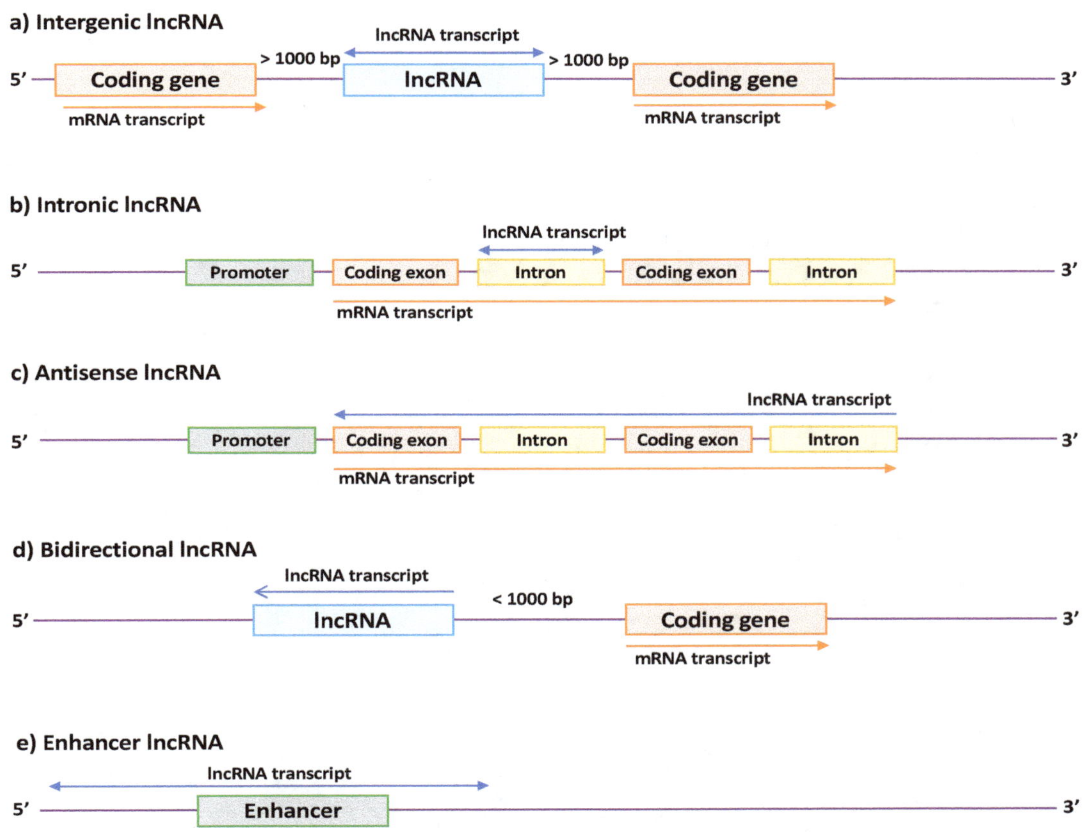

Figure 2. Classification of long non-coding RNAs (lncRNAs) according to their genomic location. (**a**) Intergenic lncRNAs are located between two coding genes; (**b**) intronic lncRNAs are transcribed entirely from introns of protein-coding genes; (**c**) antisense lncRNAs are transcribed from the antisense strand of a coding gene and overlap at least one exon; (**d**) bidirectional lncRNAs are localized within 1 kb of the promoter of a coding gene and oriented in the other direction; (**e**) enhancer lncRNAs are located in enhancer regions associated with a coding gene. Arrows indicate the direction of transcription.

3. miRNAs Implicated in Renal Fibrosis

Among the various classes of ncRNAs, miRNAs have first retained the attention of the scientific community. Many studies that focused on miRNAs in renal fibrosis have been published and allowed the identification of about thirty miRNAs with either an anti-fibrotic or pro-fibrotic effect, also called "fibromiRs" [4,40]. While Table 1 outlines publications highlighting the major role of miRNAs in renal fibrosis, we will describe more precisely the role of few particularly well-characterized miRNAs.

Table 1. Summary of miRNAs involved in renal fibrosis.

Regulation	miRNA	Models	Gene Target	References
Up	miR-21	Renal tissues from kidney transplanted patients Renal tissues from patients with IgA nephropathy Renal tissues from patients with Alport Syndrome UUO mouse model DN mouse model Ichemia reperfusion mouse model RPTEC cells Mesangial cells	PTEN, SMAD7, PPARA, PDCD4, BCL2, PHD2, MKK3, RECK, TIMP3, THSP1, RAB11A	[41–63]
	miR-22	DN rat model RPTEC cells	PTEN	[64]
	miR-135a	Serum and renal tissues from patients with DN DN mouse model Mesangial cells	TRPC1	[65]
	miR-150	renal tissue from patients with lupus nephritis RPTEC cells Mesangial cells	SOCS1	[66]
	miR-155	UUO mouse model RPTEC cells	PDE3A	[67,68]
	miR-184	UUO mouse models RPTEC cells	HIF1AN	[69]
	miR-214	UUO mouse model DN mouse model RPTEC cells Mesangial cells	DKK3, CDH1, PTEN	[70–72]
	miR-215	DN mouse model Mesangial cells	CTNNBIP1	[73]
	miR-216a	DN mouse model Mesangial cells	YBX1	[74]
	miR-324	Rat model of nephropathy (Munich Wistar Fromter rats) RPTEC cells	PREP	[75]
	miR-433	UUO mouse model RPTEC cells	AZIN1	[76]
	miR-1207	RPTEC cells Mesangial cells	G6PD, PMEPAI1, PDK1, SMAD7	[77]

Table 1. *Cont.*

Regulation	miRNA	Models	Gene Target	References
Down	let-7 family	DN mouse model RPTEC cells	HMGA2, TGFBR1	[78,79]
	miR-29 family	UUO mouse model Adenine gavage in mice Chronic renal failure rat model (5/6e nephrectomy) DN mouse model RPTEC cells Endothelial cells Podcytes HEK293 treated with ochratoxin A Renal tissues from kidney transplanted patients	COL, FN1, AGT, ADAM12, ADAM19, PIK3R2	[80–88]
	miR-30	UUO mouse model DN mouse model RPTEC cells	CTGF, KLF11, UCP2	[89–91]
	miR-34 family	UUO mouse model RPTEC cells	NOTCH1/JAG1	[92]
	miR-152	RPTEC cells	HPIP	[93]
	miR-181	UUO mouse model	EGR1	[94]
	miR-194	Ischemia reperfusion mouse model RPTEC cells	RHEB	[95]
	miR-200 family	UUO mouse model Adenine gavage in mice RPTEC cells	ZEB1/2, ETS1	[96–102]
	miR-455	DN rat model RPTEC cells Mesangial cells	ROCK2	[103]
Down/Up (controversial)	miR-192	UUO mouse model DN mouse model IgA nephropathy mouse model RPTEC cells	ZEB1/2	[104–109]

Abbreviations: UUO (ureteral unilateral obstruction); RPTEC (renal proximal tubular epithelial cells); DN (diabetic nephropathy).

3.1. miR-21

A large number of studies have emphasized the role of miR-21 in tissue fibrosis, notably in pulmonary [110], cardiac [111] or renal fibrosis [42]. The miR-21 gene locus is located within the *TMEM49* gene coding for Vacuole Membrane Protein 1 [112]. Interestingly, while miR-21 is one of the most highly expressed miRNAs in the healthy kidney [11], studies suggest that loss of miR-21 has no effect on development or healthy tissue function. This could be explained by its sequestration into an intracellular compartment. Nevertheless, in various stress conditions, miR-21 could be released into the cytoplasm to exert its regulatory functions [42,113]. In different experimental models such as the renal fibrosis (unilateral ureteral obstruction (UUO) mouse model, acute kidney injury (ischemia-reperfusion model) or diabetic nephropathy (*db/db* mice, streptozotocine-induced diabetes)), miR-21 is highly expressed in injured kidney regions [41,42,53,57]. Overexpression of miR-21 was also confirmed in renal allograft biopsies, in renal tissues of patients with IgA nephropathy or with Alport Syndrome exhibiting severe fibrotic injuries, particularly in regions enriched in fibroblasts/myofibroblasts, in the tubular epithelium and glomeruli [58–60]. The deleterious role of miR-21 in renal fibrosis was further explored using miR-21 null mice. Following UUO or ischemia-reperfusion injuries, miR-21$^{-/-}$ mice exhibited less fibrosis. Moreover, authors showed that miR-21 is also involved in lipid metabolism and mitochondrial redox regulation [42]. While only a limited number of miR-21 target genes have been experimentally validated, miR-21 has been demonstrated to be involved in the regulation of critical signaling pathways related to fibrogenesis such as cellular proliferation (PTEN) [61], apoptosis (PDCD4, Bcl2) [43,62,63], regulation of cellular metabolism (PPARα, PHD2) [44–46], inflammation (MKK3) [47,48], ECM components (Reck, TIMP3) [49–52], TGF-β signaling pathway (Smad7) [54], angiogenesis (Reck, THSP-1, PHD2) [46,49,50,55] and autophagy (Rab11a) [56].

3.2. miR-214

miR-214 has been shown to act as a fibromiR in several types of tissue fibrosis, including liver [114] and heart fibrosis [115]. miR-214 has been also consistently associated with renal fibrosis. It is in particular upregulated by the activation of the transcription factor TWIST in response to hypoxia in renal tubular epithelial cells [71]. Moreover, Denby et al., using miR-214 null mice and the UUO model of kidney fibrosis, showed that miR-214 promotes renal fibrosis independently of TGF-β pathway [116]. Similarly, treatment with an antagonist of miR-214 before UUO protected against fibrogenesis without blocking Smad2/Smad3 activation and TGF-β signaling [116]. Other studies have mechanistically linked miR-214 pro-fibrotic function with the targeting of DKK3 (Wnt/β -catenin pathway) [72], CDH1 (EMT) [71] or PTEN (proliferation) [70].

3.3. miR-200 Family

Members of the miR-200 family include five members organized into two clusters, miR-200b/a/429 and miR-200c/141 [117,118]. In animal models of renal fibrosis either induced by UUO or gavage with adenine, miR-200 family members are consistently downregulated [98,99]. Indeed, the anti-fibrotic role of these miRNAs is mainly associated with epithelial differentiation [100] by protecting renal tubular cells from EMT process through the direct regulation of ZEB1/2 (zinc finger E-box-Binding homeobox proteins 1/2) and Ets-1 transcription factors [81,101–103]. Of note, miR-200 family is also involved in TGF-β signaling pathway by modulating TGF-β2 [98].

3.4. *miR-29 Family*

miR-29 family is composed of three members: miR-29a, miR-29b and miR-29c [119]. Expression of miR-29abc is invariably downregulated during fibrosis and their low expression is associated with the up-regulation of ECM-related genes [80]. In fact, decreased expression of miR-29 family members is a general downstream molecular event of TGF-β signaling, which is essential for the release of ECM components by fibroblasts, as miR-29 family members directly target multiple collagen isoforms and other ECM components [81–83].

In various animal models of renal fibrosis, expression of miR-29 members is downregulated regardless of the cause of injury [84,85]. Interestingly, TGF-β inhibited miR-29 expression not only in renal fibroblasts, but also in mesangial cells, epithelial cells and podocytes [85], suggesting that miR-29abc exert also an anti-fibrotic function in non-fibroblastic renal cells. For example, both Adam12 and Adam19 represent two pro-fibrotic targets of miR-29abc in renal tubular epithelial cells [84]. Similarly, Hu et al. showed that miR-29 targets, in renal tubular epithelial cells, PIK3R2, an effector of PI3K/AKT signaling pathway involved in EMT induced by Angiotensin II [86]. Nevertheless, the precise contribution of miR-29abc during fibrosis in non-stromal cells remains to be clarified, especially as Long et al. reported an increased expression of miR-29c in both podocytes and endothelial cells in a mouse model of diabetic nephropathy [87].

3.5. *miR-192*

Data regarding the role of miR-192 in renal fibrosis are currently controversial. In fact, miR-192 is upregulated in various mouse models of CKD such as diabetic nephropathy, UUO and IgA nephropathy [105–108]. In line with this, treatment with an antagonist of miR-192 protected against fibrosis through induction of Zeb1/2 in diabetic nephropathy mouse model [105]. By contrast, other studies have reported in vitro in renal cells exposed to TGF-β, in a mouse model of diabetic nephropathy as well as in renal tissue from patients exhibiting severe renal fibrotic lesions a downregulation of miR-192 [108,109]. Overall, data highlighting the versatile role of miR-192 in renal fibrosis represent a relevant example of the complexity of miRNA regulation mechanisms.

4. Long Non-Coding RNAs Implicated in Renal Fibrosis

Even if elucidation of the role of lncRNAs is still ongoing, it is now accepted that besides their involvement in physiological processes such as organ development, immunity or homeostasis, their modulation can occur in chronic multifactorial diseases [35].

In the context of fibrosis, few examples showing their pro-fibrotic role have been documented, such as MALAT1 in cardiac fibrosis, H19 and DNM3os in lung fibrosis, and MALAT1, lnc-LFAR1 and HIF1A-AS1 in liver fibrosis [120–125]. Although studies about lncRNAs and renal fibrosis are quite recent, their number has significantly increased in recent years. In particular, emerging data show that various lncRNAs are involved in renal fibrosis by playing a pro- or anti-fibrotic role (Table 2). Although many studies have shown a deregulation of lncRNA expression, we chose to only focus on mechanistic studies.

Table 2. LncRNAs involved in kidney fibrosis.

Regulation	lncRNA	Models	Functions/Mechanisms	Consequences	References
Up	**LOC105375913**	**Renal tissue of patients with segmental glomeruloscleoris RPTEC cells**	**Binding to miR-27b and leading to Snail expression**	**Pro-fibrotic**	[126]
	LINC00667	**Renal tissue of patients with chronic renal failure Chronic renal failure rat model (partial nephrectomy) RPTEC cells**	**Binding to Ago2, targeting miR-19b-3p**	**Pro-fibrotic**	[127]
	NEAT1	DN rat model Mesangial cells		Pro-fibrotic and increase of proliferation	[128]
	Lnc-TSI (AP000695.6 or ENST00000429588.1)	**RPTEC cells UUO mouse model Ischemia-reperfusion mouse model Renal tissue of patients with IgA nephropathy**	**Synergic binding to Smad3**	**Anti-fibrotic**	[129]
	HOTAIR	**UUO rat model RPTEC cells**	**Acting as a ceRNA with miR-124: activation of Jagged1/Nocth1 signaling**	**Pro-fibrotic**	[130,131]
	LINC00963	**Chronic renal failure rat model (5/6e nephrectomy)**	**Inhibition of FoxO signaling pathway by targeting FoxO3a**	**Pro-fibrotic**	[132]
	TCONS_00088786	UUO mouse model RPTEC cells	Possibly regulation of miR-132 expression	Pro-fibrotic	[133]
	Errb4-IR (np-5318)	**UUO mouse model Anti GBM mouse model RPTEC cells DN mouse model Mesangial cells**	**Downstream of TGFb/Smad3 pathway by binding Smad7 gene Binding to miR-29b**	**Pro-fibrotic**	[134–136]
	CHCHD4P4	Stone kidney mouse model RPTEC cells		Pro-fibrotic	[137]
	TCONS_00088786	UUO rat model RPTEC cells		Pro-fibrotic	[138]
	TCONS_01496394	UUO rat model RPTEC cells		Pro-fibrotic	[138]
	ASncmtRNA-2	DN mouse model Mesangial cells		Pro-fibrotic	[139]
	LincRNA-Gm4419	**DN mouse model Mesangial cells**	**Activation of NFkB/NLRP3 pathway by interacting with p50**	**Pro-fibrotic and pro-inflammatory**	[140,141]
	H19	**UUO mouse model RPTEC cells**	**Acting as a ceRNA with miR-17 and fibronectin mRNA**	**Pro-fibrotic**	[142]

Table 2. *Cont.*

Regulation	lncRNA	Models	Functions/Mechanisms	Consequences	References
	RP23.45G16.5	UUO mouse model RPTEC cells		Pro-fibrotic	[143]
	AI662270	UUO mouse model RPTEC cells		No significative effect	[143]
	Arid2-IR (np-28496)	**UUO mouse model RPTEC cells**	**Smad3 binding site in Arid2-IR promoter Promoting NF-κB signaling**	**Pro-fibrotic and pro-inflammatory effects**	[144]
	np-17856	UUO mouse model Glomerulonephritis mouse model	Smad3 binding site	Pro-fibrotic and pro-inflammatory	[134]
	NR_033515	**Serum of patients with diabetic nephropathy Mesangial cells**	**Targeting miR-743b-5p**	**Pro-fibrotic and promotes proliferation**	[145]
	MALAT1	**DN mouse model Podocytes**	**Binding to SRSF1 Targeting by β-catenin**	**Pro-fibrotic**	[146]
	Gm5524	DN mouse model Podocytes		Autophagy increase and apoptosis decrease	[147]
	WISP1-AS1	RPTEC cells	Modulating ochratoxin-A-induced Egr-1 and E2F activities	Cell viability increase	[148]
Down	Gm15645	DN mouse model Podocytes		Autophagy decrease and apoptosis increase	[147]
	CYP4B1-PS1-001 (ENSMUST00000118753)	**DN mouse model Mesangial cells**	**Enhancing ubiquitination and degradation of nucleolin**	**Anti-fibrotic and anti-proliferative**	[149,150]
	3110045C21Rik	UUO mouse model RPTEC cells		Anti-fibrotic	[143]
	ENSMUST00000147869	DN mouse model Mesangial cells	Associated with Cyp4a12a	Anti-fibrotic and anti-proliferative	[151]
	lincRNA 1700020I24Rik (ENSMUSG00000085438)	**DN mouse model Mesangial cells**	**Binding to miR-34a-5p. Inhibition of Sirt1/ HIF-1α signal pathway by targeting miR-34a-5p.**	**Anti-fibrotic**	[152]
	MEG3	**RPTEC cells**		**Anti-fibrotic**	[153]
	ZEB1-AS1	**DN mouse model RPTEC cells**	**Promoting Zeb1 expression by binding H3K4 Methyltransferase MLL1**	**Anti-fibrotic**	[154]
	ENST00000453774.1	**Renal tissue of patients with renal fibrosis UUO mouse model RPTEC cells**		**Anti-fibrotic**	[155]

Note: Studies in bold are mechanistic studies. Abbreviations: UUO (ureteral unilateral obstruction); RPTEC (renal proximal tubular epithelial cells); DN (diabetic nephropathy)

4.1. *Errb4-IR*

LncRNA Errb4-IR (np_5318), located in the ERBB4 intron region between the first and second exons, has been associated with renal fibrosis [134,135]. In the UUO mouse model, Errb4-IR was upregulated and strongly expressed in interstitial fibroblasts and injured tubular epithelial cells. Errb4-IR upregulation was also associated with fibrotic marker expression such as α-SMA or Collagen I. Moreover, in vivo silencing of Errb4-IR in the UUO mouse model significantly decreased fibrotic injuries [135]. Feng et al. also assessed the mechanisms underlying the fibrogenic role of Errb4-IR and showed that, in addition to being induced by TGF-β/Smad3 signaling, Errb4-IR directly targets Smad7, which exerts anti-fibrotic functions [135]. The pathological role of Errb4-IR in renal fibrosis was further confirmed in the context of diabetic nephropathy [136] by demonstrating that Errb4-IR also targets miR-29b, a well-established anti-fibrotic miRNA.

4.2. *HOTAIR*

HOTAIR (HOX transcript antisense intergenic RNA), embedded in the HOXC locus, is known to drive cancerogenesis [156]. Recently, two studies have demonstrated that HOTAIR is upregulated in renal fibrosis. In the UUO rat model, HOTAIR overexpression was associated with an upregulation of fibrotic and EMT markers as well as with a downregulation of miR-124, a miRNA involved in EMT and acting as a negative regulator of Nocth1 signaling pathway [130,131]. Moreover, lentiviral-mediated overexpression of HOTAIR in UUO rats, led to more severe injuries, such as inflammation, necrosis and collagen deposits, an elevated score of renal fibrosis and an overexpression of fibrotic markers compared to UUO alone. Mechanistically, it has been shown that HOTAIR activates the Notch1/Jagged1 signaling pathway by acting as a ceRNA (competing endogenous RNA—an lncRNA–miRNA duplex which prevents binding miRNA to its target and thus the target inhibition) with miR-124, which targets Notch1 and JAG1, and thereby promotes renal fibrosis [157,158].

4.3. *Gm4419*

In diabetic nephropathy, lincRNA Gm4419 was found to be involved in renal fibrosis. More precisely, in mesangial cells in high glucose conditions, overexpression of GM4419 was associated with fibrosis, inflammation and cell proliferation. Authors demonstrated that the NF-κB signaling pathway, which plays an important role in fibrogenesis and inflammation [140], was activated by GM4419 by interacting with its subunit p50. Moreover, p50 and GM4419 could have a synergistic effect in the inflammatory pathway [141].

5. New Therapeutic Targets and Innovative Biomarkers

5.1. *New Therapeutic Targets*

To date, the lack of specific anti-fibrotic therapies remains a critical need in clinical practice. As ncRNAs are involved in many critical pathogenic processes driving renal fibrosis, they represent attractive therapeutic targets. Currently, two strategies can be applied to manipulate ncRNA expression levels: The first relies on restoring the expression of a ncRNA when its level is decreased, the second is related to inhibiting the function of a ncRNA when its expression is increased.

5.1.1. miRNAs as Therapeutic Targets

To restore miRNA function, miRNA mimics or pre-miRNA have been developed. A modified synthetic RNA is introduced into cells as a duplex consisting of one strand identical to the mature miRNA of interest (guide strand) and the second antisense strand with a lower stability [159]. In addition, chemical modifications such as 2′-Fluoro bases have been developed to increase the stability of the guide strand without interfering with the RISC complex [160]. Other modifications include the use of 5′-O-methyl bases on the second strand to limit its incorporation into RISC complex [161]. Finally, addition of cholesterol-like molecules improves the duplex cellular internalization [159]. Although the use of such tools is widely developed for in vitro models, their application in vivo is hampered by delivery [11]. Other approaches involved gene therapy techniques, using notably AAV-mediated miRNA delivery (adeno-associated virus). Indeed, AAVs allow the restoration of the physiological expression level of miRNA with low toxicity and without integration into the genome in a specific tissue or cellular type [159,162].

Such strategies have been successfully applied in preclinical mouse models of tissue fibrosis, including bleomycin-induced lung fibrosis, but still need to be evaluated in the context of kidney fibrosis [163]. The renal tissue is indeed accessible to AAV gene delivery by different routes, including injection through the renal artery, injection into the parenchyma and retrograde injection via the ureter.

Concerning miRNA inhibition, several strategies have been developed, especially antisense oligonucleotides (termed antimiRs) which are widely used in preclinical models of tissue fibrosis and have also entered clinical trials [164]. These molecules are also chemically modified in order to improve their affinity, pharmacokinetics, stability and cellular entrance. The major modifications include the addition on the ribose of particular groups such as 2′O-Methyl, 2′O-Methoxyethyl or 2′-Fluoro and also inclusion of bicyclic structures which lock the ribose into its preferred 3′ endo conformation and increase base-pairing affinity such as methylene bridging group, also known as LNA (locked nucleic acid). Such ribose modifications allow a reduction in the size of antimiRs without loss of affinity and specificity. Finally, backbone modifications such as phosphorothioate linkages or the addition of morpholino structures enhance nuclease resistance [165].

Finally, target site blockers (TSB) inhibit miRNA function by specifically preventing interaction between a miRNA and its target [166,167]. One advantage of this strategy relies on its specificity, as it does not affect expression of the other target genes, and thus reduces the risk of side effects.

In the context of renal fibrosis, proof-of-concept for miRNA targeting has been demonstrated for several fibromiRs. In particular, results indicated that miR-214 antagonism was associated with less fibrotic lesions in the UUO mouse model [116]. In addition, an miR-21 antagonism injection prevented fibrotic injuries in UUO [42], diabetic nephropathy [168] or Alport [169] mouse models. Moreover, Regulus Therapeutics has developed a phase II clinical trial with a miR-21 antagonist in patients with Alport syndrome (RG-012; Regulus Therapeutics Inc.; clinical trial: NCT02855268). This drug candidate has currently received the orphan drug status from the FDA and the European Commission for the treatment of this rare disease.

5.1.2. lncRNAs as Therapeutic Targets

LncRNA deregulation is also viewed as an important driver of renal fibrosis, suggesting their potential value as therapeutic targets. Given their extensive secondary structures and their localization in nuclear and/or cytoplasmic compartments [15,34], pharmacological modulation of lncRNAs is more complex and, until recently, the options for targeting lncRNAs were limited. Moreover, the low conservation of lncRNAs between species is a major obstacle for preclinical validation [39,170]. However, recently, conceptual and technological advances in antisense oligonucleotide therapy offer new pharmacological options to modulate the expression or the function of lncRNAs. For example, the development of technologies including GapmeR-mediated lncRNA silencing, CRISPR inhibition or aptamers directed against lncRNA secondary structure represent novel opportunities to improve lncRNA knowledge and clinical translation [171].

In the context of renal fibrosis, lncRNA modulation remains an almost unexplored area. However, Kato et al. have used GapmeRs, an antisense oligonucleotide technology that induces target degradation in the nuclear compartment by recruiting RNAse H [172], in a mouse model of diabetic nephropathy. Interestingly, injection of such GapmeRs against lnc-MGG induced a decreased expression of profibrotic genes (TGF-β1, Col1a2, Col4a1, Ctgf) and prevented glomerular fibrosis, podocyte death and hypertrophy in diabetic mice [173]. Otherwise, few studies have investigated the opportunity to downregulate lncRNA expression using short hairpin RNAs (shRNAs) by delivery of plasmids or through viral or bacterial vectors in vivo [174]. Indeed, targeting of Errb4-IR was shown to improve renal fibrosis in the *db/db* mouse model [136]. Moreover, in a UUO mouse model, Arid2-IR was also successfully inhibited by a shRNA [144].

6. Biomarkers

Histological examination of biopsied tissue is considered the reference method for the diagnosis and staging of kidney fibrosis [8]. However, as percutaneous tissue sampling of either native kidney or allograft remains associated with patient discomfort, risk for complications, histopathological interpretation variability and high cost [175], the development of alternative non-invasive diagnostic or prognostic biomarkers is an important clinical issue [176]. Interestingly, ncRNAs that have been extensively reported to be dysregulated in fibrotic tissues, have also been detected in a large panel of human biological fluids including serum, plasma and urine [177–179].

6.1. *miRNAs*

In order to discover relevant biomarkers, miRNA profiling in several biofluids has been performed. Urine is a particularly interesting matrix to explore kidney function, even if miRNAs in urine are less abundant than in plasma or serum, since RNase activity has been reported to be quite high in urine [180]. Cardenas-Gonzalez et al. have screened more than 2000 urinary miRNAs from patients with CKD. In particular, this study demonstrated that downregulation of miR-2861, miR-1915-3p and miR-4532 was associated with a poorer renal function, interstitial fibrosis and tubular atrophy in diabetic nephropathy [181]. Another study profiled more than 1800 miRNAs in urine samples from patients with acute kidney injury. Among the 378 detected miRNAs, 19 were upregulated in patients with acute kidney injury, including miR-21, miR-200c and miR-423 [182]. Sonoda et al. showed that miR-9a, miR-141, miR-200a, miR-200c and miR-429 from exosomes in rat urine were upregulated following ischemia-reperfusion injury [183]. Moreover, Khurana et al. identified nine upregulated miRNAs (let-7c-5p, miR-222–3p, miR-27a-3p, miR-27b-3p, miR-296-5p, miR-31-5p, miR-3687, miR-6769b-5p and miR-877-3p) and seven downregulated miRNAs (miR-133a, miR-133b, miR-15a-5p, miR-181a-5p, miR-34a-5p, miR-181c-5p and miR1-2) in urine exosomes from patients with CKD compared to healthy controls [184]. Finally, other studies showed that dysregulation of urinary miR-29c, miR-21 and miR-200b was correlated with renal fibrotic injuries in patients with CKD or in renal transplanted patients [185–187]. Altogether, these data indicate that detection of miRNAs in the urine could reflect the degree of the renal aggression [188].

Finally, miRNAs were also detectable in serum and, more specifically, in renal transplanted patients serum level expression of miR-21 was found to be associated with the severity of renal fibrosis injuries [58,189,190]. While promising, the clinical use of circulating miRNAs as biomarkers remains tempered by quality control and normalization issues. For example, hemolysis needs to be perfectly avoided since miRNAs can be released from blood cells, thus affecting the amount of detected circulating miRNAs [191]. Furthermore, no standard endogenous control to normalize circulating miRNA levels has been clearly established and this concern is still debated [192,193]. The development of new technologies such as digital PCR (dPCR) are particularly interesting as this approach allows an absolute quantification without internal normalization [194,195].

6.2. *lncRNAs*

Although the expression of many lncRNAs has been evaluated in the context of fibrosis, their validation as biomarkers is at an earlier stage than miRNAs. Nevertheless, identifying novel lncRNAs as biomarkers is of great interest, since lncRNAs are highly stable in biofluids, especially when they are included in exosomes or in apoptotic bodies [179] and could be present in extracellular vesicles [196]. In renal fibrosis, Sun et al. compared the lncRNA profile in renal tissues and urines of UUO rats. Seven lncRNAs (five upregulated and two downregulated) were similarly modulated in renal tissues and urine. In addition, several conserved Smad3 binding motifs were identified in the sequence of the five upregulated lncRNAs [138]. Altogether, these results raise the possibility of using urinary lncRNAs as non-invasive biomarkers of renal fibrosis. Otherwise, Gao et al. found that in the serum of patients with diabetic nephropathy, the upregulation of lncRNA NR_033515 was correlated with NGAL and KIM1 serum levels, and the severity of the disease [145]. While both of these studies highlighted the potential of lncRNAs as non-invasive biomarkers for renal fibrosis, further studies are clearly required for the robust identification and validation of diagnostic and prognostic biomarkers.

7. Future Directions

NcRNAs, including the well-known miRNAs and the emerging lncRNAs, have been described to be implicated in a large number of physiological and pathological processes (Figure 3). In particular, their modulation between normal and fibrotic renal tissues not only strongly suggests that ncRNAs are involved in the development and the progression of kidney fibrosis, but also that ncRNAs may represent promising biomarkers. However, in contrast to miRNAs, the underlying mechanisms of most of the identified lncRNAs are yet to be determined. Considering both technological advances and rising scientific enthusiasm in lncRNA biology, we foresee that major discoveries will soon be achieved regarding the role of lncRNAs in kidney fibrosis.

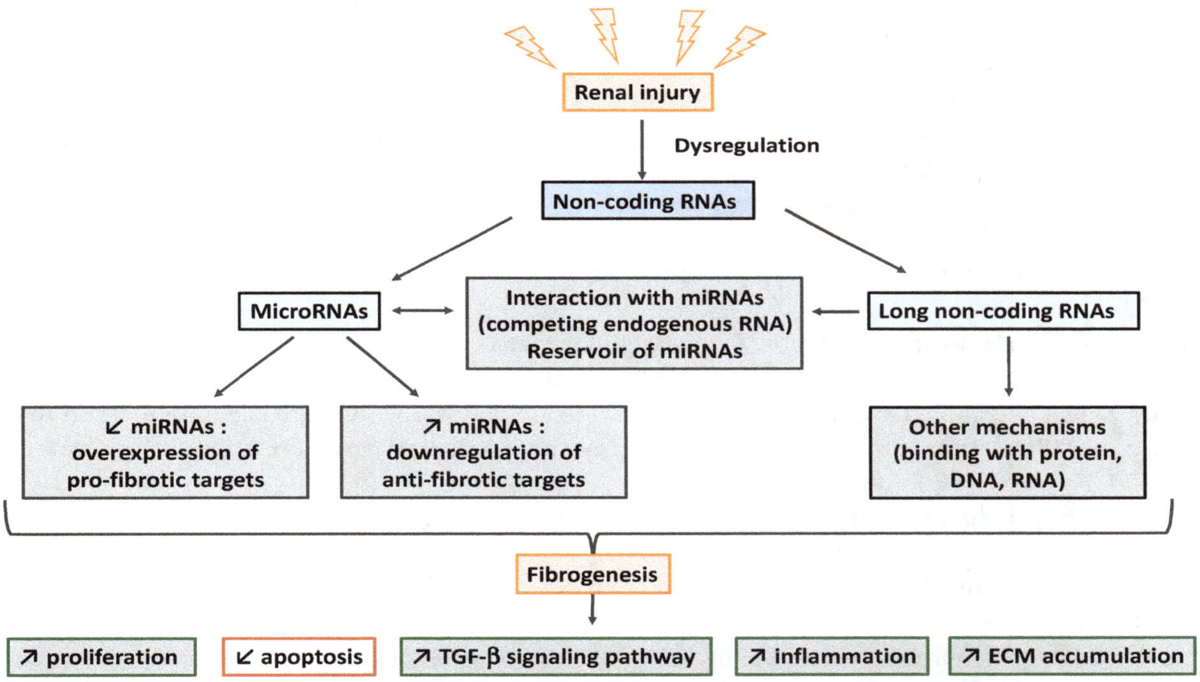

Figure 3. General mechanisms of non-coding RNAs involved in kidney fibrosis.

The proof of concept of ncRNA expression modulation to treat fibroproliferative disorders has been elegantly demonstrated. Clinical translation of these potential new therapeutic targets should be considered a research priority and will undoubtedly represent a gold mine of new therapeutic targets that may lead to the development of novel anti-fibrotics.

Author Contributions: Original draft preparation, C.V.d.H.; writing, C.V.d.H. and C.C.; review and editing, C.V.d.H., C.C., N.P. and F.G.

Abbreviations

AAV	Adeno-associated-virus
ceRNA	Competing endogenous RNA
CKD	Chronic kidney disease
DN	Diabetic nephropathy
ECM	Extracellular matrix
FDA	Food and Drug Administration
HOTAIR	HOX transcript antisense intergenic RNA
lncRNA	Long non-coding RNA
miRNA	microRNA
ncRNA	non-coding RNA
RISC	RNA-induced silencing complex
RPTEC	Renal proximal tubular epithelial cell
shRNA	Short hairpin RNA
UUO	Ureteral unilateral obstruction

References

1. Jha, V.; Garcia-Garcia, G.; Iseki, K.; Li, Z.; Naicker, S.; Plattner, B.; Saran, R.; Wang, A.Y.-M.; Yang, C.-W. Chronic kidney disease: Global dimension and perspectives. *Lancet* **2013**, *382*, 260–272. [CrossRef]
2. Klinkhammer, B.M.; Goldschmeding, R.; Floege, J.; Boor, P. Treatment of renal fibrosis—turning challenges into opportunities. *Adv. Chronic Kidney Dis.* **2017**, *24*, 117–129. [CrossRef]
3. Friedman, S.L.; Sheppard, D.; Duffield, J.S.; Violette, S. Therapy for fibrotic diseases: Nearing the starting line. *Sci. Transl. Med.* **2013**, *5*, 167sr1. [CrossRef]
4. Pottier, N.; Cauffiez, C.; Perrais, M.; Barbry, P.; Mari, B. FibromiRs: Translating molecular discoveries into new anti-fibrotic drugs. *Trends Pharmacol. Sci.* **2014**, *35*, 119–126. [CrossRef] [PubMed]
5. Gurtner, G.C.; Werner, S.; Barrandon, Y.; Longaker, M.T. Wound repair and regeneration. *Nature* **2008**, *453*, 314–321. [CrossRef]
6. Lu, P.; Takai, K.; Weaver, V.M.; Werb, Z. Extracellular matrix degradation and remodeling in development and disease. *Cold Spring Harb. Perspect. Biol.* **2011**, *3*, a005058. [CrossRef]
7. Levey, A.S.; Bosch, J.P.; Lewis, J.B.; Greene, T.; Rogers, N.; Roth, D. A more accurate method to estimate glomerular filtration rate from serum creatinine: A new prediction equation. *Ann. Intern. Med.* **1999**, *130*, 461–470. [CrossRef] [PubMed]
8. Berchtold, L.; Friedli, I.; Vallée, J.-P.; Moll, S.; Martin, P.-Y.; de Seigneux, S. Diagnosis and assessment of renal fibrosis: The state of the art. *Swiss Med. Wkly.* **2017**, *147*, w14442.
9. Chung, A.C.-K.; Lan, H.Y. MicroRNAs in renal fibrosis. *Front. Physiol.* **2015**, *6*, 50. [CrossRef] [PubMed]
10. Van der Hauwaert, C.; Savary, G.; Hennino, M.-F.; Pottier, N.; Glowacki, F.; Cauffiez, C. Implication des microARN dans la fibrose rénale. *Nephrol. Ther.* **2015**, *11*, 474–482. [CrossRef] [PubMed]
11. Gomez, I.G.; Nakagawa, N.; Duffield, J.S. MicroRNAs as novel therapeutic targets to treat kidney injury and fibrosis. *Am. J. Physiol. Renal Physiol.* **2016**, *310*, F931–F944. [CrossRef]
12. Moghaddas Sani, H.; Hejazian, M.; Hosseinian Khatibi, S.M.; Ardalan, M.; Zununi Vahed, S. Long non-coding RNAs: An essential emerging field in kidney pathogenesis. *Biomed. Pharmacother.* **2018**, *99*, 755–765. [CrossRef]
13. Jiang, X.; Zhang, F. Long noncoding RNA: A new contributor and potential therapeutic target in fibrosis. *Epigenomics* **2017**, *9*, 1233–1241. [CrossRef]
14. Cech, T.R.; Steitz, J.A. The noncoding RNA revolution—Trashing old rules to forge new ones. *Cell* **2014**, *157*, 77–94. [CrossRef]
15. Esteller, M. Non-coding RNAs in human disease. *Nat. Rev. Genet.* **2011**, *12*, 861–874. [CrossRef]
16. Ulitsky, I.; Bartel, D.P. lincRNAs: Genomics, evolution, and mechanisms. *Cell* **2013**, *154*, 26–46. [CrossRef]
17. Shi, X.; Sun, M.; Liu, H.; Yao, Y.; Song, Y. Long non-coding RNAs: A new frontier in the study of human diseases. *Cancer Lett.* **2013**, *339*, 159–166. [CrossRef] [PubMed]
18. Kozomara, A.; Birgaoanu, M.; Griffiths-Jones, S. miRBase: From microRNA sequences to function. *Nucleic Acids Res.* **2019**, *47*, D155–D162. [CrossRef]

19. Bartel, D.P. MicroRNAs: Target recognition and regulatory functions. *Cell* **2009**, *136*, 215–233. [CrossRef] [PubMed]
20. Croce, C.M.; Calin, G.A. miRNAs, Cancer, and stem cell division. *Cell* **2005**, *122*, 6–7. [CrossRef]
21. Small, E.M.; Olson, E.N. Pervasive roles of microRNAs in cardiovascular biology. *Nature* **2011**, *469*, 336–342. [CrossRef]
22. Li, G.; Zhou, R.; Zhang, Q.; Jiang, B.; Wu, Q.; Wang, C. Fibroproliferative effect of microRNA-21 in hypertrophic scar derived fibroblasts. *Exp. Cell Res.* **2016**, *345*, 93–99. [CrossRef] [PubMed]
23. Bowen, T.; Jenkins, R.H.; Fraser, D.J. MicroRNAs, transforming growth factor beta-1, and tissue fibrosis. *J. Pathol.* **2013**, *229*, 274–285. [CrossRef]
24. Corcoran, D.L.; Pandit, K.V.; Gordon, B.; Bhattacharjee, A.; Kaminski, N.; Benos, P.V. Features of mammalian microRNA promoters emerge from polymerase II chromatin immunoprecipitation data. *PLoS ONE* **2009**, *4*, e5279. [CrossRef]
25. Baskerville, S.; Bartel, D.P. Microarray profiling of microRNAs reveals frequent coexpression with neighboring miRNAs and host genes. *RNA* **2005**, *11*, 241–247. [CrossRef]
26. Ozsolak, F.; Poling, L.L.; Wang, Z.; Liu, H.; Liu, X.S.; Roeder, R.G.; Zhang, X.; Song, J.S.; Fisher, D.E. Chromatin structure analyses identify miRNA promoters. *Genes Dev.* **2008**, *22*, 3172–3183. [CrossRef] [PubMed]
27. Park, J.-E.; Heo, I.; Tian, Y.; Simanshu, D.K.; Chang, H.; Jee, D.; Patel, D.J.; Kim, V.N. Dicer recognizes the 5′ end of RNA for efficient and accurate processing. *Nature* **2011**, *475*, 201–205. [CrossRef]
28. Su, H.; Trombly, M.I.; Chen, J.; Wang, X. Essential and overlapping functions for mammalian Argonautes in microRNA silencing. *Genes Dev.* **2009**, *23*, 304–317. [CrossRef]
29. Liu, X.; Jin, D.-Y.; McManus, M.T.; Mourelatos, Z. Precursor microRNA-programmed silencing complex assembly pathways in mammals. *Mol. Cell* **2012**, *46*, 507–517. [CrossRef]
30. Jonas, S.; Izaurralde, E. Towards a molecular understanding of microRNA-mediated gene silencing. *Nat. Rev. Genet.* **2015**, *16*, 421–433. [CrossRef] [PubMed]
31. Frankish, A.; Diekhans, M.; Ferreira, A.-M.; Johnson, R.; Jungreis, I.; Loveland, J.; Mudge, J.M.; Sisu, C.; Wright, J.; Armstrong, J.; et al. GENCODE reference annotation for the human and mouse genomes. *Nucleic Acids Res.* **2019**, *47*, D766–D773. [CrossRef]
32. Quinn, J.J.; Chang, H.Y. Unique features of long non-coding RNA biogenesis and function. *Nat. Rev. Genet.* **2016**, *17*, 47–62. [CrossRef]
33. Bunch, H. Gene regulation of mammalian long non-coding RNA. *Mol. Genet. Genomics* **2018**, *293*, 1–15. [CrossRef] [PubMed]
34. Chen, L.-L. Linking long noncoding RNA localization and function. *Trends Biochem. Sci.* **2016**, *41*, 761–772. [CrossRef]
35. Kung, J.T.Y.; Colognori, D.; Lee, J.T. Long noncoding RNAs: Past, present, and future. *Genetics* **2013**, *193*, 651–669. [CrossRef]
36. Derrien, T.; Johnson, R.; Bussotti, G.; Tanzer, A.; Djebali, S.; Tilgner, H.; Guernec, G.; Martin, D.; Merkel, A.; Knowles, D.G.; et al. The GENCODE v7 catalog of human long noncoding RNAs: Analysis of their gene structure, evolution, and expression. *Genome Res.* **2012**, *22*, 1775–1789. [CrossRef]
37. Devaux, Y.; Zangrando, J.; Schroen, B.; Creemers, E.E.; Pedrazzini, T.; Chang, C.-P.; Dorn, G.W.; Thum, T.; Heymans, S.; Cardiolinc Network. Long noncoding RNAs in cardiac development and ageing. *Nat. Rev. Cardiol.* **2015**, *12*, 415–425.
38. Ward, M.; McEwan, C.; Mills, J.D.; Janitz, M. Conservation and tissue-specific transcription patterns of long noncoding RNAs. *J. Hum. Transcript.* **2015**, *1*, 2–9. [CrossRef]
39. Ulitsky, I. Evolution to the rescue: Using comparative genomics to understand long non-coding RNAs. *Nat. Rev. Genet.* **2016**, *17*, 601–614. [CrossRef] [PubMed]
40. Lv, W.; Fan, F.; Wang, Y.; Gonzalez-Fernandez, E.; Wang, C.; Yang, L.; Booz, G.W.; Roman, R.J. Therapeutic potential of microRNAs for the treatment of renal fibrosis and CKD. *Physiol. Genomics* **2018**, *50*, 20–34. [CrossRef] [PubMed]
41. Zarjou, A.; Yang, S.; Abraham, E.; Agarwal, A.; Liu, G. Identification of a microRNA signature in renal fibrosis: Role of miR-21. *Am. J. Physiol. Renal Physiol.* **2011**, *301*, F793–F801. [CrossRef]
42. Chau, B.N.; Xin, C.; Hartner, J.; Ren, S.; Castano, A.P.; Linn, G.; Li, J.; Tran, P.T.; Kaimal, V.; Huang, X.; et al. MicroRNA-21 promotes fibrosis of the kidney by silencing metabolic pathways. *Sci. Transl. Med.* **2012**, *4*, ra18–ra121. [CrossRef]

43. Dong, J.; Zhao, Y.-P.; Zhou, L.; Zhang, T.-P.; Chen, G. Bcl-2 upregulation induced by miR-21 Via a direct interaction is associated with apoptosis and chemoresistance in MIA PaCa-2 pancreatic cancer cells. *Arch. Med. Res.* **2011**, *42*, 8–14. [CrossRef]
44. Zhou, J.; Wang, K.-C.; Wu, W.; Subramaniam, S.; Shyy, J.Y.-J.; Chiu, J.-J.; Li, J.Y.-S.; Chien, S. MicroRNA-21 targets peroxisome proliferators-activated receptor- in an autoregulatory loop to modulate flow-induced endothelial inflammation. *Proc. Natl. Acad. Sci. USA* **2011**, *108*, 10355–10360. [CrossRef]
45. Zhang, K.; Han, L.; Chen, L.; Shi, Z.; Yang, M.; Ren, Y.; Chen, L.; Zhang, J.; Pu, P.; Kang, C. Blockage of a miR-21/EGFR regulatory feedback loop augments anti-EGFR therapy in glioblastomas. *Cancer Lett.* **2014**, *342*, 139–149. [CrossRef]
46. Jiao, X.; Xu, X.; Fang, Y.; Zhang, H.; Liang, M.; Teng, J.; Ding, X. miR-21 Contributes to renal protection by targeting prolyl hydroxylase domain protein 2 in delayed ischaemic preconditioning. *Nephrology* **2017**, *22*, 366–373. [CrossRef]
47. Xu, G.; Zhang, Y.; Wei, J.; Jia, W.; Ge, Z.; Zhang, Z.; Liu, X. MicroRNA-21 promotes hepatocellular carcinoma HepG2 cell proliferation through repression of mitogen-activated protein kinase-kinase 3. *BMC Cancer* **2013**, *13*, 469. [CrossRef]
48. Li, Z.; Deng, X.; Kang, Z.; Wang, Y.; Xia, T.; Ding, N.; Yin, Y. Elevation of miR-21, through targeting MKK3, may be involved in ischemia pretreatment protection from ischemia–reperfusion induced kidney injury. *J. Nephrol.* **2016**, *29*, 27–36. [CrossRef]
49. Zhou, L.; Yang, Z.-X.; Song, W.-J.; Li, Q.-J.; Yang, F.; Wang, D.-S.; Zhang, N.; Dou, K.-F. MicroRNA-21 regulates the migration and invasion of a stem-like population in hepatocellular carcinoma. *Int. J. Oncol.* **2013**, *43*, 661–669. [CrossRef]
50. Zhang, Z.; Li, Z.; Gao, C.; Chen, P.; Chen, J.; Liu, W.; Xiao, S.; Lu, H. miR-21 Plays a pivotal role in gastric cancer pathogenesis and progression. *Lab. Investig.* **2008**, *88*, 1358–1366. [CrossRef]
51. Wang, N.; Zhang, C.; He, J.; Duan, X.; Wang, Y.; Ji, X.; Zang, W.; Li, M.; Ma, Y.; Wang, T.; et al. miR-21 Down-regulation suppresses cell growth, invasion and induces cell apoptosis by targeting FASL, TIMP3, and RECK genes in esophageal carcinoma. *Dig. Dis. Sci.* **2013**, *58*, 1863–1870. [CrossRef]
52. Hu, J.; Ni, S.; Cao, Y.; Zhang, T.; Wu, T.; Yin, X.; Lang, Y.; Lu, H. The angiogenic effect of microRNA-21 targeting TIMP3 through the regulation of MMP2 and MMP9. *PLoS ONE* **2016**, *11*, e0149537. [CrossRef]
53. Zhong, X.; Chung, A.C.K.; Chen, H.Y.; Dong, Y.; Meng, X.M.; Li, R.; Yang, W.; Hou, F.F.; Lan, H.Y. miR-21 Is a key therapeutic target for renal injury in a mouse model of type 2 diabetes. *Diabetologia* **2013**, *56*, 663–674. [CrossRef]
54. Wang, J.-Y.; Gao, Y.-B.; Zhang, N.; Zou, D.-W.; Wang, P.; Zhu, Z.-Y.; Li, J.-Y.; Zhou, S.-N.; Wang, S.-C.; Wang, Y.-Y.; et al. miR-21 Overexpression enhances TGF-β1-induced epithelial-to-mesenchymal transition by target smad7 and aggravates renal damage in diabetic nephropathy. *Mol. Cell. Endocrinol.* **2014**, *392*, 163–172. [CrossRef]
55. Xu, X.; Song, N.; Zhang, X.; Jiao, X.; Hu, J.; Liang, M.; Teng, J.; Ding, X. Renal protection mediated by hypoxia inducible factor-1α depends on proangiogenesis function of miR-21 by targeting thrombospondin 1. *Transplantation* **2017**, *101*, 1811–1819. [CrossRef]
56. Liu, X.; Hong, Q.; Wang, Z.; Yu, Y.; Zou, X.; Xu, L. MiR-21 inhibits autophagy by targeting Rab11a in renal ischemia/reperfusion. *Exp. Cell Res.* **2015**, *338*, 64–69. [CrossRef]
57. Lai, J.Y.; Luo, J.; O'Connor, C.; Jing, X.; Nair, V.; Ju, W.; Randolph, A.; Ben-Dov, I.Z.; Matar, R.N.; Briskin, D.; et al. MicroRNA-21 in glomerular injury. *J. Am. Soc. Nephrol.* **2015**, *26*, 805–816. [CrossRef]
58. Glowacki, F.; Savary, G.; Gnemmi, V.; Buob, D.; Van der Hauwaert, C.; Lo-Guidice, J.-M.; Bouyé, S.; Hazzan, M.; Pottier, N.; Perrais, M.; et al. Increased circulating miR-21 levels are associated with kidney fibrosis. *PLoS ONE* **2013**, *8*, e58014. [CrossRef]
59. Hennino, M.-F.; Buob, D.; Van der Hauwaert, C.; Gnemmi, V.; Jomaa, Z.; Pottier, N.; Savary, G.; Drumez, E.; Noël, C.; Cauffiez, C.; et al. miR-21-5p Renal expression is associated with fibrosis and renal survival in patients with IgA nephropathy. *Sci. Rep.* **2016**, *6*, 27209. [CrossRef]
60. Guo, J.; Song, W.; Boulanger, J.; Xu, E.Y.; Wang, F.; Zhang, Y.; He, Q.; Wang, S.; Yang, L.; Pryce, C.; et al. Dysregulated expression of microRNA-21 and disease related genes in human patients and mouse model of alport syndrome. *Hum. Gene Ther.* **2019**. [CrossRef]

61. Dey, N.; Ghosh-Choudhury, N.; Kasinath, B.S.; Choudhury, G.G. TGFβ-stimulated microrna-21 utilizes PTEN to orchestrate AKT/mTORC1 signaling for mesangial cell hypertrophy and matrix expansion. *PLoS ONE* **2012**, *7*, e42316. [CrossRef]
62. Cheng, Y.; Zhu, P.; Yang, J.; Liu, X.; Dong, S.; Wang, X.; Chun, B.; Zhuang, J.; Zhang, C. Ischaemic preconditioning-regulated miR-21 protects heart against ischaemia/reperfusion injury via anti-apoptosis through its target PDCD4. *Cardiovasc. Res.* **2010**, *87*, 431–439. [CrossRef]
63. Sims, E.K.; Lakhter, A.J.; Anderson-Baucum, E.; Kono, T.; Tong, X.; Evans-Molina, C. MicroRNA 21 targets BCL2 mRNA to increase apoptosis in rat and human beta cells. *Diabetologia* **2017**, *60*, 1057–1065. [CrossRef] [PubMed]
64. Zhang, Y.; Zhao, S.; Wu, D.; Liu, X.; Shi, M.; Wang, Y.; Zhang, F.; Ding, J.; Xiao, Y.; Guo, B. MicroRNA-22 promotes renal tubulointerstitial fibrosis by targeting PTEN and suppressing autophagy in diabetic nephropathy. *J. Diabetes Res.* **2018**, *2018*, 1–11. [CrossRef] [PubMed]
65. He, F.; Peng, F.; Xia, X.; Zhao, C.; Luo, Q.; Guan, W.; Li, Z.; Yu, X.; Huang, F. MiR-135a promotes renal fibrosis in diabetic nephropathy by regulating TRPC1. *Diabetologia* **2014**, *57*, 1726–1736. [CrossRef] [PubMed]
66. Zhou, H.; Hasni, S.A.; Perez, P.; Tandon, M.; Jang, S.-I.; Zheng, C.; Kopp, J.B.; Austin, H.; Balow, J.E.; Alevizos, I.; et al. miR-150 Promotes renal fibrosis in lupus nephritis by downregulating SOCS1. *J. Am. Soc. Nephrol.* **2013**, *24*, 1073–1087. [CrossRef] [PubMed]
67. Xi, W.; Zhao, X.; Wu, M.; Jia, W.; Li, H. Lack of microRNA-155 ameliorates renal fibrosis by targeting PDE3A/TGF-β1/Smad signaling in mice with obstructive nephropathy. *Cell Biol. Int.* **2018**, *42*, 1523–1532. [CrossRef]
68. XIE, S.; CHEN, H.; LI, F.; WANG, S.; GUO, J. Hypoxia-induced microRNA-155 promotes fibrosis in proximal tubule cells. *Mol. Med. Rep.* **2015**, *11*, 4555–4560. [CrossRef] [PubMed]
69. Chen, B. The miRNA-184 drives renal fibrosis by targeting HIF1AN in vitro and in vivo. *Int. Urol. Nephrol.* **2019**, *51*, 543–550. [CrossRef]
70. Bera, A.; Das, F.; Ghosh-Choudhury, N.; Mariappan, M.M.; Kasinath, B.S.; Ghosh Choudhury, G. Reciprocal regulation of miR-214 and PTEN by high glucose regulates renal glomerular mesangial and proximal tubular epithelial cell hypertrophy and matrix expansion. *Am. J. Physiol. Physiol.* **2017**, *313*, C430–C447. [CrossRef]
71. Liu, M.; Liu, L.; Bai, M.; Zhang, L.; Ma, F.; Yang, X.; Sun, S. Hypoxia-induced activation of Twist/miR-214/E-cadherin axis promotes renal tubular epithelial cell mesenchymal transition and renal fibrosis. *Biochem. Biophys. Res. Commun.* **2018**, *495*, 2324–2330. [CrossRef]
72. Zhu, X.; Li, W.; Li, H. miR-214 Ameliorates acute kidney injury via targeting DKK3 and activating of Wnt/β-catenin signaling pathway. *Biol. Res.* **2018**, *51*, 31. [CrossRef]
73. Mu, J.; Pang, Q.; Guo, Y.-H.; Chen, J.-G.; Zeng, W.; Huang, Y.-J.; Zhang, J.; Feng, B. Functional implications of MicroRNA-215 in TGF-β1-induced phenotypic transition of mesangial cells by targeting CTNNBIP1. *PLoS ONE* **2013**, *8*, e58622. [CrossRef]
74. Kato, M.; Wang, L.; Putta, S.; Wang, M.; Yuan, H.; Sun, G.; Lanting, L.; Todorov, I.; Rossi, J.J.; Natarajan, R. Post-transcriptional up-regulation of Tsc-22 by Ybx1, a target of miR-216a, mediates TGF-β-induced collagen expression in kidney cells. *J. Biol. Chem.* **2010**, *285*, 34004–34015. [CrossRef]
75. Macconi, D.; Tomasoni, S.; Romagnani, P.; Trionfini, P.; Sangalli, F.; Mazzinghi, B.; Rizzo, P.; Lazzeri, E.; Abbate, M.; Remuzzi, G.; et al. MicroRNA-324-3p promotes renal fibrosis and is a target of ACE inhibition. *J. Am. Soc. Nephrol.* **2012**, *23*, 1496–1505. [CrossRef]
76. Li, R.; Chung, A.C.K.; Dong, Y.; Yang, W.; Zhong, X.; Lan, H.Y. The microRNA miR-433 promotes renal fibrosis by amplifying the TGF-β/Smad3-Azin1 pathway. *Kidney Int.* **2013**, *84*, 1129–1144. [CrossRef]
77. Alvarez, M.L.; Khosroheidari, M.; Eddy, E.; Kiefer, J. Role of MicroRNA 1207-5P and its host gene, the long non-coding RNA Pvt1, as mediators of extracellular matrix accumulation in the kidney: Implications for diabetic nephropathy. *PLoS ONE* **2013**, *8*, e77468. [CrossRef]
78. Brennan, E.P.; Nolan, K.A.; Börgeson, E.; Gough, O.S.; McEvoy, C.M.; Docherty, N.G.; Higgins, D.F.; Murphy, M.; Sadlier, D.M.; Ali-Shah, S.T.; et al. Lipoxins attenuate renal fibrosis by inducing let-7c and suppressing TGF β R1. *J. Am. Soc. Nephrol.* **2013**, *24*, 627–637. [CrossRef]
79. Wang, B.; Jha, J.C.; Hagiwara, S.; McClelland, A.D.; Jandeleit-Dahm, K.; Thomas, M.C.; Cooper, M.E.; Kantharidis, P. Transforming growth factor-β1-mediated renal fibrosis is dependent on the regulation of transforming growth factor receptor 1 expression by let-7b. *Kidney Int.* **2014**, *85*, 352–361. [CrossRef]

80. Cushing, L.; Kuang, P.; Lü, J. The role of miR-29 in pulmonary fibrosis. *Biochem. Cell Biol.* **2015**, *93*, 109–118. [CrossRef]
81. Meng, X.-M.; Tang, P.M.-K.; Li, J.; Lan, H.Y. TGF-Î²/Smad signaling in renal fibrosis. *Front. Physiol.* **2015**, *6*, 82. [CrossRef] [PubMed]
82. Van Rooij, E.; Sutherland, L.B.; Thatcher, J.E.; DiMaio, J.M.; Naseem, R.H.; Marshall, W.S.; Hill, J.A.; Olson, E.N. Dysregulation of microRNAs after myocardial infarction reveals a role of miR-29 in cardiac fibrosis. *Proc. Natl. Acad. Sci. USA* **2008**, *105*, 13027–13032. [CrossRef] [PubMed]
83. Qin, W.; Chung, A.C.K.; Huang, X.R.; Meng, X.-M.; Hui, D.S.C.; Yu, C.-M.; Sung, J.J.Y.; Lan, H.Y. TGF-β/Smad3 signaling promotes renal fibrosis by inhibiting miR-29. *J. Am. Soc. Nephrol.* **2011**, *22*, 1462–1474. [CrossRef] [PubMed]
84. Ramdas, V.; McBride, M.; Denby, L.; Baker, A.H. Canonical transforming growth factor-β signaling regulates disintegrin metalloprotease expression in experimental renal fibrosis via miR-29. *Am. J. Pathol.* **2013**, *183*, 1885–1896. [CrossRef] [PubMed]
85. Wang, B.; Komers, R.; Carew, R.; Winbanks, C.E.; Xu, B.; Herman-Edelstein, M.; Koh, P.; Thomas, M.; Jandeleit-Dahm, K.; Gregorevic, P.; et al. Suppression of microRNA-29 expression by TGF-β1 promotes collagen expression and renal fibrosis. *J. Am. Soc. Nephrol.* **2012**, *23*, 252–265. [CrossRef] [PubMed]
86. Hu, H.; Hu, S.; Xu, S.; Gao, Y.; Zeng, F.; Shui, H. miR-29b Regulates Ang II-induced EMT of rat renal tubular epithelial cells via targeting PI3K/AKT signaling pathway. *Int. J. Mol. Med.* **2018**, *42*, 453–460. [CrossRef] [PubMed]
87. Long, J.; Wang, Y.; Wang, W.; Chang, B.H.J.; Danesh, F.R. MicroRNA-29c is a signature microrna under high glucose conditions that targets sprouty homolog 1, and its in vivo knockdown prevents progression of diabetic nephropathy. *J. Biol. Chem.* **2011**, *286*, 11837–11848. [CrossRef] [PubMed]
88. Hennemeier, I.; Humpf, H.-U.; Gekle, M.; Schwerdt, G. Role of microRNA-29b in the ochratoxin a-induced enhanced collagen formation in human kidney cells. *Toxicology* **2014**, *324*, 116–122. [CrossRef] [PubMed]
89. Ben-Dov, I.Z.; Muthukumar, T.; Morozov, P.; Mueller, F.B.; Tuschl, T.; Suthanthiran, M. MicroRNA sequence profiles of human kidney allografts with or without tubulointerstitial fibrosis. *Transplantation* **2012**, *94*, 1086–1094. [CrossRef]
90. Jiang, L.; Qiu, W.; Zhou, Y.; Wen, P.; Fang, L.; Cao, H.; Zen, K.; He, W.; Zhang, C.; Dai, C.; et al. A microRNA-30e/mitochondrial uncoupling protein 2 axis mediates TGF-β1-induced tubular epithelial cell extracellular matrix production and kidney fibrosis. *Kidney Int.* **2013**, *84*, 285–296. [CrossRef] [PubMed]
91. Wang, J.; Duan, L.; Guo, T.; Gao, Y.; Tian, L.; Liu, J.; Wang, S.; Yang, J. Downregulation of miR-30c promotes renal fibrosis by target CTGF in diabetic nephropathy. *J. Diabetes Complications* **2016**, *30*, 406–414. [CrossRef]
92. Morizane, R.; Fujii, S.; Monkawa, T.; Hiratsuka, K.; Yamaguchi, S.; Homma, K.; Itoh, H. miR-34c Attenuates epithelial-mesenchymal transition and kidney fibrosis with ureteral obstruction. *Sci. Rep.* **2015**, *4*, 4578. [CrossRef]
93. Ning, Y.; Wang, X.; Wang, J.; Zeng, R.; Wang, G. miR-152 Regulates TGF-β1-induced epithelial-mesenchymal transition by targeting HPIP in tubular epithelial cells. *Mol. Med. Rep.* **2018**, *17*, 7973–7979. [CrossRef]
94. Zhang, X.; Yang, Z.; Heng, Y.; Miao, C. MicroRNA-181 exerts an inhibitory role during renal fibrosis by targeting early growth response factor-1 and attenuating the expression of profibrotic markers. *Mol. Med. Rep.* **2019**. [CrossRef]
95. Shen, Y.; Zhao, Y.; Wang, L.; Zhang, W.; Liu, C.; Yin, A. MicroRNA-194 overexpression protects against hypoxia/reperfusion-induced HK-2 cell injury through direct targeting Rheb. *J. Cell. Biochem.* **2019**, *120*, 8311–8318. [CrossRef]
96. Liu, F.; Zhang, Z.-P.; Xin, G.-D.; Guo, L.-H.; Jiang, Q.; Wang, Z.-X. miR-192 Prevents renal tubulointerstitial fibrosis in diabetic nephropathy by targeting Egr1. *Eur. Rev. Med. Pharmacol. Sci.* **2018**, *22*, 4252–4260.
97. Wang, B.; Koh, P.; Winbanks, C.; Coughlan, M.T.; McClelland, A.; Watson, A.; Jandeleit-Dahm, K.; Burns, W.C.; Thomas, M.C.; Cooper, M.E.; et al. miR-200a Prevents renal fibrogenesis through repression of TGF-β2 expression. *Diabetes* **2011**, *60*, 280–287. [CrossRef]
98. Oba, S.; Kumano, S.; Suzuki, E.; Nishimatsu, H.; Takahashi, M.; Takamori, H.; Kasuya, M.; Ogawa, Y.; Sato, K.; Kimura, K.; et al. miR-200b Precursor can ameliorate renal tubulointerstitial fibrosis. *PLoS ONE* **2010**, *5*, e13614. [CrossRef]
99. Howe, E.N.; Cochrane, D.R.; Richer, J.K. The miR-200 and miR-221/222 microRNA families: Opposing effects on epithelial identity. *J. Mammary Gland Biol. Neoplasia* **2012**, *17*, 65–77. [CrossRef]

100. Bai, J.; Xiao, X.; Zhang, X.; Cui, H.; Hao, J.; Han, J.; Cao, N. Erythropoietin inhibits hypoxia–induced epithelial-to-mesenchymal transition via upregulation of miR-200b in HK-2 cells. *Cell. Physiol. Biochem.* **2017**, *42*, 269–280. [CrossRef]
101. Xiong, M.; Jiang, L.; Zhou, Y.; Qiu, W.; Fang, L.; Tan, R.; Wen, P.; Yang, J. The miR-200 family regulates TGF-β1-induced renal tubular epithelial to mesenchymal transition through Smad pathway by targeting ZEB1 and ZEB2 expression. *Am. J. Physiol. Physiol.* **2012**, *302*, F369–F379. [CrossRef]
102. Tang, O.; Chen, X.-M.; Shen, S.; Hahn, M.; Pollock, C.A. MiRNA-200b represses transforming growth factor-β1-induced EMT and fibronectin expression in kidney proximal tubular cells. *Am. J. Physiol. Physiol.* **2013**, *304*, F1266–F1273. [CrossRef]
103. Wu, J.; Liu, J.; Ding, Y.; Zhu, M.; Lu, K.; Zhou, J.; Xie, X.; Xu, Y.; Shen, X.; Chen, Y.; et al. MiR-455-3p suppresses renal fibrosis through repression of ROCK2 expression in diabetic nephropathy. *Biochem. Biophys. Res. Commun.* **2018**, *503*, 977–983. [CrossRef]
104. Putta, S.; Lanting, L.; Sun, G.; Lawson, G.; Kato, M.; Natarajan, R. Inhibiting MicroRNA-192 ameliorates renal fibrosis in diabetic nephropathy. *J. Am. Soc. Nephrol.* **2012**, *23*, 458–469. [CrossRef]
105. Kato, M.; Zhang, J.; Wang, M.; Lanting, L.; Yuan, H.; Rossi, J.J.; Natarajan, R. MicroRNA-192 in diabetic kidney glomeruli and its function in TGF-beta-induced collagen expression via inhibition of E-box repressors. *Proc. Natl. Acad. Sci. USA* **2007**, *104*, 3432–3437. [CrossRef]
106. Chung, A.C.K.; Huang, X.R.; Meng, X.; Lan, H.Y. miR-192 Mediates TGF-β/Smad3-driven renal fibrosis. *J. Am. Soc. Nephrol.* **2010**, *21*, 1317–1325. [CrossRef]
107. Chung, A.C.K.; Dong, Y.; Yang, W.; Zhong, X.; Li, R.; Lan, H.Y. Smad7 suppresses renal fibrosis via altering expression of TGF-β/Smad3-regulated microRNAs. *Mol. Ther.* **2013**, *21*, 388–398. [CrossRef]
108. Krupa, A.; Jenkins, R.; Luo, D.D.; Lewis, A.; Phillips, A.; Fraser, D. Loss of MicroRNA-192 promotes fibrogenesis in diabetic nephropathy. *J. Am. Soc. Nephrol.* **2010**, *21*, 438–447. [CrossRef]
109. Wang, B.; Herman-Edelstein, M.; Koh, P.; Burns, W.; Jandeleit-Dahm, K.; Watson, A.; Saleem, M.; Goodall, G.J.; Twigg, S.M.; Cooper, M.E.; et al. E-cadherin expression is regulated by miR-192/215 by a mechanism that is independent of the profibrotic effects of transforming growth factor-beta. *Diabetes* **2010**, *59*, 1794–1802. [CrossRef]
110. Liu, G.; Friggeri, A.; Yang, Y.; Milosevic, J.; Ding, Q.; Thannickal, V.J.; Kaminski, N.; Abraham, E. miR-21 Mediates fibrogenic activation of pulmonary fibroblasts and lung fibrosis. *J. Exp. Med.* **2010**, *207*, 1589–1597. [CrossRef]
111. Zhou, X.; Xu, H.; Liu, Z.; Wu, Q.; Zhu, R.; Liu, J. miR-21 Promotes cardiac fibroblast-to-myofibroblast transformation and myocardial fibrosis by targeting Jagged1. *J. Cell. Mol. Med.* **2018**, *22*, 3816–3824. [CrossRef]
112. Krichevsky, A.M.; Gabriely, G. miR-21: A small multi-faceted RNA. *J. Cell. Mol. Med.* **2009**, *13*, 39–53. [CrossRef]
113. Androsavich, J.R.; Chau, B.N.; Bhat, B.; Linsley, P.S.; Walter, N.G. Disease-linked microRNA-21 exhibits drastically reduced mRNA binding and silencing activity in healthy mouse liver. *RNA* **2012**, *18*, 1510–1526. [CrossRef]
114. Ma, L.; Yang, X.; Wei, R.; Ye, T.; Zhou, J.-K.; Wen, M.; Men, R.; Li, P.; Dong, B.; Liu, L.; et al. MicroRNA-214 promotes hepatic stellate cell activation and liver fibrosis by suppressing Sufu expression. *Cell Death Dis.* **2018**, *9*, 718. [CrossRef]
115. Sun, M.; Yu, H.; Zhang, Y.; Li, Z.; Gao, W. MicroRNA-214 mediates isoproterenol-induced proliferation and collagen synthesis in cardiac fibroblasts. *Sci. Rep.* **2016**, *5*, 18351. [CrossRef]
116. Denby, L.; Ramdas, V.; Lu, R.; Conway, B.R.; Grant, J.S.; Dickinson, B.; Aurora, A.B.; McClure, J.D.; Kipgen, D.; Delles, C.; et al. MicroRNA-214 antagonism protects against renal fibrosis. *J. Am. Soc. Nephrol.* **2014**, *25*, 65–80. [CrossRef]
117. Humphries, B.; Yang, C. The microRNA-200 family: Small molecules with novel roles in cancer development, progression and therapy. *Oncotarget* **2015**, *6*, 6472–6498. [CrossRef]
118. Korpal, M.; Kang, Y. The emerging role of miR-200 family of microRNAs in epithelial-mesenchymal transition and cancer metastasis. *RNA Biol.* **2008**, *5*, 115–119. [CrossRef]
119. Kriegel, A.J.; Liu, Y.; Fang, Y.; Ding, X.; Liang, M. The miR-29 family: Genomics, cell biology, and relevance to renal and cardiovascular injury. *Physiol. Genomics* **2012**, *44*, 237–244. [CrossRef]

120. Huang, S.; Zhang, L.; Song, J.; Wang, Z.; Huang, X.; Guo, Z.; Chen, F.; Zhao, X. Long noncoding RNA MALAT1 mediates cardiac fibrosis in experimental postinfarct myocardium mice model. *J. Cell. Physiol.* **2019**, *234*, 2997–3006. [CrossRef]
121. Yu, F.; Lu, Z.; Cai, J.; Huang, K.; Chen, B.; Li, G.; Dong, P.; Zheng, J. MALAT1 functions as a competing endogenous RNA to mediate Rac1 expression by sequestering miR-101b in liver fibrosis. *Cell Cycle* **2015**, *14*, 3885–3896. [CrossRef] [PubMed]
122. Zhang, K.; Han, X.; Zhang, Z.; Zheng, L.; Hu, Z.; Yao, Q.; Cui, H.; Shu, G.; Si, M.; Li, C.; et al. The liver-enriched lnc-LFAR1 promotes liver fibrosis by activating TGFβ and Notch pathways. *Nat. Commun.* **2017**, *8*, 144. [CrossRef] [PubMed]
123. Zhang, Q.-Q.; Xu, M.-Y.; Qu, Y.; Hu, J.-J.; Li, Z.-H.; Zhang, Q.-D.; Lu, L.-G. TET3 mediates the activation of human hepatic stellate cells via modulating the expression of long non-coding RNA HIF1A-AS1. *Int. J. Clin. Exp. Pathol.* **2014**, *7*, 7744–7751.
124. Lu, Q.; Guo, Z.; Xie, W.; Jin, W.; Zhu, D.; Chen, S.; Ren, T. The lncRNA H19 mediates pulmonary fibrosis by regulating the miR-196a/COL1A1 axis. *Inflammation* **2018**, *41*, 896–903. [CrossRef]
125. Savary, G.; Dewaeles, E.; Diazzi, S.; Buscot, M.; Nottet, N.; Fassy, J.; Courcot, E.; Henaoui, I.-S.; Lemaire, J.; Martis, N.; et al. The long non-coding RNA DNM3OS is a reservoir of fibromirs with major functions in lung fibroblast response to TGF-β and pulmonary fibrosis. *Am. J. Respir. Crit. Care Med.* **2019**. [CrossRef] [PubMed]
126. Han, R.; Hu, S.; Qin, W.; Shi, J.; Zeng, C.; Bao, H.; Liu, Z. Upregulated long noncoding RNA LOC105375913 induces tubulointerstitial fibrosis in focal segmental glomerulosclerosis. *Sci. Rep.* **2019**, *9*, 716. [CrossRef] [PubMed]
127. Chen, W.; Zhou, Z.-Q.; Ren, Y.-Q.; Zhang, L.; Sun, L.-N.; Man, Y.-L.; Wang, Z.-K. Effects of long non-coding RNA LINC00667 on renal tubular epithelial cell proliferation, apoptosis and renal fibrosis via the miR-19b-3p/LINC00667/CTGF signaling pathway in chronic renal failure. *Cell. Signal.* **2019**, *54*, 102–114. [CrossRef]
128. Huang, S.; Xu, Y.; Ge, X.; Xu, B.; Peng, W.; Jiang, X.; Shen, L.; Xia, L. Long noncoding RNA NEAT1 accelerates the proliferation and fibrosis in diabetic nephropathy through activating Akt/mTOR signaling pathway. *J. Cell. Physiol.* **2019**, *234*, 11200–11207. [CrossRef]
129. Wang, P.; Luo, M.-L.; Song, E.; Zhou, Z.; Ma, T.; Wang, J.; Jia, N.; Wang, G.; Nie, S.; Liu, Y.; et al. Long noncoding RNA *lnc-TSI* inhibits renal fibrogenesis by negatively regulating the TGF-β/Smad3 pathway. *Sci. Transl. Med.* **2018**, *10*, eaat2039. [CrossRef]
130. Liang, Y.-J.; Wang, Q.-Y.; Zhou, C.-X.; Yin, Q.-Q.; He, M.; Yu, X.-T.; Cao, D.-X.; Chen, G.-Q.; He, J.-R.; Zhao, Q. MiR-124 targets Slug to regulate epithelial–mesenchymal transition and metastasis of breast cancer. *Carcinogenesis* **2013**, *34*, 713–722. [CrossRef] [PubMed]
131. Jiang, L.; Lin, T.; Xu, C.; Hu, S.; Pan, Y.; Jin, R. miR-124 Interacts with the Notch1 signalling pathway and has therapeutic potential against gastric cancer. *J. Cell. Mol. Med.* **2016**, *20*, 313–322. [CrossRef]
132. Chen, W.; Zhang, L.; Zhou, Z.-Q.; Ren, Y.-Q.; Sun, L.-N.; Man, Y.-L.; Ma, Z.-W.; Wang, Z.-K. Effects of long non-coding RNA LINC00963 on renal interstitial fibrosis and oxidative stress of rats with chronic renal failure via the foxo signaling pathway. *Cell. Physiol. Biochem.* **2018**, *46*, 815–828. [CrossRef]
133. Zhou, S.-G.; Zhang, W.; Ma, H.-J.; Guo, Z.-Y.; Xu, Y. Silencing of LncRNA TCONS_00088786 reduces renal fibrosis through miR-132. *Eur. Rev. Med. Pharmacol. Sci.* **2018**, *22*, 166–173.
134. Zhou, Q.; Chung, A.C.K.; Huang, X.R.; Dong, Y.; Yu, X.; Lan, H.Y. Identification of novel long noncoding RNAs associated with TGF-β/Smad3-mediated renal inflammation and fibrosis by RNA sequencing. *Am. J. Pathol.* **2014**, *184*, 409–417. [CrossRef]
135. Feng, M.; Tang, P.M.-K.; Huang, X.-R.; Sun, S.-F.; You, Y.-K.; Xiao, J.; Lv, L.-L.; Xu, A.-P.; Lan, H.-Y. TGF-β mediates renal fibrosis via the Smad3-Erbb4-IR long noncoding RNA axis. *Mol. Ther.* **2018**, *26*, 148–161. [CrossRef]
136. Sun, S.F.; Tang, P.M.K.; Feng, M.; Xiao, J.; Huang, X.R.; Li, P.; Ma, R.C.W.; Lan, H.Y. Novel lncRNA Erbb4-IR promotes diabetic kidney injury in *db/db* mice by targeting miR-29b. *Diabetes* **2018**, *67*, 731–744. [CrossRef]
137. Zhang, C.; Yuan, J.; Hu, H.; Chen, W.; Liu, M.; Zhang, J.; Sun, S.; Guo, Z. Long non-coding RNA CHCHD4P4 promotes epithelial-mesenchymal transition and inhibits cell proliferation in calcium oxalate-induced kidney damage. *Braz. J. Med. Biol. Res.* **2017**, *51*, e6536. [CrossRef]
138. Sun, J.; Zhang, S.; Shi, B.; Zheng, D.; Shi, J. Transcriptome identified lncRNAs associated with renal fibrosis in UUO rat model. *Front. Physiol.* **2017**, *8*, 658. [CrossRef]

139. Gao, Y.; Chen, Z.-Y.; Wang, Y.; Liu, Y.; Ma, J.-X.; Li, Y.-K. Long non-coding RNA ASncmtRNA-2 is upregulated in diabetic kidneys and high glucose-treated mesangial cells. *Exp. Ther. Med.* **2017**, *13*, 581–587. [CrossRef]
140. Zhang, H.; Sun, S.-C. NF-κB in inflammation and renal diseases. *Cell Biosci.* **2015**, *5*, 63. [CrossRef]
141. Yi, H.; Peng, R.; Zhang, L.; Sun, Y.; Peng, H.; Liu, H.; Yu, L.; Li, A.; Zhang, Y.; Jiang, W.; et al. LincRNA-Gm4419 knockdown ameliorates NF-κB/NLRP3 inflammasome-mediated inflammation in diabetic nephropathy. *Cell Death Dis.* **2017**, *8*, e2583. [CrossRef]
142. Xie, H.; Xue, J.-D.; Chao, F.; Jin, Y.-F.; Fu, Q.; Xie, H.; Xue, J.-D.; Chao, F.; Jin, Y.-F.; Fu, Q. Long non-coding RNA-H19 antagonism protects against renal fibrosis. *Oncotarget* **2016**, *7*, 51473–51481. [CrossRef]
143. Arvaniti, E.; Moulos, P.; Vakrakou, A.; Chatziantoniou, C.; Chadjichristos, C.; Kavvadas, P.; Charonis, A.; Politis, P.K. Whole-transcriptome analysis of UUO mouse model of renal fibrosis reveals new molecular players in kidney diseases. *Sci. Rep.* **2016**, *6*, 26235. [CrossRef]
144. Zhou, Q.; Huang, X.R.; Yu, J.; Yu, X.; Lan, H.Y. Long noncoding RNA Arid2-IR is a novel therapeutic target for renal inflammation. *Mol. Ther.* **2015**, *23*, 1034–1043. [CrossRef]
145. Gao, J.; Wang, W.; Wang, F.; Guo, C. LncRNA-NR_033515 promotes proliferation, fibrogenesis and epithelial-to-mesenchymal transition by targeting miR-743b-5p in diabetic nephropathy. *Biomed. Pharmacother.* **2018**, *106*, 543–552. [CrossRef]
146. Hu, M.; Wang, R.; Li, X.; Fan, M.; Lin, J.; Zhen, J.; Chen, L.; Lv, Z. LncRNA MALAT1 is dysregulated in diabetic nephropathy and involved in high glucose-induced podocyte injury via its interplay with β-catenin. *J. Cell. Mol. Med.* **2017**, *21*, 2732–2747. [CrossRef]
147. Feng, Y.; Chen, S.; Xu, J.; Zhu, Q.; Ye, X.; Ding, D.; Yao, W.; Lu, Y.; Ye, X.; Ye, X.; et al. Dysregulation of lncRNAs GM5524 and GM15645 involved in high-glucose-induced podocyte apoptosis and autophagy in diabetic nephropathy. *Mol. Med. Rep.* **2018**, *18*, 3657–3664. [CrossRef]
148. Polovic, M.; Dittmar, S.; Hennemeier, I.; Humpf, H.-U.; Seliger, B.; Fornara, P.; Theil, G.; Azinovic, P.; Nolze, A.; Köhn, M.; et al. Identification of a novel lncRNA induced by the nephrotoxin ochratoxin A and expressed in human renal tumor tissue. *Cell. Mol. Life Sci.* **2018**, *75*, 2241–2256. [CrossRef]
149. Wang, M.; Wang, S.; Yao, D.; Yan, Q.; Lu, W. A novel long non-coding RNA CYP4B1-PS1-001 regulates proliferation and fibrosis in diabetic nephropathy. *Mol. Cell. Endocrinol.* **2016**, *426*, 136–145. [CrossRef]
150. Wang, S.; Chen, X.; Wang, M.; Yao, D.; Chen, T.; Yan, Q.; Lu, W. Long non-coding RNA CYP4B1-PS1-001 inhibits proliferation and fibrosis in diabetic nephropathy by interacting with Nucleolin. *Cell. Physiol. Biochem.* **2018**, *49*, 2174–2187. [CrossRef]
151. Wang, M.; Yao, D.; Wang, S.; Yan, Q.; Lu, W. Long non-coding RNA ENSMUST00000147869 protects mesangial cells from proliferation and fibrosis induced by diabetic nephropathy. *Endocrine* **2016**, *54*, 81–92. [CrossRef]
152. Li, A.; Peng, R.; Sun, Y.; Liu, H.; Peng, H.; Zhang, Z. LincRNA 1700020I14Rik alleviates cell proliferation and fibrosis in diabetic nephropathy via miR-34a-5p/Sirt1/HIF-1α signaling. *Cell Death Dis.* **2018**, *9*, 461. [CrossRef]
153. Xue, R.; Li, Y.; Li, X.; Ma, J.; An, C.; Ma, Z. miR-185 Affected the EMT, cell viability and proliferation via DNMT1/MEG3 pathway in TGF-β1-induced renal fibrosis. *Cell Biol. Int.* **2018**. [CrossRef] [PubMed]
154. Wang, J.; Pang, J.; Li, H.; Long, J.; Fang, F.; Chen, J.; Zhu, X.; Xiang, X.; Zhang, D. lncRNA ZEB1-AS1 was suppressed by p53 for renal fibrosis in diabetic nephropathy. *Mol. Ther. Nucleic Acids* **2018**, *12*, 741–750. [CrossRef] [PubMed]
155. Xiao, X.; Yuan, Q.; Chen, Y.; Huang, Z.; Fang, X.; Zhang, H.; Peng, L.; Xiao, P. LncRNA ENST00000453774.1 contributes to oxidative stress defense dependent on autophagy mediation to reduce extracellular matrix and alleviate renal fibrosis. *J. Cell. Physiol.* **2018**, *234*, 9130–9143. [CrossRef]
156. Hajjari, M.; Salavaty, A. HOTAIR: An oncogenic long non-coding RNA in different cancers. *Cancer Biol. Med.* **2015**, *12*, 1–9.
157. Zhou, H.; Gao, L.; Yu, Z.; Hong, S.; Zhang, Z.; Qiu, Z. LncRNA HOTAIR promotes renal interstitial fibrosis by regulating Notch1 pathway via the modulation of miR-124. *Nephrology* **2018**. [CrossRef] [PubMed]
158. Zhou, H.; Qiu, Z.-Z.; Yu, Z.-H.; Gao, L.; He, J.-M.; Zhang, Z.-W.; Zheng, J. Paeonol reverses promoting effect of the HOTAIR/miR-124/Notch1 axis on renal interstitial fibrosis in a rat model. *J. Cell. Physiol.* **2019**. [CrossRef]
159. Van Rooij, E.; Kauppinen, S. Development of microRNA therapeutics is coming of age. *EMBO Mol. Med.* **2014**, *6*, 851–864. [CrossRef]
160. Chiu, Y.-L.; Rana, T.M. siRNA function in RNAi: A chemical modification analysis. *RNA* **2003**, *9*, 1034–1048.

[CrossRef] [PubMed]
161. Chen, P.Y.; Weinmann, L.; Gaidatzis, D.; Pei, Y.; Zavolan, M.; Tuschl, T.; Meister, G. Strand-specific 5′-O-methylation of siRNA duplexes controls guide strand selection and targeting specificity. *RNA* **2008**, *14*, 263–274. [CrossRef]
162. Michelfelder, S.; Trepel, M. Adeno-associated viral vectors and their redirection to cell-type specific receptors. *Adv. Genet.* **2009**, *67*, 29–60. [PubMed]
163. Montgomery, R.L.; Yu, G.; Latimer, P.A.; Stack, C.; Robinson, K.; Dalby, C.M.; Kaminski, N.; van Rooij, E. MicroRNA mimicry blocks pulmonary fibrosis. *EMBO Mol. Med.* **2014**, *6*, 1347–1356. [CrossRef] [PubMed]
164. Chakraborty, C.; Sharma, A.R.; Sharma, G.; Doss, C.G.P.; Lee, S.-S. Therapeutic miRNA and siRNA: Moving from bench to clinic as next generation medicine. *Mol. Ther. Nucleic Acids* **2017**, *8*, 132–143. [CrossRef] [PubMed]
165. Lennox, K.A.; Behlke, M.A. Chemical modification and design of anti-miRNA oligonucleotides. *Gene Ther.* **2011**, *18*, 1111–1120. [CrossRef] [PubMed]
166. Louloupi, A.; Ørom, U.A.V. Inhibiting pri-miRNA processing with target site blockers. *Methods Mol. Biol.* **2018**, *1823*, 63–68. [PubMed]
167. Knauss, J.L.; Bian, S.; Sun, T. Plasmid-based target protectors allow specific blockade of miRNA silencing activity in mammalian developmental systems. *Front. Cell. Neurosci.* **2013**, *7*, 163. [CrossRef] [PubMed]
168. Kölling, M.; Kaucsar, T.; Schauerte, C.; Hübner, A.; Dettling, A.; Park, J.-K.; Busch, M.; Wulff, X.; Meier, M.; Scherf, K.; et al. Therapeutic miR-21 silencing ameliorates diabetic kidney disease in mice. *Mol. Ther.* **2017**, *25*, 165–180. [CrossRef]
169. Gomez, I.G.; MacKenna, D.A.; Johnson, B.G.; Kaimal, V.; Roach, A.M.; Ren, S.; Nakagawa, N.; Xin, C.; Newitt, R.; Pandya, S.; et al. Anti–microRNA-21 oligonucleotides prevent Alport nephropathy progression by stimulating metabolic pathways. *J. Clin. Invest.* **2015**, *125*, 141–156. [CrossRef] [PubMed]
170. Creemers, E.E.; van Rooij, E. Function and therapeutic potential of noncoding RNAs in cardiac fibrosis. *Circ. Res.* **2016**, *118*, 108–118. [CrossRef]
171. Bonetti, A.; Carninci, P. From bench to bedside: The long journey of long non-coding RNAs. *Curr. Opin. Syst. Biol.* **2017**, *3*, 119–124. [CrossRef]
172. Hagedorn, P.H.; Pontoppidan, M.; Bisgaard, T.S.; Berrera, M.; Dieckmann, A.; Ebeling, M.; Møller, M.R.; Hudlebusch, H.; Jensen, M.L.; Hansen, H.F.; et al. Identifying and avoiding off-target effects of RNase H-dependent antisense oligonucleotides in mice. *Nucleic Acids Res.* **2018**, *46*, 5366–5380. [CrossRef]
173. Kato, M.; Wang, M.; Chen, Z.; Bhatt, K.; Oh, H.J.; Lanting, L.; Deshpande, S.; Jia, Y.; Lai, J.Y.C.; O'Connor, C.L.; et al. An endoplasmic reticulum stress-regulated lncRNA hosting a microRNA megacluster induces early features of diabetic nephropathy. *Nat. Commun.* **2016**, *7*, 12864. [CrossRef]
174. Li, C.H.; Chen, Y. Targeting long non-coding RNAs in cancers: Progress and prospects. *Int. J. Biochem. Cell Biol.* **2013**, *45*, 1895–1910. [CrossRef]
175. Prasad, N.; Kumar, S.; Manjunath, R.; Bhadauria, D.; Kaul, A.; Sharma, R.K.; Gupta, A.; Lal, H.; Jain, M.; Agrawal, V. Real-time ultrasound-guided percutaneous renal biopsy with needle guide by nephrologists decreases post-biopsy complications. *Clin. Kidney J.* **2015**, *8*, 151–156. [CrossRef]
176. Schwab, S.; Marwitz, T.; Woitas, R.P. The role of prognostic assessment with biomarkers in chronic kidney disease: A narrative review. *J. Lab. Precis. Med.* **2018**, *3*, 12. [CrossRef]
177. Weber, J.A.; Baxter, D.H.; Zhang, S.; Huang, D.Y.; How Huang, K.; Jen Lee, M.; Galas, D.J.; Wang, K. The microRNA spectrum in 12 body fluids. *Clin. Chem.* **2010**, *56*, 1733–1741. [CrossRef]
178. Mitchell, P.S.; Parkin, R.K.; Kroh, E.M.; Fritz, B.R.; Wyman, S.K.; Pogosova-Agadjanyan, E.L.; Peterson, A.; Noteboom, J.; O'Briant, K.C.; Allen, A.; et al. Circulating microRNAs as stable blood-based markers for cancer detection. *Proc. Natl. Acad. Sci. USA* **2008**, *105*, 10513–10518. [CrossRef]
179. Bolha, L.; Ravnik-Glavač, M.; Glavač, D. Long noncoding RNAs as biomarkers in cancer. *Dis. Markers* **2017**, *2017*, 7243968. [CrossRef]
180. Cheng, L.; Sun, X.; Scicluna, B.J.; Coleman, B.M.; Hill, A.F. Characterization and deep sequencing analysis of exosomal and non-exosomal miRNA in human urine. *Kidney Int.* **2014**, *86*, 433–444. [CrossRef]
181. Cardenas-Gonzalez, M.; Srivastava, A.; Pavkovic, M.; Bijol, V.; Rennke, H.G.; Stillman, I.E.; Zhang, X.; Parikh, S.; Rovin, B.H.; Afkarian, M.; et al. Identification, confirmation, and replication of novel urinary microRNA biomarkers in lupus nephritis and diabetic nephropathy. *Clin. Chem.* **2017**, *63*, 1515–1526. [CrossRef] [PubMed]
182. Ramachandran, K.; Saikumar, J.; Bijol, V.; Koyner, J.L.; Qian, J.; Betensky, R.A.; Waikar, S.S.; Vaidya, V.S.

Human miRNome profiling identifies microRNAs differentially present in the urine after kidney injury. *Clin. Chem.* **2013**, *59*, 1742–1752. [CrossRef] [PubMed]
183. Sonoda, H.; Lee, B.R.; Park, K.-H.; Nihalani, D.; Yoon, J.-H.; Ikeda, M.; Kwon, S.-H. miRNA Profiling of urinary exosomes to assess the progression of acute kidney injury. *Sci. Rep.* **2019**, *9*, 4692. [CrossRef] [PubMed]
184. Khurana, R.; Ranches, G.; Schafferer, S.; Lukasser, M.; Rudnicki, M.; Mayer, G.; Hüttenhofer, A. Identification of urinary exosomal noncoding RNAs as novel biomarkers in chronic kidney disease. *RNA* **2017**, *23*, 142–152. [CrossRef]
185. Chen, C.; Lu, C.; Qian, Y.; Li, H.; Tan, Y.; Cai, L.; Weng, H. Urinary miR-21 as a potential biomarker of hypertensive kidney injury and fibrosis. *Sci. Rep.* **2017**, *7*, 17737. [CrossRef] [PubMed]
186. Lv, L.-L.; Cao, Y.-H.; Ni, H.-F.; Xu, M.; Liu, D.; Liu, H.; Chen, P.-S.; Liu, B.-C. MicroRNA-29c in urinary exosome/microvesicle as a biomarker of renal fibrosis. *Am. J. Physiol. Physiol.* **2013**, *305*, F1220–F1227. [CrossRef]
187. Zununi Vahed, S.; Omidi, Y.; Ardalan, M.; Samadi, N. Dysregulation of urinary miR-21 and miR-200b associated with interstitial fibrosis and tubular atrophy (IFTA) in renal transplant recipients. *Clin. Biochem.* **2017**, *50*, 32–39. [CrossRef]
188. Zhou, H.; Cheruvanky, A.; Hu, X.; Matsumoto, T.; Hiramatsu, N.; Cho, M.E.; Berger, A.; Leelahavanichkul, A.; Doi, K.; Chawla, L.S.; et al. Urinary exosomal transcription factors, a new class of biomarkers for renal disease. *Kidney Int.* **2008**, *74*, 613–621. [CrossRef]
189. Zununi Vahed, S.; Poursadegh Zonouzi, A.; Ghanbarian, H.; Ghojazadeh, M.; Samadi, N.; Ardalan, M. Upregulated expression of circulating microRNAs in kidney transplant recipients with interstitial fibrosis and tubular atrophy. *Iran. J. Kidney Dis.* **2017**, *11*, 309–318.
190. Muralidharan, J.; Ramezani, A.; Hubal, M.; Knoblach, S.; Shrivastav, S.; Karandish, S.; Scott, R.; Maxwell, N.; Ozturk, S.; Beddhu, S.; et al. Extracellular microRNA signature in chronic kidney disease. *Am. J. Physiol. Renal Physiol.* **2017**, *312*, F982–F991. [CrossRef]
191. Poel, D.; Buffart, T.E.; Oosterling-Jansen, J.; Verheul, H.M.; Voortman, J. Evaluation of several methodological challenges in circulating miRNA qPCR studies in patients with head and neck cancer. *Exp. Mol. Med.* **2018**, *50*, e454. [CrossRef]
192. Nair, V.S.; Pritchard, C.C.; Tewari, M.; Ioannidis, J.P.A. Design and analysis for studying microRNAs in human disease: A primer on -omic technologies. *Am. J. Epidemiol.* **2014**, *180*, 140–152. [CrossRef]
193. Haider, B.A.; Baras, A.S.; McCall, M.N.; Hertel, J.A.; Cornish, T.C.; Halushka, M.K. A critical evaluation of microRNA biomarkers in non-neoplastic disease. *PLoS ONE* **2014**, *9*, e89565. [CrossRef]
194. Ma, J.; Li, N.; Guarnera, M.; Jiang, F. Quantification of plasma miRNAs by digital PCR for cancer diagnosis. *Biomark. Insights* **2013**, *8*, 127–136. [CrossRef]
195. Hindson, C.M.; Chevillet, J.R.; Briggs, H.A.; Gallichotte, E.N.; Ruf, I.K.; Hindson, B.J.; Vessella, R.L.; Tewari, M. Absolute quantification by droplet digital PCR versus analog real-time PCR. *Nat. Methods* **2013**, *10*, 1003–1005. [CrossRef]
196. Mohankumar, S.; Patel, T. Extracellular vesicle long noncoding RNA as potential biomarkers of liver cancer. *Brief. Funct. Genomics* **2016**, *15*, 249–256. [CrossRef]

10

Cell Death in the Kidney

Giovanna Priante *, Lisa Gianesello, Monica Ceol, Dorella Del Prete and Franca Anglani

Kidney Histomorphology and Molecular Biology Laboratory, Clinical Nephrology, Department of Medicine - DIMED, University of Padua, via Giustiniani 2, 35128 Padova, Italy

* Correspondence: giovanna.priante@unipd.it

Abstract: Apoptotic cell death is usually a response to the cell's microenvironment. In the kidney, apoptosis contributes to parenchymal cell loss in the course of acute and chronic renal injury, but does not trigger an inflammatory response. What distinguishes necrosis from apoptosis is the rupture of the plasma membrane, so necrotic cell death is accompanied by the release of unprocessed intracellular content, including cellular organelles, which are highly immunogenic proteins. The relative contribution of apoptosis and necrosis to injury varies, depending on the severity of the insult. Regulated cell death may result from immunologically silent apoptosis or from immunogenic necrosis. Recent advances have enhanced the most revolutionary concept of regulated necrosis. Several modalities of regulated necrosis have been described, such as necroptosis, ferroptosis, pyroptosis, and mitochondrial permeability transition-dependent regulated necrosis. We review the different modalities of apoptosis, necrosis, and regulated necrosis in kidney injury, focusing particularly on evidence implicating cell death in ectopic renal calcification. We also review the evidence for the role of cell death in kidney injury, which may pave the way for new therapeutic opportunities.

Keywords: apoptosis; necrosis; regulated necrosis; kidney injury; tubular injury; glomerular injury

---

1. Introduction

While naturally occurring cell death had already been observed many years ago, it was long considered a passive phenomenon and seen as an unavoidable endpoint of biological systems. Cells can remain stationary, supporting the relationships between an organ's structure and function, or they can proliferate, sometimes becoming hypertrophic, or they can die. Regulation of the homeostatic balance between cell proliferation and cell death is important to the development and maintenance of multicellular organisms.

The historical concept of programmed cell death has been associated with apoptosis because it is considered a form of suicide, based on a genetic mechanism. Any cell death other than apoptosis has generally been called "accidental cell death" [1]. Necrosis has consequently been described as accidental cell death [2] rather than as the result of definite pathways. The classic definition of necrosis is not really appropriate, because it does not always indicate a particular form of cell death. The term is often used to refer to changes secondary to cell death by any mechanism, including apoptosis. Many insults induce apoptosis at lower doses and necrosis at higher doses. Depending on the stimulus, apoptosis and necrosis could lie on a continuum of cell death, so the two forms are not mutually exclusive, and can coexist in many pathological conditions.

Cell death by apoptosis usually occurs in response to the cell's microenvironment, and it is as fundamental to cellular and tissue physiology as cell division and differentiation. Attention to this form of cell death was prompted primarily by its crucial role in the normal embryonic development of higher vertebrates and in maintaining normal tissue homeostasis [3–6] by controlling cell numbers and eliminating nonfunctioning, damaged, or misplaced cells. As a result, and given that there are both pro- and anti-cell-death genes, the apoptotic pathway has been equated to programmed cell death (PCD). PCD is described as cell death occurring at a definite point in time during physiological development, based on an embedded genetic program that works like a clock. Because most examples of PCD happen by apoptosis, and apoptosis appears to be programmed by molecular events in the cell, the two terms are often used interchangeably. A now well-accepted concept of PCD includes clear examples that are not apoptosis, however [7–9]. Indeed, PCD can result in either a lytic or a nonlytic morphology, depending on the signaling pathway, whereas apoptosis is a nonlytic and typically immunologically silent form of cell death. Programmed lytic cell death is highly inflammatory, and necrosis is distinguished from apoptosis because of the related inflammatory response due to the rupture of the plasma membrane and release of intracellular content, including cellular organelles and highly immunogenic proteins (Figure 1).

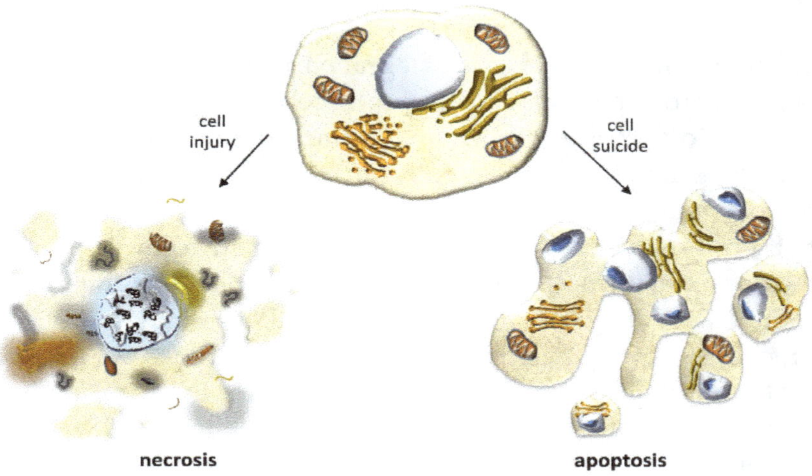

Loss of membrane integrity	Membrane blebbing, no loss of integrity
Begins with swelling of cytoplasm and mitochondria; ends with total cell lysis	Begins with shrinking of cytoplasm and condensation of nucleus; ends with the cell fragmentation into smaller bodies
Blebs form and the structure of the nucleus changes; no organelles are located in the blebs	The nucleus breaks apart, and DNA breaks into small regular pieces. The organelles are located in the blebs
The cell membrane breaks and releases the cell contents.	The cell membrane breaks into several apoptotic bodies.

Figure 1. Changes in cell morphology that distinguish apoptosis from necrosis.

It has now been established that necrosis is not an accidental, passive, unregulated form of cell death, but like apoptosis, it can be governed by a "regulated" mechanism, meaning a death with the classic morphological features of necrosis but genetically determined [5,10,11].

At a molecular level, the best-characterized pathway of regulated necrosis (RN) is necroptosis, a receptor-interacting protein kinase (RIPK)-based necrotic cell death [9,12–15]. Several other specialized forms of regulated necrosis have been described, however, such as ferroptosis [16], pyroptosis [17], parthanatos [18,19], mitochondrial permeability transition-dependent regulated necrosis (MPT-RN) [20], pyronecrosis [21,22], and NETosis, a process based on the rapid release of so-called neutrophil extracellular traps (NETs) [23]. All of these cell death pathways occur independently of an RIPK, or they can occur in the presence of RIPK inhibitors, often highlighting overlapping functions and pathways. Thus, cell death, be it by apoptosis or necrosis, is now considered to be regulated cell death (RCD) rather than a PCD. RCD implies an active participation of the cell in its own death through the activation of a genetically encoded death program, which specifies the means for starting a process that leads to the point of no return. Autophagy is a newly described, highly regulated cell death typified by the markers of a specific pathway [24], and it is as necessary as apoptosis for keeping the kidney healthy.

It is very important to be aware that every cell is "programmed" to die in response to an appropriate stimulus. Disruption of the signaling pathways or aberrant triggering of the processes that regulate physiological cell death due to extracellular causes, infections, toxins and toxicants, gene mutations, etc., may lead to abnormal cell functioning, which can become manifest in a wide array of human diseases. Gaining further insight into cell death mechanisms and a better understanding of the molecular processes involved will lead to a better characterization of a disease's etiology and pathogenesis. Cell death pathways can also be manipulated, targeting their clinical management as a way to develop new treatment approaches.

2. Kidney Injury and Cell Death

Although the term apoptosis was first introduced in the early 1970s by Kerr et al. [25], Glucksmann et al. had already described the morphological alterations associated with the process in kidney cells in the early 1950s [26].

It is now well accepted that apoptosis is an integral part of normal kidney functioning. As in other tissues, there is no inflammatory response in apoptotic cells, and their smaller fragments (apoptotic bodies) in the kidney providing these bodies are promptly ingested by neighboring cells and are degraded in lysosomes or eliminated via the tubular lumen. In fact, various types of cells may be involved in this tissue maintenance process, including epithelial cells. Phagocytes recognize and engulf apoptotic cells before their membrane is damaged, protecting surrounding tissues and cells from the damaging effects of the release of intracellular contents. If apoptotic cells are not ingested by phagocytes or epithelia, however, the cells proceed to a necrotic phase (called secondary necrosis), and their contents can spill into the extracellular space, causing inflammation and leading to inflammation-mediated kidney injury. Attempts to interfere with apoptosis (by certain caspase inhibitors, for instance) may trigger necrosis and consequent inflammation-mediated kidney injury [27].

The rate of apoptosis in the kidney is particularly intense in the developmental age [28–31]. Given the complexity of the renal microenvironment, cell death in the kidney is decoded in terms of the organ as a whole, not separately by its tubular, glomerular, interstitial, or endothelial compartments. Like all complex organisms, moreover, the kidney needs a physiological cell death modality: cell proliferation and cell death are strictly linked to keep the overall number of cells constant, eliminating cells that are damaged or no longer necessary at each stage of development, based on endogenous or exogenous factors. Developing kidneys are known not only to contain apoptotic cells [28,32], but also to express high levels of several apoptosis-related genes [33–39].

The mature mammalian kidney is a quiescent organ with little or no mitotic activity, and little or no apoptosis has been found in adult human kidneys. Thus, the nephrogenesis process (the formation of new nephrons) is limited to the period of embryonic development in humans. However, the mature kidney is capable of cellular proliferation, and in certain circumstances renal cells (like differentiated neurons) can divide. Several observations now point to the existence of adult kidney stem cells being implicated in both homeostatic tissue maintenance and functional recovery after injury [40–48].

In the case of injury in the adult kidney, cell death may occur in different compartments (the tubular and glomerular) and different types of cells, including the proximal and distal tubular cells and endothelial and glomerular cells [27]. Renal cell death is central to the pathophysiology of renal diseases. Renal cell loss is rarely a consequence of apoptosis, but rather of regulated necrosis, or simply the flushing of detached living cells.

Several common renal insults have been shown to disrupt kidney autophagy, including ischemia, toxic injury, and inflammation. Dysregulated, excessive, or defective autophagy is implicated in numerous disease states. Dysregulated autophagy leads to chronic inflammation and autoimmune diseases. Excessive autophagy can contribute to the expansion of malignant cells in renal cell cancer. Insufficient autophagy is a result of renal ischemia and facilitates cell death [49]. The death rate of renal cells might be abnormally high in nephropathies, promoting cell loss, as in acute tubular necrosis (ATN), acute rejection, necrotizing glomerulonephritis, or renal atrophy. Conversely, the cell death rate may drop (with an abnormal accumulation of cells) in cases of proliferative glomerulonephritis, polycystic renal disease, and neoplasia, for instance [50–53].

2.1. Tubular Cell Injury

Cell death in renal disease has been investigated primarily through the mechanism of tubular damages. In acute renal failure, cell death may be a direct consequence of exposure to harmful stimuli. Many renal insults, such as toxic injury or ischemia, mainly affect tubular epithelial cells and the metabolically very active proximal tubular segment in particular. Tubules are responsible for the reabsorption and secretion of several solutes, and injury to this nephron segment is the main mediator of acute kidney injury (AKI), which determines a rapid decline in renal function.

Apoptosis increases in the event of an acute unilateral ureteral obstruction (UUO) due to a physical obstruction or congenital anomalies. This causes renal growth impairment and tubular atrophy, primarily in the distal tubular epithelium, but also in the proximal renal tubules, resulting in hydronephrosis and renal failure [54–59]. Stretching, ischemia, and oxidative stress following ureteral obstruction are primary causes of tubular cell apoptosis. Increased apoptosis also activates cell infiltration, interstitial cell proliferation, and interstitial fibrosis [59–61]. Intriguingly, mild injury triggers apoptosis, and tubulointerstitial atrophy after UUO results from cell deletion by apoptosis. This leads to phagocytosis of the apoptotic bodies by neighboring tubular cells and direct apoptotic cell shedding into the tubular lumen, reestablishing homeostasis. When injury is severe, however, necrosis is more likely to be the dominant model of cell loss [61–64].

Renal ischemia followed by reperfusion (I/R) initiates apoptosis in the proximal tubular cells [27, 65–67]. I/R injury is known to be caused by ischemia, and then recovery of the blood flow unexpectedly worsens the damage. Renal tubular epithelial cell apoptosis is the key pathophysiological alteration occurring in I/R, and it defines the extent of the damage to kidney function. I/R injury is related to several inflammatory reactions, among which endothelial cell activation, the expression of adhesion molecules, the adhesion, aggregation and activation of leukocytes and platelets, the production of oxygen free radicals, and cellular calcium increase, as well as with the apoptosis mediated by these processes. AKI caused by I/R is a clinical syndrome that prompts kidney dysfunction and leads to a high mortality rate [68,69].

The consecutively hypoxic and oxidative stress evoked by renal I/R has been shown to enhance autophagy in several rodent models. The role of autophagy after renal I/R injury is still debated, however, and both protective and detrimental properties have been proposed [70].

Apoptosis seems to be common in post-transplant acute and chronic renal failure due to I/R injury [71–77]. In acute rejection, apoptosis occurs in the renal tubular epithelium, leading to tubular atrophy [78]. Chronic renal allograft rejection develops gradually, suggesting persistent low-grade injury, with a sustained and irreversible loss of renal function accompanied by clinical signs of proteinuria and hypertension [79,80].

During chronic kidney disease (CKD), the depletion of tubular cells by apoptosis gradually increases, contributing to the tubular atrophy and renal fibrosis associated with the progression of CKD [56,81–85]. Necrosis occurs in CKD as well, and the relative involvement of the two death mechanisms in cell loss depends on the balance of regulatory events. The dynamics of cell death during the early and intermediate stages of CKD have remained unclear, however. In an animal model that mimicked the progression of CKD in humans (rats undergoing subtotal nephrectomy), the authors demonstrated that both necrosis and apoptosis caused tubular injury. Since the RIPK3-regulated pathway was predominant with respect to the caspase-3 regulated pathway, the authors concluded that necrosis was the primary mechanism mediating renal tubular epithelial cell loss in the early and intermediate stages of chronic renal damage [86].

Tubular atrophy and tubular epithelial cell apoptosis have a role in diabetic kidney disease, although vascular and glomerular injuries are considered the main features of this condition [87–89]. Hyperglycemia triggers the generation of free radicals and oxidative stress in the tubular cells, and reactive oxygen species (ROS) are well-known important mediators of several biological responses, including proliferation, extracellular matrix deposition, and apoptosis [90].

Evidence of apoptosis has also been found in toxic renal exposure. The large luminal membrane surface area of proximal tubular cells makes them particularly susceptible to toxicants. Both toxicants and natural toxins are associated with altered renal apoptosis and affect several cellular factors. Studies with arsenic trioxide showed that low quantities of this agent prompted Bax/Bak-dependent apoptosis, while higher doses triggered MPT and apoptotic/necrotic cell death [91]. Thes studies showed that different cell death modalities may coexist within the same injury and that interference with specific signaling pathways or critical cell functions might result in cell killing by a distinct process. Various heavy metals induce apoptosis in renal cells via diverse mechanisms and molecular pathways [92–98]. For example, free cadmium accumulates in mitochondria, blocking the respiratory chain and culminating in mitochondrial dysfunction and the release of free radicals, which triggers caspase cascade and apoptosis. Antineoplastic agents are among the drugs that can trigger renal epithelial cell apoptosis. Cisplatin induces apoptosis in already low concentrations, resulting in cell loss, and this effect appears to be mediated by the generation of ROS. Oxidative damage to mitochondrial lipids and proteins increases with caspase-3 activity [27,99–101]. Moreover, the disruption of intracellular Ca^{2+} homeostasis or the induction of mild oxidative stress might mediate the apoptosis-inducing effects of these chemicals. In rat renal proximal tubules, cytochalasin D and dithiothreitol also caused apoptosis with associated cytoskeletal disorganization [102,103]. Antibiotics may have the potential to induce apoptosis, too. Gentamicin was found to induce apoptosis in renal distal tubules in the acute phase of injury and in the proximal tubules during the recovery phase [104,105]. Natural toxins from contaminated food and water supplies also pose a potential risk of renal apoptosis [106].

2.2. *Glomerular Cell Injury*

Cell death has also been documented in the diseased glomerulus [107–111]. Harrison et al. [107] were the first to report finding apoptotic bodies in human glomerulonephritis based on light and electron microscopy of kidney biopsies.

Apoptosis in glomerulonephritis appears to reduce hypercellularity during the repair process, controlling the size of the glomerular population and clearing excess cells. Apoptosis is required for the recovery of normal glomerular function [109,110,112,113]. In an experimental model of glomerulonephritis, however, the number of apoptotic glomerular cells was found to increase with the progression of glomerulosclerosis [114]. Apoptotic cell accumulation in the glomeruli has also been found to correlate with the glomerular sclerosis index and apoptotic index (the number of apoptotic cells divided by the number of normal cells) and with a decline in kidney function [114,115]. These results suggest that apoptosis is one of the mechanisms of glomerular cell depletion during progressive glomerulosclerosis.

In proliferative glomerulonephritis, on the other hand, the lack of a compensatory increase in cell death gives rise to an accumulation of cells, with glomerular hypercellularity due to mesangial and endocapillary cell proliferation [108,116–119]. During the chronic proliferative stage of systemic lupus erythematosus (SLE), apoptotic cells' number declines, while the number of proliferating cells increases, resulting in an imbalance in tissue homeostasis. An impaired removal of apoptotic bodies also indirectly contributes to the pathogenesis of SLE. Histone-bound DNA complexes, which have high affinity for the glomerular basement membrane, are carried out from apoptotic cells and accumulated in the glomerulus, triggering an immune response and causing glomerular damage [120–129].

In crescentic glomerulonephritis (CGN), disease progression is related to fibrosis of the glomerular crescents and renal interstitium. A number of different cell types, such as epithelial cells, fibroblasts, monocytes and macrophages, have been involved in the development of glomerular crescents and their progression to fibrosis. Proliferating macrophages as well as proliferating parietal epithelial cells seem to be the master contributors to this type of lesion [130–132], however, indicating that the glomerular proliferative index is more important than apoptosis alone in CGN.

Idiopathic nephrotic syndrome is the result of podocyte impairment. Basement membrane denuding and podocyte detachment and loss have been implicated in several human nephrotic syndromes, including focal and segmental glomerulosclerosis, minimal change disease, glomerulonephritis, and diabetic nephropathy [133–136]. Remarkably, not only resident glomerular cells but also infiltrating leukocytes might be eliminated by apoptosis in the glomeruli. Indeed, apoptotic bodies have been found to be particularly prominent in glomeruli containing numerous neutrophils, proving that apoptosis is a homeostatic mechanism that enables hypercellular glomeruli to return to normal [108–110,137,138].

2.3. Necrosis/Regulated Necrosis and the Kidney

Renal cortical necrosis is the death of tissue in the outer portion of the kidney (cortex) resulting from the blockage of the small arteries supplying blood to the cortex, and it causes AKI. The cause is usually a significantly diminished renal arterial perfusion secondary to vascular spasm, microvascular injury, or intravascular coagulation. Renal cortical necrosis is generally extensive, though focal and localized forms do occur. In most cases, the medulla, the juxtamedullary cortex, and a thin rim of subcapsular cortex are spared [139].

Renal papillary necrosis is a disorder in which all or part of the renal papillae die. It is characterized by coagulative necrosis of the renal medullary pyramids and papillae brought on by several associated conditions and toxins synergistically promoting the onset of ischemia. Renal papillary necrosis can lead to secondary infection of desquamated necrotic foci, stone formation, and/or the separation and eventual sloughing of papillae, resulting in acute urinary tract obstruction. The clinical course of renal papillary necrosis depends on the degree of vascular impairment, the presence of associated causal factors, the patient's general health, any bilateral involvement, and specifically, the number of papillae affected [140].

The biochemical signaling pathways that trigger necrosis have been investigated in detail in recent years. It is now clear that RN is a genetically driven process that strongly contributes to the pathophysiology of kidney injury.

Cell death by RN involves RIPK pathway-mediated rupture of the plasma membrane caused by a complement-related membrane attack complex, exotoxins, or cytotoxic T cells. Necrotic cell death is thus accompanied by the release of immunogenic cellular components collectively known as damage-associated molecular patterns (DAMPs) [141,142], which cause severe tissue damage, leading to systemic inflammation and organ injury or failure. Immune cell necrosis (i.e., NETosis or pyroptosis) is another component of necrotic renal lesions. This means that any causal factors triggering the RN signal pathways and the release of inflammatory mediators could be mutually enhancing and self-amplifying, leading to further renal cell loss, kidney atrophy, and scarring. The extremely proinflammatory effect of necrosis is very important in the kidney transplantation setting and in AKI, when inflammation occurs mostly together with renal cell necrosis (necroinflammation), as in necrotizing glomerulonephritis, thrombotic microangiopathy, and ATN [143,144]. RN modalities such as necroptosis, ferroptosis, parthanatos, and MPT-RN may be mechanistically distinct, but their damage to tubular segments and multicellular functional units may be synchronized, because otherwise they would only kill single cells in the tubular compartment [67,145–148]. Interestingly, the localization of tubular injury may differ in the several forms of renal damage. For example, tubular injury is variable in ischemic lesions, acting on short pieces of the proximal straight tubule and focal areas of the ascending limb of Henle's loop. In toxic forms, tubular damage is more continuous along all segments of the proximal tubule.

In the early phases of I/R injury, reduced oxygen supply to metabolically active tubular epithelial cells lowers oxidative metabolism and depletes cell supplies of high-energy phosphate compounds. Reperfusion restores the oxygen supply and improves oxygen radical formation, resulting in mitochondrial impairment. Neutrophil infiltration participates in this process via NET formation and further histone release into the extracellular space due to tubular cell necrosis [143,149]. The innate immune response arises soon after I/R injury and involves neutrophils, natural killer cells, and macrophages. Together with the tubular epithelial cells, macrophages produce proinflammatory cytokines, thus contributing to injury. The histones released kill more tubular cells through direct cytotoxic effects, possibly interfering with normal mitochondrial function or altering lysosome function, thus resulting in cell membrane alteration and disorganized protein synthesis. The mechanism of histone cytotoxicity is probably due to the polycationic nature of histones and their capacity to bind to the anionic moiety cell walls [149]. Moreover, histones that are immunologically inert when they are within the nucleus exert DAMP effects once released into the extracellular space [143]. Concomitant with the injury, there is shedding of viable and necrotic cells into the tubular lumen, and as the lesion progresses, cell proliferation could also intensify in an effort to replace neighboring cells and repair tubular cell injury [150].

In immune complex diseases such as crescent glomerulonephritis, renal vasculitis, or antiglomerular basement membrane disease, cell necrosis triggers massive glomerular inflammation with cytokine and chemokine expression, together with the release of dangerous intracellular molecules. The influx of neutrophils accelerates this process, with a subsequent inflammatory response (NETosis) in the capillaries of the glomerular tuft. This loop triggers a massive parietal epithelial cell hyperplasia, followed by basement membrane rupture and plasma leakage from disrupted glomerular capillaries and then crescent formation [151–154].

In either tubular or glomerular injury, a mild form of the same insult can lead to apoptosis, while a severe form can lead to necrosis. The pathway followed by the cell therefore depends on both the nature and the severity of the insult, sometimes evolving from an apoptotic to a necrotic form of cell death.

2.4. Cell Death and Crystal Nephropathies

The kidney is susceptible to crystal formation, as mineral secretion and urine concentration favor supersaturation, which can give rise to several acute and chronic kidney disorders related to crystal deposition or formation inside the kidney, referred to as crystal or crystalline nephropathies and renal stone disease [155–160].

Tubular crystallopathies result from precipitates inside the tubular lumen. The dynamics of crystal deposition determine the outcomes of kidney injury, i.e., AKI or CKD. A sudden onset of crystal formation causes cell necrosis and inflammation leading to AKI, whereas a chronic dynamic of crystal formation causes plugs in distal tubules or collecting ducts, leading to persistent tubule obstruction and hence CKD.

Apart from the urine concentration of both minerals and regulators of crystallization, the different types of crystal-induced renal disease are determined not only by the physicochemical properties of the crystals but also by the type of signaling pathway triggered by the crystals. Once crystals have formed in the tubular lumen, they contribute to kidney injury mainly through a direct or indirect cytotoxic effect, the underlying molecular mechanisms of which are largely unknown. Furthermore, crystals elicit inflammation and inflammation-driven cell necrosis in an auto-amplifying loop that is referred to as necroinflammation [143].

Calcium oxalate, calcium phosphate, and other crystals of various composition are known to be capable of inducing cell death, especially in renal proximal tubule cells [155]. Their effect might depend on their size. Nanosized crystals primarily cause apoptotic cell death, whereas micron-sized crystals cause necrotic cell death. Nanosized crystals may be internalized and transferred into lysosomes, thus causing damage that can trigger apoptosis. Alternatively, crystals can pass through pores into the nucleus, prompting DNA cleavage into regular fragments, an important characteristic of apoptotic cell death.

Micron-sized crystals on cells may cause irregular injury of the cell membrane and local strong physical stress, resulting in necrotic cell death. Released inflammatory factors by necrotic cells lead to cell membrane rupture that in turn causes an imbalance in cell osmotic pressure and consequently the sudden massive destruction of lysosomes accompanied by hydrolytic enzyme release [157].

Various crystals can also enter cells via a process of phagocytosis [159,161]. Phagosomes fuse with lysosomes in an attempt to digest the crystals. However, either amorphous calcium released by lysosomes into the cytosol or indigestible lysosome particles trigger necroptosis.

Crystals deposited in the kidneys act as intrarenal DAMPs, promoting intrarenal inflammation and contributing to further tubular injury and subsequent renal dysfunction [100,162]. These molecules can activate Toll-like receptors, which results in inflammasome activation in immune renal cells. Tubular cell necroptosis or ferroptosis due to calcium oxalate internalization can contribute to promoting inflammation [147,148]. Crystal-induced DAMPs also include histones that in large amounts are released into extracellular space by necrotic cells. Due to their strong basic charge, histones can potentially disrupt plasma membranes of neighboring intact cells, a process that increases the number of dying tubular cells and thus aggravates kidney injury [149,160].

The importance of cell death in pathological soft tissue calcification is well documented [163]. Such calcifications usually consist of calcium phosphate salts (including hydroxyapatite), but they sometimes contain calcium oxalates, too, as in calcium nephrolithiasis. In the kidney, the presence of necrotic tubular cells has been associated with renal cortical calcification, a rare condition usually due to severe cortex destruction and any condition causing acute and prolonged shock [164]. The role of cell death in the more common medullary nephrocalcinosis - microscopic renal crystal deposition in the tubular lumen (intratubular nephrocalcinosis) or interstitium (interstitial nephrocalcinosis) -, frequently associated with nephrolithiasis remains unclear. In two in vitro models of nephrocalcinosis obtained by exposing wild-type or Glial cell-derived neurotrophic factor (GDNF)-silenced human renal tubular cells to an osteogenic medium, it was recently shown that apoptosis and necroptosis respectively triggered renal cell calcification even before calcium phosphate crystal deposition [165,166] and mimicked vascular cell calcification [167–170]. The authors speculated that if cell death is an important event in the pathogenesis of renal ectopic calcification, any damage that shifts the balance between cell survival and cell death toward the latter could (in conjunction with a particular renal milieu) give rise to interstitial nephrocalcinosis and ultimately to kidney stones [171].

3. Targeting Renal Cell Death

In the undeniably complex picture of the mechanisms involved in cell death, under certain conditions, markers of apoptosis and necrosis may be found simultaneously, meaning that more than one cell death mechanism can be activated at the same time [146,172–174]. While there may be signs of different cell death pathways being involved, one pathway is usually the fastest and most effective. It is important to understand the interplay between different cell death pathways, especially with a view toward targeting these pathways for therapeutic purposes.

Elucidating the precise mechanisms behind cell death is essential to the development of new drugs. Numerous cellular factors have been proposed to regulate cell death response following a variety of induction mechanisms in numerous cell types, but the role of many of these factors depends both on the signal triggering a given cell death process and on the type of cell in which the response is induced.

Apoptosis and RN are characterized by distinct morphological, cell biological, and biochemical features. These two forms of cell death can occur at the same time in the same kidney compartment. They are not mutually exclusive and coexist in many renal pathological conditions [27,67,175]. The occurrence of either may depend on the intensity of the triggering events. For instance, renal ischemia may kill cells by either apoptosis or necrosis. The proportion of cells killed by each mechanism may also vary from one individual to another, because a part of the cell population predetermined to die by apoptosis might be rescued by interference with the genetic program, or apoptotic cells and their debris might be rapidly removed by phagocytes. Alternatively, apoptosis may cause secondary necrosis, as in prolonged kidney injury, in which case the plasma membrane of apoptotic cells may break down, thus acquiring a necrotic morphology.

Apoptosis occurs in three different phases: Initiation, effector, and final. The initiation phase is dependent upon stimuli, and two pathways can be identified, either extrinsic or intrinsic. In the extrinsic (death receptor-mediated) pathway, the ligation of death receptors determines the enrolment and activation of caspase-8. Caspase-8 further activates downstream caspases leading to apoptosis. Caspase-8 also triggers the intrinsic pathway to intensify the apoptotic cascade and inhibits necroptosis (Figure 2). In the intrinsic (mitochondrial) pathway, pro-apoptotic Bcl-2 family proteins Bax and

Bak create pores on the mitochondrial outer membrane, determining the release of apoptogenic factors, such as Cytochrome *c* (Cyt C). In the cytosol, Cyt C binds to and stimulates conformational modifications in the adaptor protein Apaf-1, thus leading to the enrolment and activation of caspase-9. Caspase-9 further activates executioner caspases to elicit apoptosis. Notably, other components of the Bcl-2 protein family, such as Bcl-xL and Bcl-2, prevents pore formation in healthy cells by binding to Bax and Bak. Initiating factors include Tumor necrosis factor (TNF) receptors and ligands, growth factors, and changes in the extracellular matrix. Oxidative stress plays an important role in renal apoptosis. Either by acting as signal transduction molecules or by directly causing cellular damage, ROS activate apoptosis at multiple steps in the cell death pathway and lead to the damage of cellular macromolecules, including DNA, proteins, and lipids [27,91] (Figure 2).

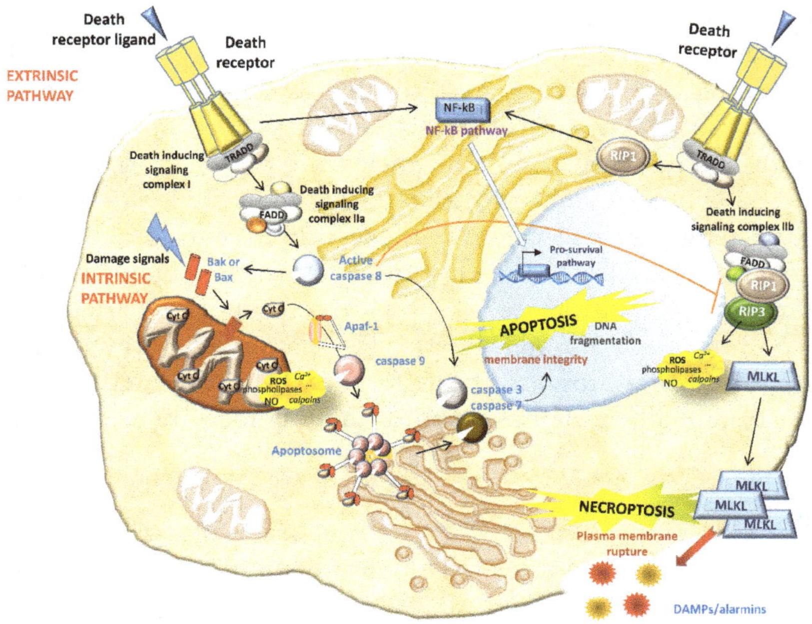

Figure 2. Overview of key molecular pathways of apoptosis and necroptosis. Apoptosis can start via intrinsic pathways (perturbation of intracellular homeostasis) or extrinsic pathways (death receptor binding). In the former case, cell stress leads directly (or via mediators, such as Bax and Bak) to mitochondrial outer membrane permeabilization, resulting in the release of apoptogenic factors, including Cytochrome *c*, which binds Apaf-1 to stimulate caspase-9 via apoptosomes. Bcl-2-related proteins induce apoptosis (e.g., Bax) or protect against it (e.g., Bcl-2). As for the extrinsic pathway, death receptor binding guides the recruitment of adapter proteins such as TRADD (TNFR-associated death domain), forming complex I. While complex I promotes cell survival via NF-κB activation, its transition to a secondary cytosolic complex, complex II, mediates cell death. Complex II is formed through the association of complex I with FADD (Fas-associated death domain). The formation of complex IIa promotes the activation of apoptosis in a caspase-8-dependent manner. Upon inhibition of caspase 8, complex IIb promotes necroptosis. Caspase-8 or caspase-9 activation subsequently triggers executioner caspases, such as caspase-3, -6, and -7. The cleavage of receptor-interacting protein kinase (RIPK) 1 and 3 by caspase-8 leads to apoptosis, whereas their phosphorylation triggers necroptosis in conditions of caspase-8 inhibition. RIPK1 and RIPK3 activation in turn causes the recruitment of the executioner mixed-lineage kinase domain-like protein (MLKL), which is phosphorylated by RIPK3 and initiates structural changes, leading to its insertion into the plasma membrane and channel formation. MLK channels increase Na^+ influx, osmotic pressure, and membrane rupture, ending in cell death. Membrane rupture promotes the release of intracellular contents and endogenous damage-associated molecular patterns (DAMPs) and/or preformed proinflammatory molecules (alarmins). Through RIPK1 kinase activity, a wide range of necrotic mediators are activated in the execution phase of necrotic cell death, including reactive oxygen species (ROS), calcium (Ca^{2+}), calpains, cathepsins, phospholipases, and ceramide.

In the final phase, which is common in extrinsic and intrinsic pathways, apoptotic cells show cytoplasmic shrinkage, chromatin condensation (pyknosis), nuclear fragmentation (karyorrhexis), and plasma membrane blebbing, culminating with the formation of apoptotic bodies. Since initiators and effectors of apoptosis are often unique to a particular cell or induction mode and take action upstream from the final common phase, cells committed to an apoptotic pathway may be rescued by specific therapeutic interventions. Several therapies targeting the apoptotic pathway have shown beneficial effects in many in vitro and in vivo models. Caspase inhibitors, such as z-VAD (z-Val-Ala-Asp fluoromethyl ketone), reduced apoptosis and improved organ function in several AKI models [176, 177]. TDZD-8 (4-benzyl-2-methyl-1,2,4-thiadiazolidine-3,5-dione), a pharmacological inhibitor of the powerful proapoptotic kinase GSK3β (glycogen synthase kinase 3 beta), reduces proximal tubular epithelial cell apoptosis and has positive influences on the kidney by inhibiting inflammation and increasing renal cell proliferation [178,179]: This makes it a rational option in human trials designed to prevent or treat AKI (Figure 3).

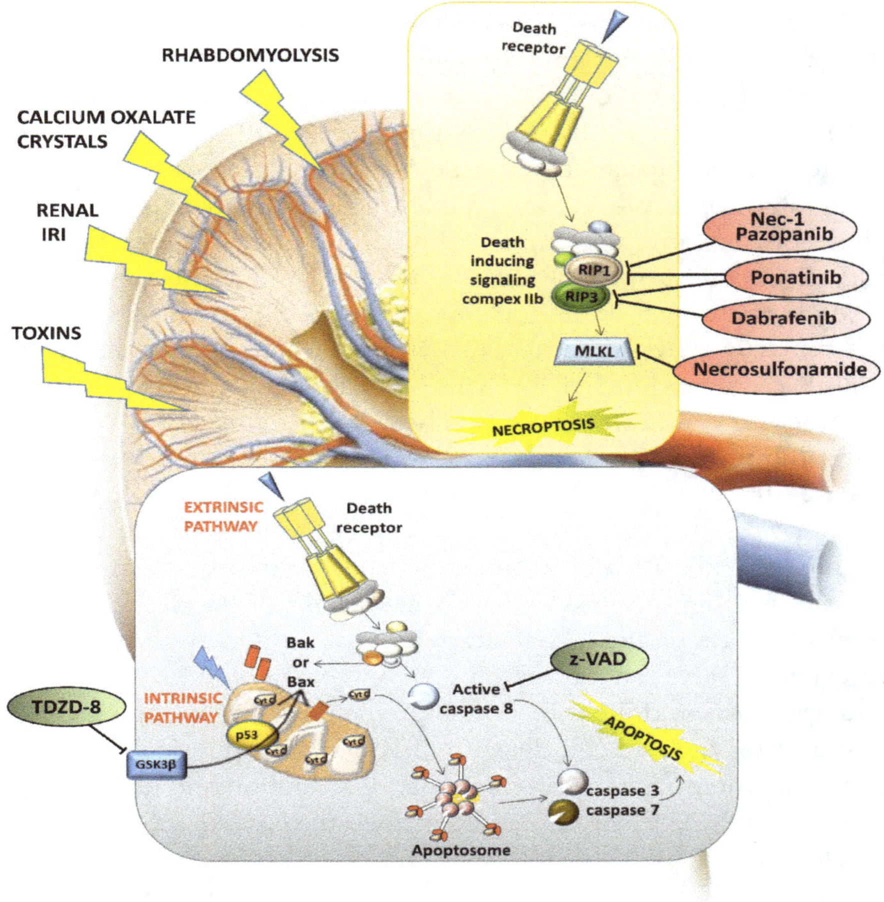

Figure 3. Targeting apoptosis and necroptosis in kidney lesions. Different kidney lesions activate different cell death modalities: z-VAD (z-Val-Ala-Asp fluoromethyl ketone) has been found to protect renal function, and the effect of the pan-caspase inhibitor z-VAD on experimental renal ischemia-reperfusion (I/R) injury was to reduce serum urea levels, thereby preventing inflammation. TDZD-8 (4-benzyl-2-methyl-1,2,4-thiadiazolidine-3,5-dione) has been found to inhibit ischemia-induced activation of GSK3β (glycogen synthase kinase 3 beta), Bax, and caspase 3, thus ameliorating tubular and epithelial cell damage and significantly protecting renal function.

RN may interact with apoptosis at various molecular and cellular levels, but both forms of cell death involve pathological changes in the mitochondria. In renal and other cells, the mitochondria are crucial sites for integrating intrinsic and extrinsic apoptotic signals. Bax, a known classic pro-apoptotic protein taking effect via mitochondrial membrane permeabilization, has been shown to regulate

MPT-RN as well, again by affecting mitochondrial dynamics [180]. It is important to bear in mind, however, that mitochondria are not involved in some RN pathways [20]. Necroptosis is generally considered a mitochondrion-independent form of RN. Very recent studies, however, have shown that in TNF-induced necroptosis, ROS induction was RIPK3-dependent and well correlated with necroptosis. Using mitochondrial respiration inhibitors and mitochondrial depletion, the authors showed that a TNF-induced increment of aerobic respiration accounted for ROS induction in necroptosis [181]. As they are the point where cell injury and death converge, the mitochondria may be promising targets for therapy.

Similarly to extrinsic apoptosis, necroptosis begins with the activation of death receptors such as Fas and TNF-α receptor 1 (Figure 2). Provided that caspase-8 (a key inhibitor of necrosis) is inactive, RIPK1 activates RIPK3, which in turn activates the mixed-lineage kinase domain-like protein (MLKL). MLKL oligomerizes and translocates to the plasma membrane, determining membrane rupture. RIPK1 is thought to be essential to necrosis induced by the Fas ligand and TNF- α. Necrostatin-1 (Nec-1) is an RIPK1 inhibitor that prevents the death of TNF-α-treated Fas-associated death domain (FADD)-deficient cells [182,183] (Figure 3). In addition to Nec-1, a number of necroptosis inhibitors have been reported [184–192], and some of them have been approved by the Food and drug administration (FDA), such as dabrafenib (a selective RIPK3 inhibitor), pazopanib (for RIPK1), and ponatinib (for both RIPK1 and RIPK3) [189,190] (Figure 3). In light of the multiple initiating pathways upstream, manipulating downstream necroptosis mediators such as MLKL may be more effective [182] (Figure 3). Although necroptosis inhibitors have been used in clinical trials, there are several issues to consider. These drugs may be useful, given their current clinical use as anticancer agents, but whether their toxicity-related side effects are admissible for patients with necroptosis-associated renal diseases remains to be seen. Many necroptosis inhibitors have yet to be extensively explored, so the efficacy and safety of these potential drugs should be further validated. Necroptosis also prompts the release of unprocessed intracellular contents, such as DAMPs or various preformed proinflammatory molecules (alarmins) stored inside the cell [142,193–195]. These proinflammatory molecules activate innate immunity, prompting the production of more proinflammatory cytokines and consequently more necrosis in renal tissue. If not opposed at an early stage, this self-amplifying process can lead to systemic inflammation and remote organ injury or even organ failure. In theory, the RN pathways can therefore be targeted therapeutically to block these inflammatory agents, and this should suffice to slow and even cancel RN [16,182,196–198]. It is essential to consider a combination of therapies capable of blocking multiple regulated cell death pathways, either simultaneously or at different time points, to ensure cell survival and renal function.

Necroptosis and apoptosis undoubtedly coexist in the pathophysiological process of AKI. Despite the limitations of separating the two cell death pathways, therapeutic interventions that primarily inhibit apoptosis have the potential to minimize renal dysfunction and accelerate recovery after AKI. The effectiveness of anti-apoptosis therapies has confirmed the contribution of apoptosis to AKI, which should not be neglected. Preclinical studies have identified several pathways resulting in RN that could be modulated successfully in AKI in vivo by drugs or interventions targeting the molecular pathways. In practice, specific therapies need to intercept events occurring upstream from cell death, so early intervention is essential. Unfortunately, this strategy might not be feasible in a large proportion of cases, because AKI is usually asymptomatic in the early stage.

4. Conclusions

Despite the difficulties of classifying cell death modalities in categorized patterns, great efforts have been made in recent years to do so in kidney injury. The description of new regulated cell death modalities, the realization that they may coexist in the same organ, and the discovery of inhibitors of the various types of cell death have raised hopes for therapeutic interventions in diseases characterized by massive cell death, such as AKI. Unfortunately, there have been no changes in clinical practice to date because it is difficult to translate these results into clinical trials in the absence of convincing preclinical evidence.

Author Contributions: G.P., L.G., M.C., D.D.P., and F.A. contributed to the literature review and critically reviewed manuscript drafting, each author in his/her specific field of expertise. G.P. conceived of the manuscript structure, wrote the manuscript, and prepared the table and figures. F.A. conceived of the manuscript structure, supervised its writing, and thoroughly reviewed all content.

References

1. Bessis, M. Studies on cell agony and death: An attempt at classification. In *Ciba Foundation Symposium - Cellular Injury*; de Reuck, A.V.S., Knight, J., Eds.; J&A Churchill: London, UK, 1964; ISBN 978-04-7072-277-0.
2. Green, D.R. *Means to an End: Apoptosis and Other Cell Death Mechanisms*, 1st ed.; Cold Spring Harbor Laboratory Press: Cold Spring Harbor, NY, USA, 2010; ISBN 978-08-7969-888-1.
3. Lynch, M.P.; Nawaz, S.; Gerschenson, L.E. Evidence for soluble factors regulating cell death and cell proliferation in primary cultures of rabbit endometrial cells grown on collagen. *Proc. Natl. Acad. Sci. USA* **1986**, *83*, 4784–4788. [CrossRef] [PubMed]
4. Fuchs, Y.; Steller, H. Programmed cell death in animal development and disease. *Cell* **2011**, *147*, 742–758. [CrossRef] [PubMed]
5. Galluzzi, L.; Bravo-San Pedro, J.M.; Vitale, I.; Aaronson, S.A.; Abrams, J.M.; Adam, D.; Alnemri, E.S.; Altucci, L.; Andrews, D.; Annicchiarico-Petruzzelli, M.; et al. Essential versus accessory aspects of cell death: Recommendations of the NCCD 2015. *Cell Death Differ.* **2015**, *22*, 58–73. [CrossRef] [PubMed]
6. Green, D.R. *Cell Death: Apoptosis and Other Means to an End*, 2nd ed.; Cold Spring Harbor Laboratory Press: Cold Spring Harbor, NY, USA, 2018; ISBN 978-16-2182-214-1.
7. Schwartz, L.M.; Smith, S.W.; Jones, M.E.; Osborne, B.A. Do all programmed cell deaths occur via apoptosis? *Proc. Natl Acad. Sci. USA* **1993**, *90*, 980–984. [CrossRef] [PubMed]
8. Taylor, R.C.; Cullen, S.P.; Martin, S.J. Apoptosis: Controlled demolition at the cellular level. *Nat. Rev. Mol. Cell Biol.* **2008**, *9*, 231–241. [CrossRef] [PubMed]
9. Jorgensen, I.; Rayamajhi, M.; Miao, E.A. Programmed cell death as a defence against infection. *Nat. Rev. Immunol.* **2017**, *17*, 151–164. [CrossRef] [PubMed]
10. Vanden Berghe, T.; Linkermann, A.; Jouan-Lanhouet, S.; Walczak, H.; Vandenabeele, P. Regulated necrosis: The expanding network of non-apoptotic cell death pathways. *Nat. Rev. Mol. Cell Biol* **2014**, *15*, 135–147. [CrossRef]
11. Galluzzi, L.; Kepp, O.; Krautwald, S.; Kroemer, G.; Linkermann, A. Molecular mechanisms of regulated necrosis. *Semin Cell Dev. Biol.* **2014**, *35*, 24–32. [CrossRef]
12. Tait, S.W.; Oberst, A.; Quarato, G.; Milasta, S.; Haller, M.; Wang, R.; Karvela, M.; Ichim, G.; Yatim, N.; Albert, M.L.; et al. Widespread mitochondrial depletion via mitophagy does not compromise necroptosis. *Cell Reports* **2013**, *5*, 878–885. [CrossRef]
13. Vanden Berghe, T.; Hassannia, B.; Vandenabeele, P. An outline of necrosome triggers. *Cell Mol. Life Sci.* **2016**, *73*, 2137–2152. [CrossRef]
14. Dillon, C.P.; Tummers, B.; Baran, K.; Green, D.R. Developmental checkpoints guarded by regulated necrosis. *Cell Mol. Life Sci.* **2016**, *73*, 2125–2136. [CrossRef] [PubMed]
15. Dondelinger, Y.; Darding, M.; Bertrand, M.J.M.; Walczak, H. Poly-ubiquitination in TNFR1-mediated necroptosis. *Cell Mol. Life Sci.* **2016**, *73*, 2165–2176. [CrossRef] [PubMed]
16. Dixon, S.J.; Lemberg, K.M.; Lamprecht, M.R.; Skouta, R.; Zaitsev, E.M.; Gleason, C.E.; Patel, D.N.; Bauer, A.J.; Cantley, A.M.; Yang, W.S.; et al. Ferroptosis: An iron-dependent form of nonapoptotic cell death. *Cell* **2012**, *149*, 1060–1072. [CrossRef] [PubMed]
17. Jorgensen, I.; Miao, E.A. Pyroptotic cell death defends against intracellular pathogens. *Immunol. Rev.* **2015**, *265*, 130–142. [CrossRef] [PubMed]
18. Andrabi, S.A.; Dawson, T.L.; Dawson, V.L. Mitochondrial and nuclear cross talk in cell death: Parthanatos. *Ann. NY Acad. Sci.* **2008**, *1147*, 233–241. [CrossRef] [PubMed]
19. Gibson, B.; Kraus, W. New insights into the molecular and cellular functions of poly(ADP-ribose) and PARPs. *Nature Rev. Mol. Cell Biol.* **2012**, *13*, 411–424. [CrossRef]

20. Galluzzi, L.; Kepp, O.; Kroemer, G. Mitochondrial regulation of cell death: A phylogenetically conserved control. *Microb. Cell* **2016**, *3*, 101–108. [CrossRef]
21. Cookson, B.T.; Brennan, M.A. Pro-inflammatory programmed cell death. *Trends Microbiol* **2001**, *9*, 113–114. [CrossRef]
22. Fink, S.L.; Cookson, B.T. Caspase-1-dependent pore formation during pyroptosis leads to osmotic lysis of infected host macrophages. *Cell Microbiol.* **2006**, *8*, 1812–1825. [CrossRef]
23. Remijsen, Q.; Kuijpers, T.W.; Wirawan, E.; Lippens, S.; Vandenabeele, P.; Vanden Berghe, T. Dying for a cause: NETosis, mechanisms behind an antimicrobial cell death modality. *Cell Death Differ.* **2011**, *18*, 581–588. [CrossRef]
24. Galluzzi, L.; Maiuri, M.C.; Vitale, I.; Zischka, H.; Castedo, M.; Zitvogel, L.; Kroemer, G. Cell death modalities: Classification and pathophysiological implications. *Cell Death Differ.* **2007**, *147*, 1237–1243. [CrossRef] [PubMed]
25. Kerr, J.F.; Wyllie, A.H.; Currie, A.R. Apoptosis: A basic biological phenomenon with wide-ranging implications in tissue kinetics. *Br. J. Cancer* **1972**, *26*, 239–257. [CrossRef] [PubMed]
26. Glucksmann, A. Cell deaths in normal verebrate ontogeny. *Biol. Rev.* **1951**, *26*, 59–86. [CrossRef] [PubMed]
27. Havasi, A.; Borkan, S.C. Apoptosis and acute kidney injury. *Kidney Int.* **2011**, *80*, 29–40. [CrossRef]
28. Koseki, C.; Herzlinger, D.; al-Awqati, Q. Apoptosis in metanephric development. *J. Cell Biol.* **1992**, *119*, 1327–1333. [CrossRef]
29. Meier, P.; Finch, A.; Evan, G. Apoptosis in development. *Nature* **2000**, *407*, 796–801. [CrossRef]
30. Bard, J.B. Growth and death in the developing mammalian kidney: Signals, receptors and conversations. *Bioessays* **2002**, *24*, 72–82. [CrossRef]
31. Bouchard, M. Transcriptional control of kidney development. *Differentiation* **2004**, *72*, 295–306. [CrossRef]
32. Coles, H.S.R.; Burne, J.F.; Raff, M.C. Large scale normal cell death in the developing rat kidney and its reduction by epidermal growth factor. *Development* **1993**, *118*, 777–784.
33. Lebrun, D.P.; Warncke, R.A.; Cleary, M.L. Expression of bcl-2 in fetal tissues suggests a role in morphogenesis. *Am. J. Pathol.* **1993**, *142*, 743–753.
34. Lu, Q.L.; Poulsom, R.; Wong, L.; Hanby, A.M. Bcl-2 expression in adult and embryonic non hematopietic tissues. *J. Pathol.* **1993**, *169*, 431–437. [CrossRef] [PubMed]
35. Saifudeen, Z.; Dipp, S.; El-Dahr, S.S. A role for p53 in terminal epithelial cell differentiation. *J. Clin. Invest.* **2002**, *109*, 1021–1030. [CrossRef] [PubMed]
36. Ewings, K.E.; Wiggins, C.M.; Cook, S.J. Bim and the pro-survival Bcl-2 proteins: Opposites attract, ERK repels. *Cell Cycle* **2007**, *6*, 2236–2240. [CrossRef] [PubMed]
37. Saifudeen, Z.; Dipp, S.; Stefkova, J.; Yao, X.; Lookabaugh, S.; El-Dahr, S.S. p53 regulates metanephric development. *J. Am. Soc. Nephrol.* **2009**, *20*, 2328–2337. [CrossRef] [PubMed]
38. El-Dahr, S.; Hilliard, S.; Aboudehen, K.; Saifudeen, Z. The MDM2-p53 pathway: Multiple roles in kidney evelopment. *Pediatr. Nephrol.* **2014**, *29*, 621–627. [CrossRef] [PubMed]
39. Ho, J. The regulation of apoptosis in kidney development: Implications for nephron number and pattern? *Front. Pediatr.* **2014**, *2*, 128. [CrossRef] [PubMed]
40. Bussolati, B.; Bruno, S.; Grange, C.; Buttiglieri, S.; Deregibus, M.C.; Cantino, D.; Camussi, G. Isolation of renal progenitor cells from adult human kidney. *Am. J. Pathol.* **2005**, *166*, 545–555. [CrossRef]
41. Kitamura, S.; Yamasaki, Y.; Kinomura, M.; Sugaya, T.; Sugiyama, H.; Maeshima, Y.; Makino, H. Establishment and characterization of renal progenitor like cells from S3 segment of nephron in rat adult kidney. *FASEB J.* **2005**, *19*, 1789–1797. [CrossRef]
42. Dekel, B.; Zangi, L.; Shezen, E.; Reich-Zeliger, S.; Eventov-Friedman, S.; Katchman, H.; Jacob-Hirsch, J.; Amariglio, N.; Rechavi, G.; Margalit, R.; et al. Isolation and characterization of non tubular sca-1+lin_multipotent stem/progenitor cells from adult mouse kidney. *J. Am. Soc. Nephrol.* **2006**, *17*, 3300–3314. [CrossRef]
43. Gupta, S.; Verfaillie, C.; Chmielewski, D.; Kren, S.; Eidman, K.; Connaire, J.; Heremans, Y.; Lund, T.; Blackstad, M.; Jiang, Y.; et al. Isolation and characterization of kidney-derived stem cells. *J. Am. Soc. Nephrol.* **2006**, *17*, 3028–3040. [CrossRef]
44. Maeshima, A.; Sakurai, H.; Nigam, S.K. Adult kidney tubular cell population showing phenotypic plasticity, tubulogenic capacity, and integration capability into developing kidney. *J. Am. Soc. Nephrol.* **2006**, *17*, 188–198. [CrossRef] [PubMed]

45. Humphreys, B.D.; Bonventre, J.V. Mesenchymal Stem Cells in Acute Kidney Injury. *Annu Rev. Med.* **2008**, *59*, 311–325. [CrossRef] [PubMed]
46. Chou, Y.H.; Pan, S.Y.; Yang, C.H.; Lin, S.L. Stem cells and kidney regeneration. *J. Formos Med. Assoc.* **2014**, *113*, 201–209. [CrossRef] [PubMed]
47. Lam, A.Q.; Bonventre, J.V. Regenerating the nephron with human pluripotent stem cells. *Curr Opin Organ. Transplant.* **2015**, *20*, 187–192. [CrossRef] [PubMed]
48. Thomasova, D.; Anders, H.J. Cell cycle control in the kidney. *Nephrol Dial. Transplant.* **2015**, *30*, 1622–1630. [CrossRef] [PubMed]
49. Havasi, A.; Dong, Z. Autophagy and Tubular Cell Death in the Kidney. *Semin. Nephrol.* **2016**, *36*, 174–188. [CrossRef]
50. Gobe, G.C.; Axeisen, R.A. Genesís of renal tubular atrophy in experimental hydronephrosis in the rat. *Lab. Invest.* **1987**, *56*, 273–281.
51. Gobe, G.C.; Axelson, R.A.; Searle, J.W. Cellular events in experimental unilateral ischemic renal atrophy and in regeneration after contralateral nephrectomy. *Lab. Invest.* **1990**, *63*, 770–779.
52. Todd, D.; Yang, G.; Brown, R.W.; Cao, J.; D'Agati, V.; Thompson, T.S.; Truong, L.D. Apoptosis in renal cell carcinoma: Detection by in situ end-labeling of fragmented DNA and correlation with other prognostic factors. *Hum. Pathol.* **1996**, *27*, 1012–1017. [CrossRef]
53. Tannapfel, A.; Hahn, H.A.; Katalinic, A.; Fietkau, R.J.; Kuhn, R.; Wittekind, C.W. Incidence of apoptosis, cell proliferation and p53 expression in renal cell carcinomas. *Anticancer Res.* **1997**, *17*, 1155–1162.
54. Kennedy, W.A., II; Stenberg, A.; Lackgren, G.; Hensle, T.W.; Sawczuk, I.S. Renal tubular apoptosis after partial ureteral obstruction. *J. Urol.* **1994**, *152*, 658–664. [CrossRef]
55. Truong, L.D.; Petrusevska, G.; Yang, G.; Gurpinar, T.; Shappell, S.; Lechago, J.; Rouse, D.; Suki, W.N. Cell apoptosis and proliferation in experimental chronic obstructive uropathy. *Kidney Int.* **1996**, *50*, 200–207. [CrossRef] [PubMed]
56. Kennedy, W.A., 2nd; Buttyan, R.; Garcia-Montes, E.; D'Agati, V.; Olsson, C.A.; Sawczuk, I.S. Epidermal growth factor suppresses renal tubular apoptosis following ureteral obstruction. *Urology* **1997**, *49*, 973–980. [CrossRef]
57. Klahr, S.; Morrissey, J. Obstructive nephropathy and renal fibrosis. *Am. J. Physiol. Renal Physiol.* **2002**, *283*, F861–F875. [CrossRef] [PubMed]
58. Jang, H.S.; Padanilam, B.J. Simultaneous deletion of Bax and Bak is required to prevent apoptosis and interstitial fibrosis in obstructive nephropathy. *Am. J. Physiol Renal Physiol.* **2015**, *309*, F540–F550. [CrossRef] [PubMed]
59. Nilsson, L.; Madsen, K.; Krag, S.; Frokiaer, J.; Jensen, B.L.; Norregaard, R. Disruption of cyclooxygenase type 2 exacerbates apoptosis and renal damage during obstructive nephropathy. *Am. J. Physiol. Renal Physiol.* **2015**, *309*, F1035–F1048. [CrossRef]
60. Docherty, N.G.; O'Sullivan, O.E.; Healy, D.A.; Fitzpatrick, J.M.; Watson, R.W. Evidence that inhibition of tubular cell apoptosis protects against renal damage and development of fibrosis following ureteric obstruction. *Am. J. Physiol. Renal Physiol. 2006* **2006**, *290*, F4–F13. [CrossRef]
61. Mei, W.; Peng, Z.; Lu, M.; Liu, C.; Deng, Z.; Xiao, Y.; Liu, J.; He, Y.; Yuan, Q.; Yuan, X.; et al. Peroxiredoxin 1 inhibits the oxidative stress induced apoptosis in renal tubulointerstitial fibrosis. *Nephrology* **2015**, *20*, 832–842. [CrossRef]
62. Saikumar, P.; Venkatachalam, M.A. Role of apoptosis in hypoxic/ischemic damage in the kidney. *Semin Nephrol.* **2003**, *23*, 511–521. [CrossRef]
63. Luo, S.; Rubinsztein, D.C. Apoptosis blocks Beclin 1-dependent autophagosome synthesis: An effect rescued by Bcl-xL. *Cell Death Differ.* **2010**, *17*, 268–277. [CrossRef]
64. Xu, Y.; Ruan, S.; Wu, X.; Chen, H.; Zheng, K.; Fu, B. Autophagy and apoptosis in tubular cells following unilateral ureteral obstruction are associated with mitochondrial oxidative stress. *Int. J. Mol. Med.* **2013**, *31*, 628–636. [CrossRef] [PubMed]
65. Schumer, M.; Colombel, M.C.; Sawczuk, I.S.; Gobé, G.; Connor, J.; O'Toole, K.M.; Olsson, C.A.; Wise, G.J.; Buttyan, R. Morphologic, biochemical, and molecular evidence of apoptosis during the reperfusion phase after brief periods of renal ischemia. *Am. J. Pathol.* **1992**, *140*, 831–838. [PubMed]
66. Price, P.M.; Hodeify, R. A possible mechanism of renal cell death after ischemia/reperfusion. *Kidney Int.* **2012**, *81*, 720–721. [CrossRef] [PubMed]

67. Linkermann, A.; Chen, G.; Dong, G.; Kunzendorf, U.; Krautwald, S.; Dong, Z. Regulated cell death in AKI. *J. Am. Soc. Nephrol.* **2014**, *25*, 2689–2701. [CrossRef] [PubMed]
68. Hoste, E.A.; Clermont, G.; Kersten, A.; Venkataraman, R.; Angus, D.C.; De Bacquer, D.; Kellum, J.A. RIFLE criteria for acute kidney injury are associated with hospital mortality in critically ill patients: A cohort analysis. *Crit Care* **2006**, *10*, R73:1-73-10. [CrossRef] [PubMed]
69. Kellum, J.A.; Unruh, M.L.; Murugan, R. Acute kidney injury. *BMJ Clin. Evid.* **2011**, *2011*, 2001:1–2001:36. [CrossRef] [PubMed]
70. Decuypere, J.P.; Ceulemans, L.J.; Agostinis, P.; Monbaliu, D.; Naesens, M.; Pirenne, J.; Jochmans, I. Autophagy and the Kidney: Implications for Ischemia-Reperfusion Injury and Therapy. *Am. J. Kidney Dis.* **2015**, *66*, 699–709. [CrossRef] [PubMed]
71. Olsen, S.; Burdick, J.F.; Keown, P.A.; Wallace, A.C.; Racussen, L.C.; Solez, K. Primary acute renal failure ("acute tubular necrosis") in the transplanted kidney: Morphology and pathogenesis. *Medicine (Baltimore)* **1989**, *68*, 173–187. [CrossRef]
72. Ito, H.; Kasagi, N.; Shomori, K.; Osaki, M.; Adachi, H. Apoptosis in the human allografted kidney. Analysis by terminal deoxynucleotidyl transferase-mediated DUTP-botin nick end labeling. *Transplantation* **1995**, *60*, 794–798. [CrossRef] [PubMed]
73. Kato, S.; Akasaka, Y.; Kawamura, S. Fas antigen expression and its relationship with apoptosis in transplanted kidney. *Pathol. Int.* **1997**, *47*, 230–237. [CrossRef]
74. Seron, D.; Moreso, F.; Bover, J.; Condom, E.; Gil-Vernet, S.; Canas, C.; Fulladosa, X.; Torras, J.; Carrera, M.; Grinyo, J.M.; et al. Early protocol renal allograft biopsies and graft outcome. *Kidney Int.* **1997**, *51*, 310–316. [CrossRef] [PubMed]
75. Castaneda, M.P.; Swiatecka-Urban, A.; Mitsnefes, M.M.; Feuerstein, D.; Kaskel, F.J.; Tellis, V.; Devarajan, P. Activation of mitochondrial apoptotic pathways in human renal allografts after ischemiareperfusion injury. *Transplantation* **2003**, *76*, 50–54. [CrossRef] [PubMed]
76. Sanz, A.B.; Santamaría, B.; Ruiz-Ortega, M.; Egido, J.; Ortiz, A. Mechanisms of Renal Apoptosis in Health and Disease. *J. Am. Soc. Nephrol.* **2008**, *19*, 1634–1642. [CrossRef] [PubMed]
77. Pallet, N.; Dieudé, M.; Cailhier, J.; Hébert, M. The Molecular Legacy of Apoptosis in Transplantation. *Am. J. Transplant.* **2012**, *12*, 1378–1384. [CrossRef] [PubMed]
78. Bonegio, R.; Lieberthal, W. Role of apoptosis in the pathogenesis of acute renal failure. *Curr. Opin. Nephrol. Hypertens* **2002**, *11*, 301–308. [CrossRef] [PubMed]
79. Foster, M.C.; Wenham, P.W.; Rowe, P.A.; Burden, R.P.; Morgan, A.G.; Cotton, R.E.; Blamey, R.W. The late results of renal transplantation and the importance of chronic rejection as a cause of graft loss. *Ann. R Coll Surg. Engl.* **1989**, *71*, 44–47. [PubMed]
80. Laine, J.; Etelamaki, P.; Holmberg, C.; Dunkel, L. Apoptotic cell death in human chronic renal allograft rejection. *Transplantation* **1997**, *63*, 101–105. [CrossRef]
81. Thomas, G.L.; Yang, B.; Wagner, B.E.; Savill., J.; El Nahas, A.M. Cellular apoptosis and proliferation in experimental renal fibrosis. *Nephrol Dial. Transplant.* **1998**, *13*, 2216–2226. [CrossRef]
82. Schelling, J.R.; Nkemere, N.; Kopp, J.B.; Cleveland, R.P. Fas-dependent fratricidal apoptosis is a mechanism of tubular epithelial cell deletion in chronic renal failure. *Lab. Invest.* **1998**, *78*, 813–824.
83. Khan, S.; Cleveland, R.P.; Koch, C.J.; Schelling, J.R. Hypoxia induces renal tubular epithelial cell apoptosis in chronic renal disease. *Lab. Invest.* **1999**, *79*, 1089–1099.
84. Choi, Y.J.; Baranowska-Daca, E.; Nguyen, V.; Kpji, T.; Ballantyne, C.M.; Sheikh-Hamand, D.; Suki, W.N.; Truong, L.D. Mechanism of chronic obstructive uropathy: Increased expression of apoptosis-promoting molecules. *Kidney Int. 2000 58*, 1481–1491. [CrossRef]
85. Yang, B.; Johnson, T.S.; Thomas, G.L.; Watson, P.F.; Wagner, B.; Skill, N.J.; Haylor, J.L.; El Nahas, A.M. Expression of apoptosis related genes and proteins in experimental chronic renal scarring. *J. Am. Soc. Nephrol.* **2001**, *12*, 275–288. [PubMed]
86. Zhu, Y.; Cui, H.; Xia, Y.; Gan, H. RIPK3-Mediated Necroptosis and Apoptosis Contributes toRenal Tubular Cell Progressive Loss and ChronicKidney Disease Progression in Rats. *PLoS ONE* **2016**, *11*, e0156729. [CrossRef]
87. Barnes, D.J.; Pinto, J.R.; Davison, A.M.; Cameron, J.S.; Grunfeld, J.P.; Kerr, D.N.S.; Ritz, E.; Viberti, G.C. The patient with diabetes mellitus. In *Oxford Textbook of Clinical Nephrology*, 2nd ed.; Turner, N., Turner, N.N., Lameire, N., Goldsmith, D.J., Winearls, C.G., Himmelfarb, J., Remuzzi, G., Eds.; Oxford university Press: Oxford, UK, 1998; pp. 723–775. ISBN 978-01-9959-254-8.

88. Bamri-Ezzine, S.; Ao, Z.J.; Londoño, I.; Gingras, D.; Bendayan, M. Apoptosis of Tubular Epithelial Cells in Glycogen Nephrosis During Diabetes. *Lab. Invest.* **2003**, *83*, 1069–1080. [CrossRef] [PubMed]
89. Habib, S.L. Diabetes and renal tubular cell apoptosis. *World J. Diabetes* **2013**, *4*, 27–30. [CrossRef] [PubMed]
90. Martindale, J.L.; Holbrook, N.J. Cellular response to oxidative stress: Signaling for suicide and survival. *J. Cell Physiol.* **2002**, *192*, 1–15. [CrossRef] [PubMed]
91. Orrenius, S.; Nicotera, P.; . Zhivotovsky, B. Cell Death Mechanisms and Their Implications in Toxicology. *Toxicological Sci.* **2011**, *119*, 3–19. [CrossRef]
92. Hamada, T.; Nakano, S.; Iwai, S.; Tanimoto, A.; Ariyoshi, K.; Koide, O. Pathological study on beagles after long-term oral administration of cadmium. *Toxicol. Pathol.* **1991**, *19*, 138–147. [CrossRef]
93. Hamada, T.; Tanimoto, A.; Iwai, S.; Fujiwara, H.; Sasaguri, Y. Cytopathological changes induced by cadmium-exposure in canine proximal tubular cells: A cytochemical and ultrastructural study. *Nephron* **1994**, *68*, 104–111. [CrossRef]
94. Duncan-Achanzar, K.B.; Jones, J.T.; Burke, M.F.; Carter, D.E.; Laird, H.E., II. Inorganic mercury chloride-induced apoptosis in the cultured porcine renal cell line LLC-PK1. *J. Pharmacol. Exp. Ther.* **1996**, *277*, 1726–1732.
95. Nath, K.A.; Croatt, A.J.; Likely, S.; Behrens, T.W.; Warden, D. Renal oxidant injury and oxidant response induced by mercury. *Kidney Int.* **1996**, *50*, 1032–1043. [CrossRef] [PubMed]
96. Sabath, E.; Robles-Osorio, M.L. Renal health and the environment: Heavy metal nephrotoxicity. *Nefrologia* **2012**, *32*, 279–286. [CrossRef] [PubMed]
97. Yuan, G.; Dai, S.; Yin, Z.; Lu, H.; Jia, R.; Xu, J.; Song, X.; Li, L.; Shu, Y.; Zhao, X.; et al. Sub-chronic lead and cadmium co-induce apoptosis protein expression in liver and kidney of rats. *Int J. Clin. Exp. Pathol.* **2014**, *7*, 2905–2914. [PubMed]
98. Eid, R.A. Apoptosis of Rat Renal Cells by Organophosphate Pesticide, Quinalphos: Ultrastructural Study. *Saudi J. Kidney Dis. Transpl.* **2017**, *28*, 725–736. [PubMed]
99. Lieberthal, W.; Triaca, V.; Levine, J. Mechanisms of death induced by cisplatin in proximal tubular epithelial cells: Apoptosis vs. necrosis. *Am. J. Physiol.* **1996**, *270*, F700–F708. [CrossRef] [PubMed]
100. Miller, R.P.; Tadagavadi, R.K.; Ramesh, G.; Reeves, W.B. Mechanisms of Cisplatin Nephrotoxicity. *Toxins (Basel)* **2010**, *2*, 2490–2518. [CrossRef] [PubMed]
101. Ortiz, A.; Lorz, C.; Catalán, M.P.; Danoff, T.M.; Yamasaki, Y.; Egido, J.; Neilson, E.G. Expression of apoptosis regulatory proteins in tubular epithelium stressed in culture or following acute renal failure. *Kidney Int.* **2000**, *57*, 969–981. [CrossRef]
102. Van de Water, B.; Kruidering, M.; Nagelkerke, J.F. F-actin disorganization in apoptotic cell death of cultured rat renal proximal tubular cells. *Am. J. Physiol.* **1996**, *270*, F593–F603. [CrossRef]
103. Desouza, M.; Gunning, P.W.; Stehn, J.R. The actin cytoskeleton as a sensor and mediator of apoptosis. *Bioarchitecture* **2012**, *2*, 75–87. [CrossRef]
104. Nouwen, E.J.; Verstrepen, W.A.; Buyssens, N.; Zhu, M.Q.; De Broe, M.E. Hyperplasia, hypertrophy, and phenotypic alterations in the distal nephron after acute proximal tubular injury in the rat. *Lab. Invest.* **1994**, *70*, 479–493.
105. Abuelezz, S.A.; Hendawy, N.; Abdel Gawad, S. Alleviation of renal mitochondrial dysfunction and apoptosis underlies the protective effect of sitagliptin in gentamicin-induced nephrotoxicity. *J. Pharm. Pharmacol.* **2016**, *68*, 523–532. [CrossRef] [PubMed]
106. Vervaet, B.A.; D'Haese, P.C.; Verhulst, A. Environmental toxin-induced acute kidney injury. *Clin. Kidney J.* **2017**, *10*, 747–758. [CrossRef] [PubMed]
107. Harrison, D.J. Cell death in the diseased glomerulus. *Histopathology* **1998**, *12*, 679–683. [CrossRef]
108. Savill, J.; Smith, J.; Sarraf, C.; Ren, Y.; Abbott, F.; Rees, A. Glomerular mesangial cells and inflammatory macrophages ingest neutrophils undergoing apoptosis. *Kidney Int.* **1992**, *42*, 924–936. [CrossRef] [PubMed]
109. Baker, A.J.; Mooney, A.; Hughes, J.; Lombardi, D.; Johnson, R.J.; Savill, J. Mesangial cell apoptosis: The major mechanism for resolution of glomerular hypercellularity in experimental mesangial proliferative nephritis. *J. Clin. Invest.* **1994**, *94*, 2105–2116. [CrossRef] [PubMed]
110. Shimizu, A.; Kitamura, H.; Masuda, Y.; Ishizaki, M.; Sugisaki, Y.; Yamanaka, N. Apoptosis in the repair process of experimental proliferative glomerulonephritis. *Kidney Int.* **1995**, *47*, 114–121. [CrossRef] [PubMed]
111. Jung, D.S.; Lee, S.H.; Kwak, S.J.; Li, J.J.; Kim, D.H.; Nam, B.Y.; Kang, H.Y.; Chang, T.I.; Park, J.T.; Han, S.H.; et al. Apoptosis occurs differentially according to glomerular size in diabetic kidney disease. *Nephrol Dial. Transplant.* **2012**, *27*, 259–266. [CrossRef] [PubMed]

112. Savill, J. Apoptosis and the kidney. *J. Am. Soc. Nephrol* **1994**, *5*, 12–21.
113. Takemura, T.; Murakami, K.; Miyazato, H.; Yagi, K.; Yoshioka, K. Expression of Fas antigen and Bcl-2 in human glomerulonephritis. *Kidney Int* **1995**, *48*, 1886–1892. [CrossRef]
114. Sugiyama, H.; Kashihara, N.; Makino, H.; Yamasaki, Y.; Ota, A. Apoptosis in glomerular sclerosis. *Kidney Int* **1996**, *49*, 103–111. [CrossRef]
115. Shimizu, A.; Kitamura, H.; Masuda, Y.; Ishizaki, M.; Sugisaki, Y.; Yamanaka, N. Glomerular capillary regeneration and endothelial cell apoptosis in both reversible and progressive models of glomerulonephritis. *Contrib Nephrol* **1996**, *118*, 29–40. [PubMed]
116. Shimizu, A.; Masuda, Y.; Kitamura, H.; Ishizaki, M.; Sugisaki, Y.; Yamanaka, N. Apoptosis in progressive crescentic glomerulonephritis. *Lab. Invest.* **1996**, *74*, 941–951. [PubMed]
117. Soto, H.; Mosquera, J.; Rodriguez, I.B.; Henriquez, L.A.; Roche, C.; Pinto, A. Apoptosis in proliferative glomerulonephritis: Decreased apoptosis expression in lupus nephritis. *Nephrol Dial. Transplant.* **1997**, *12*, 273–280. [CrossRef] [PubMed]
118. Savill, J. Regulation of glomerular cell number by apoptosis. *Kidney Int* **1999**, *56*, 1216–1222. [CrossRef] [PubMed]
119. Ruiz, P.; Soares, M.F. Acute postinfectious glomerulonephritis: An immune response gone bad? *Hum. Pathol* **2003**, *34*, 1–2. [CrossRef] [PubMed]
120. Schmiedeke, T.M.; Stockl, F.W.; Weber, R.; Sugisaki, Y.; Batsford, S.R.; Vogt, A. Histones have high affinity for the glomerular basement membrane. Relevance for immune complex formation in lupus nephritis. *J. Exp. Med.* **1989**, *169*, 1879–1894. [CrossRef] [PubMed]
121. Vogt, A.; Schmiedeke, T.; Stockl, F.; Sugisaki, Y.; Mertz, A.; Batsford, S. The role of cationic proteins in the pathogenesis of immune complex glomerulonephritis. *Nephrol Dial. Transplant.* **1990**, *5*, 6–9. [CrossRef]
122. Schmiedeke, T.; Stoeckl, F.; Muller, S.; Sugisaki, Y.; Batsford, S.; Woitas, R.; Vogt, A. Glomerular immune deposits in murine lupus models may contain histones. *Clin. Exp. Immunol* **1992**, *90*, 453–458. [CrossRef]
123. Stockl, F.; Muller, S.; Batsford, S.; Schmiedeke, T.; Waldherr, R.; Andrassy, K.; Sugisaki, Y.; Nakabayashi, K.; Nagasawa, T.; Rodriguez- Iturbe, B.; et al. A role for histones and ubiquitin in lupus nephritis? *Clin. Nephrol* **1994**, *41*, 10–17.
124. Kuenkele, S.; Beyer, T.D.; Voll, R.E.; Kalden, J.R.; Herrmann, M. Impaired clearance of apoptotic cells in systemic lupus erythematosus: Challenge of T and B cell tolerance. *Curr Rheumatol Rep.* **2003**, *5*, 175–177. [CrossRef]
125. Dieker, J.W.; van der Vlag, J.; Berden, J.H. Deranged removal of apoptotic cells: Its role in the genesis of lupus. *Nephrol Dial. Transplant.* **2004**, *19*, 282–285. [CrossRef] [PubMed]
126. Gaipl, U.S.; Voll, R.E.; Sheriff, A.; Franz, S.; Kalden, J.R.; Herrmann, M. Impaired clearance of dying cells in systemic lupus erythematosus. *Autoimmun Rev.* **2005**, *4*, 189–194. [CrossRef] [PubMed]
127. Kalaaji, M.; Mortensen, E.; Jorgensen, L.; Olsen, R.; Rekvig, O.P. Nephritogenic lupus antibodies recognize glomerular basement membrane-associated chromatin fragments released from apoptotic intraglomerular cells. *Am. J. Pathol* **2006**, *168*, 1779–1792. [CrossRef] [PubMed]
128. Gaipl, U.S.; Sheriff, A.; Franz, S.; Munoz, L.E.; Voll, R.E.; Kalden, J.R.; Herrmann, M. Inefficient clearance of dying cells and autoreactivity. *Curr Top. Microbiol Immunol* **2006**, *305*, 161–176. [PubMed]
129. Chen, R.; Kang, R.; Fan, X.G.; Tang, D. Release and activity of histone in diseases. *Cell Death Dis* **2014**, *5*, e1370:1-1370:9. [CrossRef] [PubMed]
130. Holzman, B.L.; Wiggins, R.C. Glomerular crescent formation. *Semin Nephrol* **1991**, *11*, 346–353. [PubMed]
131. Ophascharoensuk, V.; Pippin, J.W.; Gordon, K.L.; Shankland, S.J.; Couser, W.G.; Johnson, R.J. Role of intrinsic renal cells versus infiltrating cells in glomerular crescent formation. *Kidney Int* **1998**, *54*, 416–425. [CrossRef] [PubMed]
132. Su, H.; Chen, S.; He, F.F.; Wang, Y.M.; Bondzie, P.; Zhang, C. New Insights into Glomerular Parietal Epithelial Cell Activation and Its Signaling Pathways in Glomerular Diseases. *Biomed. Res. Int* **2015**, *2015*, 318935:1–318935:8. [CrossRef] [PubMed]
133. Cohen, A.H.; Mampaso, F.; Zamboni, L. Glomerular podocyte degeneration in human renal disease. *Lab. Invest.* **1977**, *37*, 30–42. [PubMed]
134. Susztak, K.; Raff, A.C.; Schiffer, M.; Böttinger, E.P. Glucose-induced reactive oxygen species cause apoptosis of podocytes and podocyte depletion at the onset of diabetic nephropathy. *Diabetes* **2006**, *55*, 225–233. [CrossRef] [PubMed]

135. Tharaux, P.L.; Huber, T.B. How Many Ways Can a Podocyte Die? *Semin Nephrol* **2012**, *32*, 394–404. [CrossRef] [PubMed]
136. Burlaka, I.; Nilsson, L.M.; Scott, L.; Holtbäck, U.; Eklöf, A.C.; Fogo, A.B.; Brismar, H.; Aperia, A. Prevention of apoptosis averts glomerular tubular disconnection and podocyte loss in proteinuric. kidney disease. *Kidney Int* **2016**, *90*, 135–148. [CrossRef] [PubMed]
137. Bagchus, W.M.; Hoedemaeker, P.J.; Rozing, J.; Bakker, W.W. Glomerulonephritis induced by monoclonal anti-Thy 1.1 antibodies. A sequential histological and ultrastructural study in the rat. *Lab. Invest.* **1986**, *55*, 680–687. [PubMed]
138. Wörnle, M.; Schmid, H.; Merkle, M.; Banas, B. Effects of chemokines on proliferation and apoptosis of human mesangial cells. *BMC Nephrology* **2004**, *5*, 8:1–8:14. [CrossRef] [PubMed]
139. Prakash, J.; Singh, V.P. Changing picture of renal cortical necrosis in acute kidney injury in developing country. *World J. Nephrol* **2015**, *4*, 480–486. [CrossRef] [PubMed]
140. Brix, A.E. Renal papillary necrosis. *Toxicol Pathol* **2002**, *30*, 672–674. [CrossRef] [PubMed]
141. Kono, H.; Rock, K.L. How dying cells alert the immune system to danger. *Nat. Rev. Immunol* **2008**, *8*, 279–289. [CrossRef]
142. Kaczmarek, A.; Vandenabeele, P.; Krysko, D.V. Necroptosis: The release of damage-associated molecular patterns and its physiological relevance. *Immunity* **2013**, *38*, 209–223. [CrossRef]
143. Mulay, S.R.; Linkermann, A.; Anders, H.J. Necroinflammation in kidney disease. *J. Am. Soc. Nephrol* **2016**, *27*, 27–39. [CrossRef]
144. Sarhan, M.; von Mässenhausen, A.; Hugo, C.; Oberbauer, R.; Linkermann, A. Immunological consequences of kidney cell death. *Cell Death Dis* **2018**, *9*, 114:1–114:15. [CrossRef]
145. Linkermann, A.; Bräsen, J.H.; Himmerkus, N.; Liu, S.; Huber, T.B.; Kunzendorf, U.; Krautwald, S. Rip1 (receptor-interacting protein kinase 1) mediates necroptosis and contributes to renal ischemia/reperfusion injury. *Kidney Int* **2012**, *81*, 751–761. [CrossRef] [PubMed]
146. Linkermann, A.; Bräsen, J.H.; Darding, M.; Jin, M.K.; Sanz, A.B.; Heller, J.O.; De Zen, F.; Weinlich, R.; Ortiz, A.; Walczak, H.; et al. Two independent pathways of regulated necrosis mediate ischemia-reperfusion injury. *Proc. Natl. Acad. Sci. USA* **2013**, *110*, 12024–12029. [CrossRef] [PubMed]
147. Linkermann, A.; Skouta, R.; Himmerkus, N.; Mulay, S.R.; Dewitz, C.; De Zen, F.; Prokai, A.; Zuchtriegel, G.; Krombach, F.; Welz, P.S.; et al. Synchronized renal tubular cell death involves ferroptosis. *Proc. Natl. Acad. Sci. USA* **2014**, *111*, 16836–16841. [CrossRef] [PubMed]
148. Mulay, S.R.; Desay, J.; Kumar, S.V.R.; Eberhard, J.N.; Thomasova, D.; Romoli, S.; Grigorescu, M.; Kulkarni, O.P.; Popper, B.; Vielhauer, V.; et al. Cytotoxicity of crystals involves RIPK3- MLKL-mediated necroptosis. *Nat. Commun* **2016**, *7*, 10274:1–10274:15. [CrossRef] [PubMed]
149. Allam, R.; Kumar, S.V.; Darisipudi, M.N.; Anders, H.J. Extracellular histones in tissue injury and inflammation. *J. Mol. Med. (Berl)* **2014**, *92*, 465–472. [CrossRef] [PubMed]
150. Humphreys, B.D.; Valerius, M.T.; Kobayashi, A.; Mugford, J.W.; Soeung, S.; Duffield, J.S.; McMahon, A.P.; Bonventre, J.V. Intrinsic epithelial cells repair the kidney after injury. *Cell Stem Cell* **2008**, *2*, 284–291. [CrossRef] [PubMed]
151. Bonsib, S.M. Glomerular basement membrane necrosis and crescent organization. *Kidney Int* **1988**, *33*, 966–974. [CrossRef]
152. Smeets, B.; Angelotti, M.L.; Rizzo, P.; Dijkman, H.; Lazzeri, E.; Mooren, F.; Ballerini, L.; Parente, E.; Sagrinati, C.; Mazzinghi, B.; et al. Renal progenitor cells contribute to hyperplastic lesions of podocytopathies and crescentic glomerulonephritis. *J. Am. Soc. Nephrol* **2009**, *20*, 2593–2603. [CrossRef]
153. Schreiber, A.; Xiao, H.; Jennette, J.C.; Schneider, W.; Luft, F.C.; Kettritz, R. C5a receptor mediates neutrophil activation and ANCA-induced glomerulonephritis. *J. Am. Soc. Nephrol* **2009**, *20*, 289–298. [CrossRef]
154. Ryu, M.; Migliorini, A.; Miosge, N.; Gross, O.; Shankland, S.; Brinkkoetter, P.T.; Hagmann, H.; Romagnani, P.; Liapis, H.; Anders, H.J. Plasma leakage through glomerular basement membrane ruptures triggers the proliferation of parietal epithelial cells and crescent formation in non-inflammatory glomerular injury. *J. Pathol* **2012**, *228*, 482–494. [CrossRef]
155. Schepers, M.S.; van Ballegooijen, E.S.; Bangma, C.H.; Verkoelen, C.F. Crystals cause acute necrotic cell death in renal proximal tubule cells, but not in collecting tubule cells. *Kidney Int* **2005**, *68*, 1543–1553. [CrossRef] [PubMed]
156. Mulay, S.R.; Evan, A.; Anders, H.J. Molecular mechanisms of crystal-related kidney inflammation and injury. Implications for cholesterol embolism, crystalline nephropathies and kidney stone disease. *Nephrol Dial.*

Transplant. **2014**, *29*, 507–514. [CrossRef] [PubMed]
157. Sun, X.Y.; Ouyang, J.M. New view in cell death mode: Effect of crystal size in renal epithelial cells. *Cell Death Dis* **2015**, *6*, e2013:1-2013:3. [CrossRef] [PubMed]
158. Sun, X.Y.; Ouyang, J.M.; Yu, K. Shape-dependent cellular toxicity on renal epithelial cells and stone risk of calcium oxalate dihydrate crystals. *Sci Rep.* **2017**, *7*, 7250:1–7250:13. [CrossRef] [PubMed]
159. Honarpisheh, M.; Foresto-Neto, O.; Desai, J.; Steiger, S.; Gómez, L.A.; Popper, B.; Boor, P.; Anders, H.J.; Mulay, S.R. Phagocytosis of environmental or metabolic crystalline particles induces cytotoxicity by triggering necroptosis across a broad range of particle size and shape. *Sci Rep.* **2017**, *7*, 15523:1–15523:11. [CrossRef] [PubMed]
160. Mulay, S.R.; Anders, H.J. Crystal nephropathies: Mechanisms of crystal-induced kidney injury. *Nat. Rev. Nephrol* **2017**, *13*, 226–240. [CrossRef] [PubMed]
161. Sun, X.Y.; Gan, Q.Z.; Ouyang, J.M. Calcium oxalate toxicity in renal epithelial cells: The mediation of crystal size on cell death mode. *Cell Death Discov* **2015**, *1*, 15055:1–15055:8. [CrossRef] [PubMed]
162. Mulay, S.R.; Kulkarni, O.P.; Rupanagudi, K.V.; Migliorini, A.; Darisipudi, M.N.; Vilaysane, A.; Muruve, D.; Shi, Y.; Munro, F.; Liapis, H.; et al. Calcium oxalate crystals induce renal inflammation by NLRP3-mediated IL-1beta secretion. *J. Clin. Invest.* **2013**, *123*, 236–246. [CrossRef]
163. Kirsch, T. Determinants of pathological mineralization. *Curr Opin Rheumatol* **2006**, *18*, 174–180. [CrossRef]
164. Schepens, D.; Verswijvel, G.; Kuypers, D.; Vanrenterghem, Y. Renal cortical nephrocalcinosis. *Nephrol Dial. Transplant.* **2000**, *15*, 1080–1082. [CrossRef]
165. Priante, G.; Quaggio, F.; Gianesello, L.; Ceol, M.; Cristofaro, R.; Terrin, L.; Furlan, C.; Del Prete, D.; Anglani, F. Caspase-independent programmed cell death triggers Ca2PO4 deposition in an in vitro model of nephrocalcinosis. *Biosci Rep.* **2018**, *38*, BSR20171228:1-BSR20171228:19. [CrossRef] [PubMed]
166. Priante, G.; Ceol, M.; Gianesello, L.; Furlan, C.; Del Prete, D.; Anglani, F. Human proximal tubular cells can form calcium phosphate deposits in osteogenic culture: Role of cell death and osteoblast-like transdifferentiation. *Cell Death Discov* **2019**, *5*, 57:1–57:14. [CrossRef]
167. Proudfoot, D.; Skepper, J.N.; Hegyi, L.; Bennett, M.R.; Shanahan, C.M.; Weissberg, P.L. Apoptosis regulates human vascular calcification in vitro: Evidence for initiation of vascular calcification by apoptotic bodies. *Circ Res* **2000**, *87*, 1055–1062. [CrossRef] [PubMed]
168. Giachelli, C.M. Vascular calcification mechanisms. *J. Am. Soc. Nephrol* **2004**, *15*, 2959–2964. [CrossRef] [PubMed]
169. Evrard, S.; Delanaye, P.; Kamel, S.; Cristol, J.P.; Cavalier, E. Vascular calcification: From pathophysiology to biomarkers. *Clin. Chim Acta* **2015**, *438*, 401–414. [CrossRef] [PubMed]
170. Leopold, J.A. Vascular calcification: Mechanisms of vascular smooth muscle cell calcification. *Trends Cardiovasc Med.* **2015**, *25*, 267–274. [CrossRef]
171. Priante, G.; Mezzabotta, F.; Cristofaro, R.; Quaggio, F.; Ceol, M.; Gianesello, L.; Del Prete, D.; Anglani, F. Cell death in ectopic calcification of the kidney. *Cell Death Dis* **2019**, *10*, 466. [CrossRef]
172. Unal-Cevik, I.; Kilinç, M.; Can, A.; Gürsoy-Ozdemir, Y.; Dalkara, T. Apoptotic and necrotic death mechanisms are concomitantly activated in the same cell after cerebral ischemia. *Stroke* **2004**, *35*, 2189–2194. [CrossRef]
173. Zychlinsky, A.; Zheng, L.M.; Liu, C.; Young, J.D. Cytolytic lymphocytes induce both apoptosis and necrosis in target celis. *J. Immunol* **1991**, *146*, 393–400.
174. Vanden Berghe, T.; Vanlangenakker, N.; Parthoens, E.; Deckers, W.; Devos, M.; Festjens, N.; Guerin, C.J.; Brunk, U.T.; Declercq, W.; Vandenabeele, P. Necroptosis, necrosis and secondary necrosis converge on similar cellular disintegration features. *Cell Death Differ.* **2010**, *17*, 922–930. [CrossRef]
175. Wang, S.; Zhang, C.; Hu, L.; Yang, C. Necroptosis in acute kidney injury: A shedding light. *Cell Death Dis* **2016**, *7*, e2125:1-2125:9. [CrossRef] [PubMed]
176. Homsi, E.; Janino, P.; de Faria, J.B. Role of caspases on cell death, inflammation, and cell cycle in glycerol-induced acute renal failure. *Kidney Int* **2006**, *69*, 1385–1392. [CrossRef] [PubMed]
177. Servais, H.; Ortiz, A.; Devuyst, O.; Denamur, S.; Tulkens, P.M.; Mingeot-Leclercq, M.P. Renal cell apoptosis induced by nephrotoxic drugs: Cellular and molecular mechanisms and potential approaches to modulation. *Apoptosis* **2008**, *13*, 11–32. [CrossRef] [PubMed]
178. Nelson, P.J.; Cantley, L. GSK3beta plays dirty in acute kidney injury. *J. Am. Soc. Nephrol* **2010**, *21*, 199–200. [CrossRef] [PubMed]
179. Wang, Z.; Havasi, A.; Gall, J.; Bonegio, R.; Li, Z.; Mao, H.; Schwartz, J.H.; Borkan, S.C. GSK3beta promotes apoptosis after renal ischemic injury. *J. Am. Soc. Nephrol* **2010** *21*, 284–294. [CrossRef] [PubMed]

180. Whelan, R.S.; Konstantinidis, K.; Wei, A.C.; Chen, Y.; Reyna, D.E.; Jha, S.; Yang, Y.; Calvert, J.W.; Lindsten, T.; Thompson, C.B.; et al. Bax regulates primary necrosis through mitochondrial dynamics. *Proc. Natl. Acad. Sci. USA* **2012**, *109*, 6566–6571. [CrossRef]
181. Qiu, X.; Zhang, Y.; Han, J. RIP3 is an upregulator of aerobic metabolism and the enhanced respiration by necrosomal RIP3 feeds back on necrosome to promote necroptosis. *Cell Death & Differentiation* **2018**, *25*, 821–824.
182. Teng, X.; Degterev, A.; Jagtap, P.; Xing, X.; Choi, S.; Denu, R.; Yuan, J.; Cuny, G.D. Structure-activity relationship study of novel necroptosis inhibitors. *Bioorg Med. Chem Lett* **2005**, *15*, 5039–5044. [CrossRef]
183. Degterev, A.; Hitomi, J.; Germscheid, M.; Ch'en, I.L.; Korkina, O.; Teng, X.; Abbott, D.; Cuny, G.D.; Yuan, C.; Wagner, G.; et al. Identification of RIP1 kinase as a specific cellular target of necrostatins. *Nat. Chem Biol* **2008**, *4*, 313–321. [CrossRef]
184. Sun, L.; Wang, H.; Wang, Z.; He, S.; Chen, S.; Liao, D.; Wang, L.; Yan, J.; Liu, W.; Lei, X.; et al. Mixed lineage kinase domain-like protein mediates necrosis signaling downstream of RIP3 kinase. *Cell* **2012**, *148*, 213–227. [CrossRef]
185. Kaiser, W.J.; Sridharan, H.; Huang, C.; Mandal, P.; Upton, J.W.; Gough, P.J.; Sehon, C.A.; Marquis, R.W.; Bertin, J.; Mocarski, E.S. Toll-like receptor 3-mediated necrosis via TRIF, RIP3, and MLKL. *J. Biol Chem* **2013**, *288*, 31268–31279. [CrossRef] [PubMed]
186. Harris, P.A.; Bandyopadhyay, D.; Berger, S.B.; Campobasso, N.; Capriotti, C.A.; Cox, J.A.; Dare, L.; Finger, J.N.; Hoffman, S.J.; Kahler, K.M.; et al. Discovery of small molecule RIP1 kinase inhibitors for the treatment of pathologies associated with necroptosis. *ACS Med. Chem Lett* **2013**, *4*, 1238–1243. [CrossRef] [PubMed]
187. Hildebrand, J.M.; Tanzer, M.C.; Lucet, I.S.; Young, S.N.; Spall, S.K.; Sharma, P.; Pierotti, C.; Garnier, J.M.; Dobson, R.C.; Webb, A.I.; et al. Activation of the pseudokinase MLKL unleashes the four-helix bundle domain to induce membrane localization and necroptotic cell death. *Proc. Natl. Acad. Sci. USA* **2014**, *111*, 15072–15077. [CrossRef] [PubMed]
188. Weng, D.; Marty-Roix, R.; Ganesan, S.; Proulx, M.K.; Vladimer, G.I.; Kaiser, W.J.; Mocarski, E.S.; Pouliot, K.; Chan, F.K.; Kelliher, M.A.; et al. Caspase-8 and RIP kinases regulate bacteria-induced innate immune responses and cell death. *Proc. Natl. Acad. Sci. USA* **2014**, *111*, 7391–7396. [CrossRef] [PubMed]
189. Mandal, P.; Berger, S.B.; Pillay, S.; Moriwaki, K.; Huang, C.; Guo, H.; Lich, J.D.; Finger, J.; Kasparcova, V.; Votta, B.; et al. RIP3 induces apoptosis independent of pronecrotic kinase activity. *Mol. Cell* **2014**, *56*, 481–495. [CrossRef]
190. Li, J.X.; Feng, J.M.; Wang, Y.; Li, X.H.; Chen, X.X.; Su, Y.; Shen, Y.Y.; Chen, Y.; Xiong, B.; Yang, C.H.; et al. The B-Raf(V600E) inhibitor dabrafenib selectively inhibits RIP3 and alleviates acetaminophen-induced liver injury. *Cell Death Dis* **2014**, *5*, e1278:1-1278:11. [CrossRef]
191. Fauster, A.; Rebsamen, M.; Huber, K.V.; Bigenzahn, J.W.; Stukalov, A.; Lardeau, C.H.; Scorzoni, S.; Bruckner, M.; Gridling, M.; Parapatics, K.; et al. A cellular screen identifies ponatinib and pazopanib as inhibitors of necroptosis. *Cell Death Dis* **2015**, *6*, e1767:1-1767:10. [CrossRef]
192. Rodriguez, D.A.; Weinlich, R.; Brown, S.; Guy, C.; Fitzgerald, P.; Dillon, C.P.; Oberst, A.; Quarato, G.; Low, J.; Cripps, J.G.; et al. Characterization of RIPK3-mediated phosphorylation of the activation loop of MLKL during necroptosis. *Cell Death Differ.* **2016**, *23*, 76–88. [CrossRef]
193. Oppenheim, J.J.; Yang, D. Alarmins: Chemotactic activators of immune responses. *Curr Opin Immunol* **2005**, *17*, 359–365. [CrossRef]
194. Chan, J.K.; Roth, J.; Oppenheim, J.J.; Tracey, K.J.; Vogl, T.; Feldmann, M.; Horwood, N.; Nanchahal, J. Alarmins: Awaiting a clinical response. *J. Clin. Invest.* **2012**, *122*, 2711–2719. [CrossRef]
195. Silke, J.; Rickard, J.A.; Gerlic, M. The diverse role of RIP kinases in necroptosis and inflammation. *Nat. Immunol* **2015**, *16*, 689–697. [CrossRef] [PubMed]
196. Linkermann, A.; Hackl, M.J.; Kunzendorf, U.; Walczak, H.; Krautwald, S.; Jevnikar, A.M. Necroptosis in immunity and ischemia-reperfusion injury. *Am. J. Transplant.* **2013**, *13*, 2797–2804. [CrossRef] [PubMed]
197. Linkermann, A.; Green, D.R. Necroptosis. *N Engl J. Med.* **2014**, *370*, 455–465. [CrossRef] [PubMed]
198. Degterev, A.; Linkermann, A. Generation of small molecules to interfere with regulated necrosis. *Cell Mol. Life Sci.* **2016**, *73*, 2251–2267. [CrossRef] [PubMed]

Chemokine CXCL13 as a New Systemic Biomarker for B-Cell Involvement in Acute T Cell-Mediated Kidney Allograft Rejection

Lena Schiffer [1,2,†], Flavia Wiehler [1,†], Jan Hinrich Bräsen [3], Wilfried Gwinner [1], Robert Greite [1], Kirill Kreimann [1], Anja Thorenz [1], Katja Derlin [4], Beina Teng [1], Song Rong [1], Sibylle von Vietinghoff [1], Hermann Haller [1], Michael Mengel [5], Lars Pape [2], Christian Lerch [2], Mario Schiffer [1,6,†] and Faikah Gueler [1,*,†]

1 Nephrology, Hannover Medical School, 30625 Hannover, Germany; Schiffer.Lena@mh-hannover.de (L.S.); Wiehler.Flavia@mh-hannover.de (F.W.); Gwinner.Wilfried@mh-hannover.de (W.G.); Greite.Robert@mh-hannover.de (R.G.); Kirill.Kreimann@stud.mh-hannover.de (K.K.); athorenz@gmx.de (A.T.); teng.beina@mh-hannover.de (B.T.); rong.song@mh-hannover.de (S.R.); vonvietinghoff.sibylle@mh-hannover.de (S.v.V.); haller.hermann@mh-hannover.de (H.H.); Mario.Schiffer@uk-erlangen.de (M.S.)
2 Pediatric Nephrology, Hannover Medical School, 30625 Hannover, Germany; pape.lars@mh-hannover.de (L.P.); Lerch.christian@mh-hannover.de (C.L.)
3 Pathology, Hannover Medical School, 30625 Hannover, Germany; Braesen.Jan@mh-hannover.de
4 Radiology, Hannover Medical School, 30625 Hannover, Germany; derlin.katja@mh-hannover.de
5 Laboratory Medicine & Pathology, University of Alberta, Edmonton, AB T6G 2R3, Canada; mmengel@ualberta.ca
6 Nephrology and Hypertension, University Hospital Erlangen, 91054 Erlangen, Gerrmany
* Correspondence: gueler.faikah@mh-hannover.de
† These authors contributed equally to this work.

Abstract: The presence of B-cell clusters in allogenic T cell-mediated rejection (TCMR) of kidney allografts is linked to more severe disease entities. In this study we characterized B-cell infiltrates in patients with TCMR and examined the role of serum CXCL-13 in these patients and experimentally. CXCL-13 serum levels were analyzed in 73 kidney allograft recipients at the time of allograft biopsy. In addition, four patients were evaluated for CXCL13 levels during the first week after transplantation. ELISA was done to measure CXCL-13 serum levels. For further mechanistic understanding, a translational allogenic kidney transplant (ktx) mouse model for TCMR was studied in BalbC recipients of fully mismatched transplants with C57BL/6 donor kidneys. CXCL-13 serum levels were measured longitudinally, CD20 and CD3 composition and CXCL13 mRNA in tissue were examined by flow cytometry and kidneys were examined by histology and immunohistochemistry. We found significantly higher serum levels of the B-cell chemoattractant CXCL13 in patients with TCMR compared to controls and patients with borderline TCMR. Moreover, in patients with acute rejection within the first week after ktx, a >5-fold CXCL13 increase was measured and correlated with B-cell infiltrates in the biopsies. In line with the clinical findings, TCMR in mice correlated with increased systemic serum-CXCL13 levels. Moreover, renal allografts had significantly higher CXCL13 mRNA expression than isogenic controls and showed interstitial CD20+ B-cell clusters and CD3+ cell infiltrates accumulating in the vicinity of renal vessels. CXCL13 blood levels correlate with B-cell involvement in TCMR and might help to identify patients at risk of a more severe clinical course of rejection.

Keywords: B-cell attracting chemokine; CXCL13; kidney transplantation; allograft rejection; T cell-mediated rejection

1. Introduction

Kidney allograft rejection is the major cause for loss of graft function and may have a negative impact on long-term allograft survival. Currently, besides donor specific antibodies or non-HLA antibodies, which are linked to humoral rejection, no reliable serum markers for ktx rejection exist [1,2]. Impaired allograft function with elevated serum creatinine drives the decision to perform a biopsy. The majority (about 90%) of acute rejections, especially in the first year after ktx, are T cell-mediated [3]. However, emerging evidence has revealed that intra-graft B-cell accumulation plays an important role in T cell-mediated rejection as well and correlates with a worse outcome [4–6]. However, the mechanistic details are not completely resolved. The chemokine CXC ligand 13 (CXCL13), also known as B-cell-attracting chemokine-1 (BAC-1) or B-lymphocyte-chemoattractant (BLC), is a CXC subtype member of the chemokine superfamily. CXCL13 is particularly important in the context of leukocyte recruitment and is sufficient to induce secondary lymphoid nodes [7,8]. Besides B-cell attraction CXCL13 activates different intracellular pathways that are involved in cell survival, invasion and growth and is able to stimulate resident kidney cells to produce pro-inflammatory cytokines and chemokines [7,9–11]. In sum, these biological functions of CXCL13 have led us to hypothesize that CXCL13 may also be linked to B-cell accumulation in kidney allografts in the presence of TCMR.

Here, we were able to show that CXCL13 can be monitored systemically and is elevated in TCMR compared to borderline rejection and controls. In addition, increasing CXCL13 values in the first week after ktx were indicators for acute rejection with B-cell rich infiltrates in two more patients. Furthermore, in a murine model for TCMR after ktx with similar histological TCMR patterns as in patients, we verified systemic upregulation of CXCL13 in blood as well as on an mRNA-level in the allografts. Taken together, our data indicate that CXCL13 blood levels can function as a readily available biomarker for B-cell involvement in T cell-mediated rejection and possibly as a therapeutic target.

2. Results

2.1. B-cell Involvement in Kidney Allograft Rejection in Patients

Different morphologies have been described for renal allograft rejection. We characterized different B-cell expression patterns (Figure 1A–E) in 67 randomly selected human biopsies with TCMR and graded them as B-cell rich infiltrates if more than 30 CD20+ cells were detected per high power field (HPF) (Figure 1E).

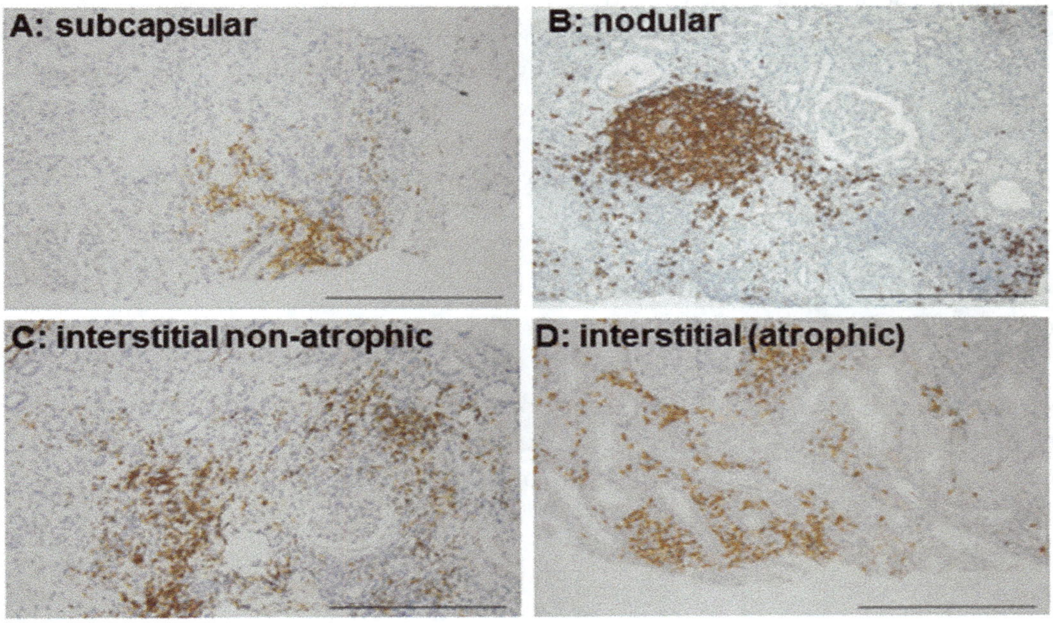

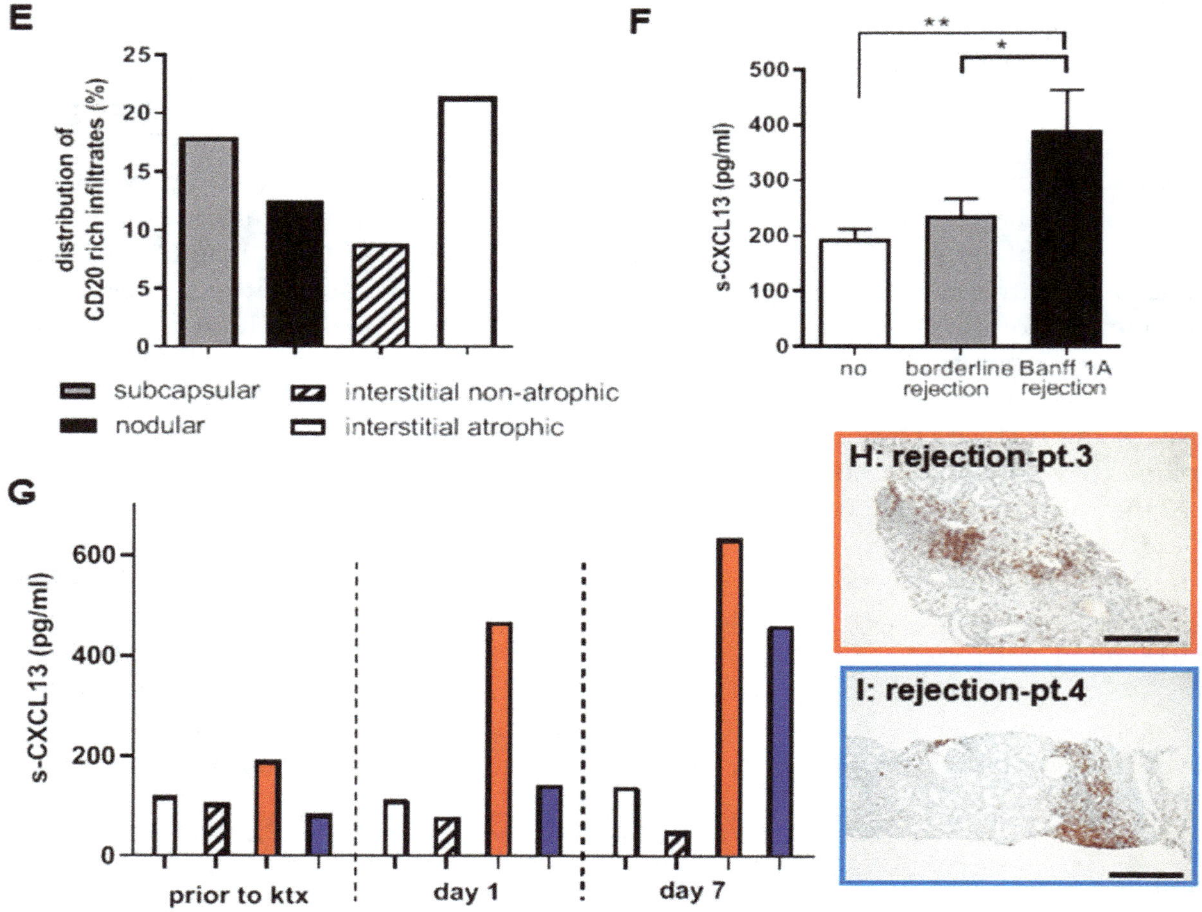

Figure 1. CD20+ cells were detected as part of inflammatory infiltrates in patient biopsies with TCMR (**A**–**D**, bar: 100 μm)) in subcapsular, tubular-interstitial (atrophic and non-atrophic) areas as well as in nodular infiltrates. In the non-rejection state, no CD20 positivity is detectable (data not shown). CD20+ cells were quantified in 67 randomly selected human biopsies with TCMR and graded as B-cell rich (>30 CD20-positive cells/hpf). In subcapsular infiltrates, 17.9%, in interstitial-nodular infiltrates, 12.5%, and in interstitial/atrophic areas, 21.4% were B-cell rich. The Banff-relevant interstitial non-atrophic areas contained 8.9% B-cell rich infiltrates (**E**). Serum CXCL13 levels are increased in patients with TCMR (Banff1a) compared to patients with borderline or no rejection (** $p = 0.01$; * $p = 0.05$) (**F**). Four patients had CXCL13 measurements during the first week after ktx (**G**). All had low levels of CXCL13 prior to ktx and two patients developed a relevant increase of CXCL13 levels up to day 7. Biopsy revealed a rejection with B-cell rich infiltrates (**H**,**I**, bar: 200 μm).

We found CD20+ rich infiltrates in 83.6% ($n = 56$) of the biopsies while only 16.4% were negative for CD20. The B-cell infiltrates were localized in the subcapsular region in 28.6% of renal biopsies, of these 17.9% contained more than 30 CD20+ cells per HPF. In 19.6% of the biopsies, interstitial-nodular infiltrates occurred, and 12.5% contained more than 30 CD20+ cells per HPF. The majority of CD20+ infiltrates was detected in interstitial/atrophic areas of biopsies (60.7%), more than 30 CD20+ cells per HPF were detected in 21.4% of the biopsies. Interestingly, the nodular infiltrates showed starry sky macrophages and signs of tertiary lymphoid organ formation (TLO) as depicted by CD3 and CD68-stains (Figure S1).

2.2. CXCL13 as a Systemic Biomarker of TCMR Rejection in Patients

Serum samples of 73 patients undergoing kidney transplant biopsies with an interval of 39–214 days after surgery (n = 28 with allograft rejection and n= 45 without rejection) were analyzed by ELISA for systemic CXCL13 expression (Figure 1F). Patient characteristics are summarized in Table 1. Serum CXCL13 was significantly higher in patients with TCMR than in the control group (rejection (n = 10 samples); mean 357.6 ±73.2 pg/mL versus controls (n = 65 samples; 211.4 ± 19 pg/mL, p = 0.006) and also higher compared to patients with borderline rejection (n= 24 samples; CXCL13: 214.2 ± 33.7 pg/mL, p = 0.06). No significant difference was observed between patients without rejection compared to borderline rejection. In four patients CXCL13 levels were measured longitudinally prior to ktx, at day 1 and 7 after surgery (Figure 1G). All patients had low initial CXCL13 levels and only the two patients with allograft rejection with B-cell rich infiltrates (Figure 1H,J) had >5-fold CXCL13 elevation. Allograft biopsy was indicated when serum-creatinine levels stayed high. Serum-creatinine decreased after anti-rejection therapy (serum-creatinine levels are shown in Figure S2).

Table 1. Patient characteristics (study 2001–2006).

Type of Rejection	Banff 1A or Higher	Borderline	No Rejection
Number of patients	9	19	45
Number of serum samples	10	24	65
Time between transplantation and biopsy (days; ±SD)	108.9 (±56.2)	110.4 (±59.0)	117.0 (±53.6)
Age at transplantation (years; ±SD)	54.1 (±19.6)	48.3 (±10.2)	54.5 (±12.6)
HLA-Mismatch (mean ± SD)	1.5 (±2.3)	1.9 (±1.6)	2.1 (±1.7)
Data available for the following number of patients	8 (9)	15 (19)	41 (45)
Creatinine level at time of biopsy (μmol/l; ±SD)	160.1 (±72.9)	194.0 (±91.8)	154.1 (±72.4)
Creatinine level after 1 year (μmol/l; ±SD)	156.4 (±41.1)	188.1 (±73.7)	142.2 (±63.9)
Creatinine level after 5 year (μmol/l; ±SD)	146.2 (±41.9)	196.9 (±91.5)	162.9 (±99.9)
Immunosuppression at time of biopsy			
Number of immunosuppressants (±SD)	2.2 (±0.6)	2.2 (±0.4)	2.6 (±0.6)
Data available for the following number of samples	10 (10)	23 (24)	62(65)
Prednisolon dose (mg; ±SD)	10.5 (±5.7)	12.2 (±5.3)	9.6 (±5.4)
Cyclosporine A	50%	91.7%	88.7%
Mycophenolat mofetil	20%	25%	59.7%
Sirolimus	0%	8.3%	16.1%
Tacrolimus	30%	4.2%	3.2%
Belatacept	20%	0%	4.8%
Number of rejections (mean ± SD)	1.2 (±0.4)	0.2 (±0.4)	0 (±0)
DSA-Status	n.d.	n.d.	n.d.

2.3. Allograft Rejection in a Translational Mouse Model for TCMR

To study CXCL13 up-regulation in more detail, we investigated a well described translational mouse model of kidney transplantation. The fully mismatched B6 to BALB/c ktx resulted in TCMR and was compared to isogenic ktx (Figure 2).

Histology at three weeks after transplantation revealed Banff 1A or higher rejection in the allografts which had severe interstitial inflammation (Figure 2A–C). The majority of infiltrating cells were CD3+ (Figure 2D–F). In addition, dense, nodular CD22+ B-cell clusters around the vessels could be identified (Figure 2G–I). By flow cytometry, significantly more CD3+ T-cells and also to a lesser extent CD19+ B-cells were observed in the allografts compared to isografts (Figure 2J). In the spleen no differences between T- and B-lymphocytes from allo- or isografts were observed. When measuring systemic CXCL13 expression, a significant increase at day 6 and 14 after ktx in allograft recipients was detected (Figure 3A).

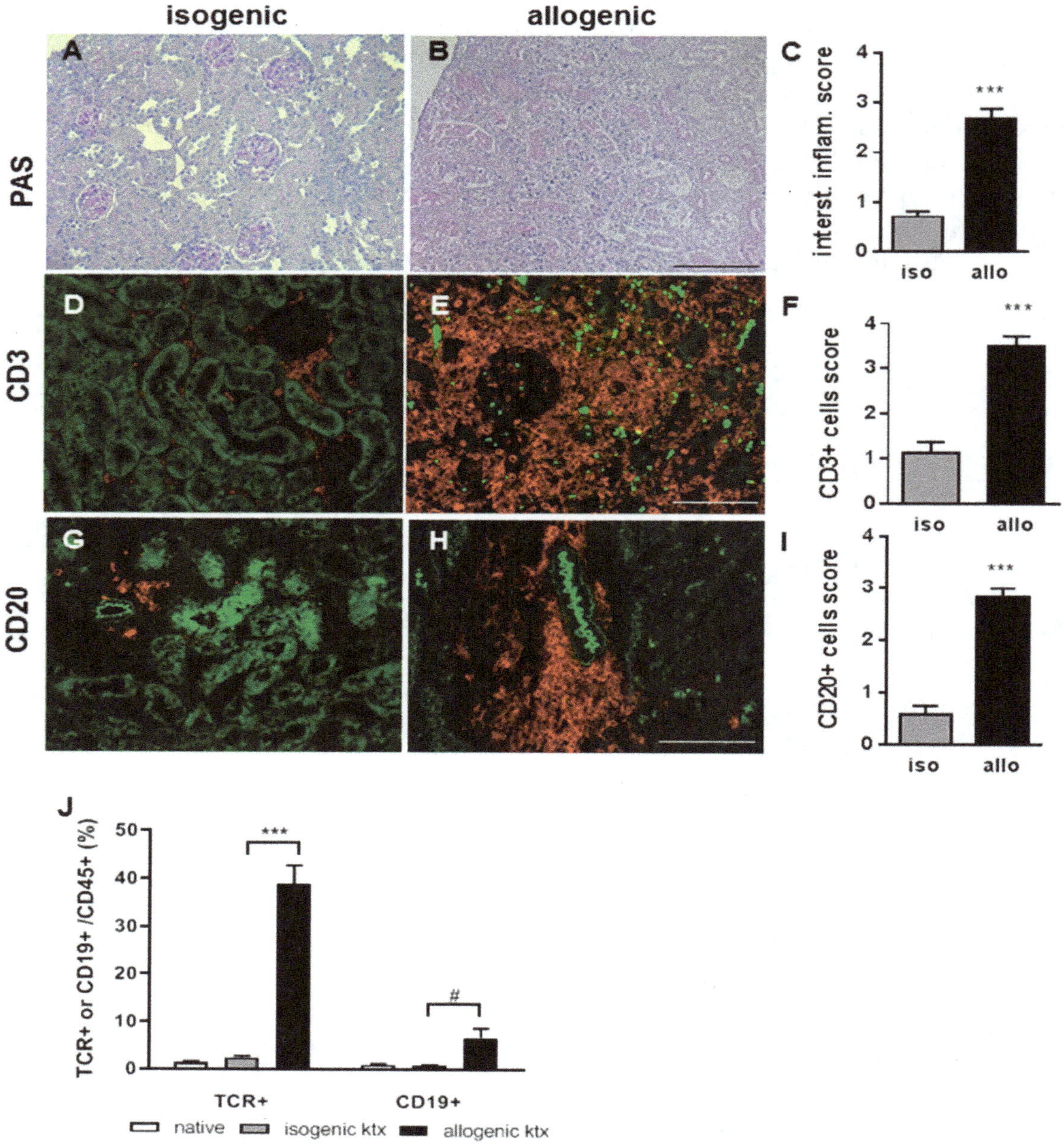

Figure 2. At three weeks after ktx, renal allograft rejection was characterized by severe inflammation and Banff 1A, and higher rejection grades in comparison to isogenic grafts without inflammation (**A–C**, representative PAS stains, bar: 200 μm). The majority of infiltration cells were CD3+ T-lymphocytes, which formed interstitial dense infiltrates and clustered around vessels and glomeruli (**D–F**, bar: 200 μm). CD20+ nodular B-cell clusters were identified with much higher cell count in allografts compared to isografts (**G–I**, bar: 100 μm). Flow cytometry of the infiltrating leukocytes of the grafts showed significantly enhanced proportion of CD3+ T-lymphocytes in allografts and also enhanced CD20+ B-lymphocytes (**J**, *** $p < 0.001$, # $p < 0.05$).

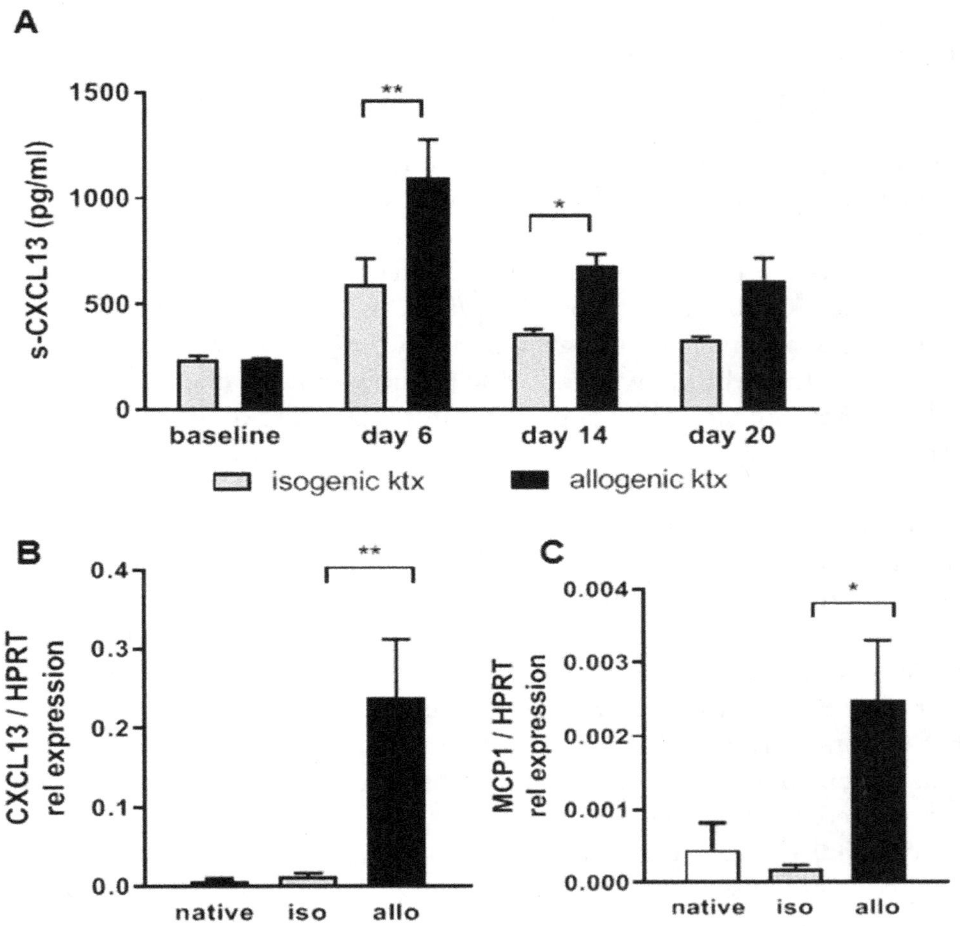

Figure 3. In the mouse ktx model, allograft recipients showed significantly increased serum CXCL13 levels towards day 6 and 14 (**A**). Rejecting kidney allografts showed significantly enhanced CXCL13 mRNA expression compared to isografts and native controls (**B**). MCP-1 mRNA was significantly up-regulated in rejecting kidneys (**C**, $n = 6$ in each group, HPRT served as house keeper, * $p < 0.05$, ** $p < 0.01$).

This was in line with the increased systemic CXCL13 levels in patients. Furthermore, in the renal tissue, significantly enhanced CXCL13 mRNA expression was detected in allografts compared to isografts (Figure 3B). As expected, the pro-inflammatory cytokine monocyte chemoattractant protein (MCP-1) was also significantly upregulated in allografts compared to isografts (Figure 3C).

3. Discussion

Kidney allograft rejection remains a major complication after transplantation along with the risk of graft loss or limited long term graft survival. The majority of rejection types in the early phase after ktx are TCMR [12]. In this context it is known that a significant proportion of TCMR cases additionally contain relevant number of B-cells in the infiltrates [13]. B-cell involvement has been linked to more severe clinical courses of allograft rejection, which were more difficult to control [13,14]. It is generally accepted that B-cells act as positive mediators of inflammation through their production of immunoglobulins and of cytokines such as IL-4 and IL-6. B-cells also support T cell activation by acting as antigen presenting cells and exacerbate renal damage through this interaction [15]. Even though the pathophysiological role is not completely resolved, the association of B-cell infiltrates and an inferior ktx outcome is beyond controversy: different clinical studies have confirmed an association of B-cell infiltrates and a worse transplant survival rate [16,17].

Previously, Steinmetz et al. described an association between CXCL13 expression and CXCR5+ and CD 20+ B-cells in acute renal transplant rejection in patients [18]. Interestingly, in the current study we were able to show that B-cells can be detected in the majority of cases with TCMR in patients. We demonstrated that B-cells were, besides localizations in the subcapsular region and the interstitium, mainly located in interstitial non-atrophic areas. Of note, the revised Banff-classification newly introduced the inflammation-interstitial fibrosis and tubular atrophy (i-IFTA) score, which recognizes inflammation within areas of fibrosis and atrophy as relevant [19].

Previously, we found that the expression of the B-cell attracting chemokine CXCL13 plays a pivotal role in patients with different B-cell mediated diseases [20]. Besides its role in B-cell homeostasis, the CXCL13/CXCR5 interaction also leads to an activation of different important intracellular pathways such as PI3K/AKT, Raf/MEK/ERK, Integrin-beta3/Scr/FAK and DOCK/Rac/JNK [7,9,10]. These pathways are involved in cell survival, invasion and growth, underlining a more complex function of CXCL13 than initially suspected. In addition, we were able to show that the chemokine CXCL13 was able to stimulate resident kidney cells to produce pro-inflammatory cytokines and chemokines [21]. These mediators lead to a neutrophil respiratory burst, indicating that CXCL13 aggravated the course of disease [21].

In the current study, we demonstrated that CXCL13 was significantly increased in the serum of patients with an acute transplant rejection. Of clinical interest, a statistically significant increase was only detected in patients with a clinically relevant rejection, but not in patients with borderline rejection [22]. In a pilot study with four patients we showed that prior to ktx, serum CXCL13 levels were low and increased due to rejection in two patients. A clinical trial is ongoing to validate CXCL13 as a biomarker for early B-cell activation and to study its relevance in the context with allograft rejection shortly after transplantation. Especially in times of organ shortage, this is of clinical interest since allograft rejections are one of the main reasons for transplant loss and early identification of patients at risk allows for early medical intervention.

The sources of CXCL13 production are not completely understood. So far, a variety of transient and non-transient cells have been shown to express CXCL13 [21,23]. Steinmetz et al. showed that CXCL13 expression is exclusively present in areas of B-cell clusters [18].

To further investigate the role of CXCL13 and B-cells in acute allograft rejection we used a well-established translational ktx mouse model of TCMR [22]. By using a non-life supporting model where one native kidney remained in situ, we were able to perform longitudinal follow up for three weeks despite ongoing TCMR. In this model, TCMR onset starts at 4–5 days after ktx and is triggered by a prolonged cold ischemia time of 60 min. Flow cytometry and immunohistochemistry showed that the main infiltrating cell type was CD3+ T-lymphocytes. However, similar to the findings in human biopsies, nodular B-cell clusters were also identified in rejecting renal allograft specimens in mice. Accordingly, enhanced CD19+ B-cell population were also identified by flow cytometry in the allografts. Interestingly, the circulating CD19+ B-cell population was reduced in allograft recipients compared to the isogenic controls. This might be explained by the fact that the B-cells were recruited into the lymphoid organs and the rejecting allograft where they form tertiary lymphoid organs [24].

Taken together, our data show that CXCL13 could serve as a relevant circulating biomarker to identify B-cell involvement in ktx recipients with TCMR and relevant B-cell involvement. CXCL13 serum levels may be a readily available surrogate marker for ktx rejection and it is tempting to speculate that CXCL13 could function as a potential therapeutic target.

4. Materials and Methods

4.1. Patient Samples

The first clinical study (2001 and 2006) was approved by the Institutional Review Board of Hannover Medical School (approval number 2765). Following informed consent, serum samples from 73 patients were collected at the time of a kidney graft biopsy. Samples for 28 patients with allograft rejection (9 patients with Bannf1A or higher and 19 with Borderline rejection) and 45 patients without rejection were collected. Some patients had repeated biopsies over time so that total sample number was ($n = 99$) (see Table 1). In addition, in an ongoing clinical study (approval number 6895) with longitudinal blood sampling prior to ktx, at day 1 and 7 after ktx we identified two patients with early rejection and two with initial function, and tested for CXCL13 levels in correlation to ktx biopsy ($n = 4$, patient characteristics are shown in Table 2). All patients had standard triple therapy with prednisolone, MMF and tacrolimus and induction therapy with basiliximab. Patient 2 had high panel reactive antibodies (77%) and received plasmapheresis at the day of ktx and afterwards. All serum samples were stored at −80°C.

Table 2. Pilot study in the early phase after ktx.

Patient Characteristics	Patient 1	Patient 2	Patient 3	Patient 4
Recipient age (years)	22	48	51	50
Hemodialysis (years)	None	6	12	12
Type of ktx	living donation	postmortal, AM-Program	postmortal	postmortal
Plasmapheresis	no	2× day 0 + 1	day 15, 16, 17	no
Delayed graft function	no	no	no	yes
Allograft biopsy (day)	n/a	n/a	10	14
In hospital stay (days)	8	8	21	14
Steroid boli for rejection treatment	n.a.	n.a.	3× 500 mg prednisolone	3× 500 mg prednisolone
Creatinine at 4 weeks after ktx (μmol/L)	145	178	162	169

4.2. CXCL13 ELISA

CXCL13 serum levels in human and mice samples were analyzed by ELISA (Quantikine Human CXCL13/BLC/BCA-1 Immunoassay Catalog Number DCX130, Quantikine Mouse CXCL13/BLC/BCA-1, Immunoassay Catalog Number MCX130), respectively, as described previously [10,20]. Color development was measured by using an ELISA reader (Tecan spectra mini, Crailsheim, Germany). The color intensity was correlated with the amounts of bound CXCL13 by comparison with internal standards.

4.3. Renal Morphology and Immunohistochemistry of Patient Allograft Biopsies

Human kidney transplant biopsies were fixed in 4% neutral buffered formaldehyde and embedded in paraffin. Two μm sections were stained for routine histochemical diagnostics (H&E, PAS, Jones Methenamine) according to standard protocols, immunohistochemical stains were performed for CD20 (Dako, clone L26, 1:500 after heat pretreatment with EDTA at pH8.4 for 16 minutes) on an automated platform (Ventana Benchmark Ultra). Normal biopsies can contain single B-cell infiltrates without any clinical relevance. Therefore, we developed a cutoff of >30 CD20+ cells per hpf for definition of relevant "B-cell rich" infiltrates. For the evaluation we used a visual analog scale that we have developed ourselves for standardized evaluation of the samples Figure S3).

4.4. Mice

Male C57Bl/6N (B6, H2b) and BALB/cAnCrl (H2d) mice (Charles River, Sulzfeld Germany) weighing 25–28 g at 10–12 weeks of age were used for all experiments. B6 mice served as donors, BALB/c mice as recipients.

4.5. Kidney Transplantation

For allogenic kidney transplantation (ktx), B6 mice served as donors and BALB/c as recipients and for isogenic controls, B6 mice served as donors and recipients. Surgeries were done in general anesthesia with isoflurane (induction 3–5% and maintenance 1.5%) by a vascular surgeon with >15 years' experience in small animal surgery. For analgesia, butorphanol (2.5 mg/kg bodyweight ip) was given prior to surgery [25]. Briefly, the kidney graft was retrieved en bloc with the renal vessels and the ureter. After left recipient nephrectomy, the kidney graft was transplanted. Vessel anastomosis with the abdominal aorta and the caval vene was done. Afterwards, the ureter was directly anastomosed into the bladder dome. Cold ischemia time was standardized to 60 min and warm ischemia time to 30 min. The prolonged cold ischemia time is needed to induce 100% allograft rejection. To overcome mortality in the allograft model, a non-live supporting model was chosen and the right native kidney remained in situ to ensure normal renal function throughout the three weeks observation time. The model has been described previously in detail by functional MRI studies [26,27]. After surgery, animals were monitored until fully awake and had free access to a standard diet (Altromin, Lippe) and tap water. Daily monitoring of physical well-being and behavior was done throughout the follow up of three weeks. Criteria for study termination were impaired food uptake, passive behavior and scrubby appearance. Animals were cared for in accordance to the national and international guidelines of animal welfare and animal protection. Ethical approval was given by the local authority (Lower Saxony Ministry for Food and Drug Safety number: 33.9-42502-04-11/0492).

4.6. Renal Morphology and Immunohistochemistry of Mouse Kidney Grafts

For mouse kidney graft histology and immunohistochemistry two μm paraffin sections were analyzed by PAS stain to define the type and degree of rejection according to the Banff classification [28]. The analysis was done without knowledge of animal group assignment by a nephropathologist with >20 years of experience. Immunohistochemistry for CD3+ T-cell (Acris Antibodies GmbH, Herford, Germany) infiltrates was done on paraffin sections. CD22+ B cells (Southern Biotech, Birmingham, AL, USA) were stained on four μm cryosections. Semi-quantitative assessment of the density of CD3+ cell infiltration was done as follows: 0 < 5 cells per view field (VF40x), 1 mild infiltration: 5–10 cells/VF, 2 moderate infiltration: 11–25 cells/VF, 3 severe: 26–50 cells/VF, 4 very severe >50 cells/VF. B-cell clusters were quantified with 0.5: single CD22+ cell, 1: B-cell cluster with 2–9 CD22+ cells, 2: B-cell cluster with 10–20 CD22+ cells, 3: B-cell cluster with >21 CD22+ cells.

4.7. Flow Cytometry

Flow cytometry of the kidney grafts, whole blood and spleen was done to characterize leukocyte subsets as described previously [27]. FACS Canto-I (BD Biosciences, San Jose, CA, USA) was used for all experiments with FACSDiva software version 6·0. Data were analyzed using WinList™ software (Verity Software House, Topsham, ME, USA). After collagen digest of the renal tissue, live death stain was done. Living leukocytes were stained by CD45+ and CD19+ B-lymphocytes and TCR+ T-lymphocytes were gated from CD11b+ cells. Quantification is given in % from CD45+ cell counts.

4.8. CXCL13 Expression in Kidney Graft Tissue

After organ retrieval, tissue was immediately fixed in RNAlater. Total mRNA was extracted using the RNeasy mini kit system (Qiagen, Hilden, Germany) and transcribed with Quiagen mini kits. For quantitative PCR (qPCR), 1 μg of DNase-treated total RNA was reverse transcribed using Superscript II Reverse transcriptase (Invitrogen, Carlsbad, CA, USA) and qPCR was performed on a Lightcycler 420 II (Roche Diagnostics, Penzberg, Germany) using FastStart Sybr-Green. Gene-specific primers for CXCL13 (Primer-sequence: fwd-TCT GGA CCA AGA rev-TGA AGA AAG TT) and monocyte chemoattractant protein-1 (MCP-1; Mm_Ccl2_1_SG QuantiTect Primer Assay QT00167832) were used. Quantification was carried out using QGene software.

4.9. Statistical Analysis

For human data we used R (Version 3.3.3) for analysis [29]. As some patients were investigated more than once, we had to account for the correlated nature of the data. We used the multgee package, which applies a generalized estimating equations (GEE) approach for correlated multinomial responses using a local odds ratios parameterization [30]. Besides, statistical analysis was performed with GraphPad Prism 6.0 (GraphPad Software, Inc., La Jolla, CA, USA). One-way ANOVA for multiple comparison was used with post-hoc Tukey correction. For comparison of two groups, T-test was done. Values are expressed as mean with standard error of mean (SEM). Significance was assumed at * $p < 0.05$, ** $p < 0.01$, *** $p < 0.001$.

Author Contributions: L.S.: Research design, result evaluation, manuscript writing; F.W.: Performed experimental work-up, result evaluation, manuscript writing, approval of the manuscript; J.H.B.: Performed histology work-up and evaluation of patient ktx biopsies, approval of the manuscript; W.G.: Participated in manuscript writing; A.T.: Participated in mouse ktx analysis, discussed and approved the manuscript; R.G.: enrolled patients for the clinical study, retrieved blood samples and discussed and approved the manuscript; K.K.: measured CXCL13 ELISA, did data analysis and approved the manuscript; K.D.: discussed and approved the manuscript; B.T.: discussed and approved the manuscript; S.R.: performed ktx in mice, approved the manuscript; S.v.V.: participated in analysis of flow cytometry data, approved the manuscript; H.H.: discussed and approved the manuscript; M.M.: Analyzed mouse kidney transplants, approved the manuscript; L.P.: Participated in statistical evaluation, approved the manuscript; C.L.: Participated in statistical evaluation, approved the manuscript; M.S.: Research design, participated in result evaluation, discussed and approved the manuscript; F.G.: designed kidney transplant mouse study, result evaluation, manuscript writing.

Acknowledgments: We thank Heike Lührs, Herle Chlebusch and Barbara Hertel for excellent technical support. We thank Patricia Schroder for critical reading of the manuscript.

Abbreviations

BCA	B-cell attracting chemokine
CXCL13	CXC ligand 13 protein
ktx	Kidney transplantation
allograft rejection	T cell-mediated rejection

References

1. Cardinal, H.; Dieude, M.; Hebert, M.J. The Emerging Importance of Non-HLA Autoantibodies in Kidney Transplant Complications. *J. Am. Soc. Nephrol.* **2017**, *28*, 400–406. [CrossRef] [PubMed]
2. Lefaucheur, C.; Viglietti, D.; Bouatou, Y.; Philippe, A.; Pievani, D.; Aubert, O.; Duong Van Huyen, J.P.; Taupin, J.L.; Glotz, D.; Legendre, C.; et al. Non-HLA agonistic anti-angiotensin II type 1 receptor antibodies induce a distinctive phenotype of antibody-mediated rejection in kidney transplant recipients. *Kidney Int.* **2019**. (Epub ahead of print). [CrossRef] [PubMed]
3. Sellares, J.; de Freitas, D.G.; Mengel, M.; Reeve, J.; Einecke, G.; Sis, B.; Hidalgo, L.G.; Famulski, K.; Matas, A.; Halloran, P.F. Understanding the causes of kidney transplant failure: The dominant role of antibody-mediated rejection and nonadherence. *Am. J. Transpl.* **2012**, *12*, 388–399. [CrossRef]
4. Mengel, M.; Gwinner, W.; Schwarz, A.; Bajeski, R.; Franz, I.; Brocker, V.; Becker, T.; Neipp, M.; Klempnauer, J.; Haller, H.; et al. Infiltrates in protocol biopsies from renal allografts. *Am. J. Transpl.* **2007**, *7*, 356–365. [CrossRef]
5. Hasegawa, J.; Honda, K.; Omoto, K.; Wakai, S.; Shirakawa, H.; Okumi, M.; Ishida, H.; Fuchinoue, S.; Hattori, M.; Tanabe, K. Clinical and Pathological Features of Plasma Cell-Rich Acute Rejection After Kidney Transplantation. *Transplantation* **2018**, *102*, 853–859. [CrossRef]
6. Kwun, J.; Manook, M.; Page, E.; Burghuber, C.; Hong, J.; Knechtle, S.J. Crosstalk Between T and B Cells in the Germinal Center After Transplantation. *Transplantation* **2017**, *101*, 704–712. [CrossRef]

7. Ansel, K.M.; Ngo, V.N.; Hyman, P.L.; Luther, S.A.; Forster, R.; Sedgwick, J.D.; Browning, J.L.; Lipp, M.; Cyster, J.G. A chemokine-driven positive feedback loop organizes lymphoid follicles. *Nature* **2000**, *406*, 309–314. [CrossRef]
8. Luther, S.A.; Ansel, K.M.; Cyster, J.G. Overlapping roles of CXCL13, interleukin 7 receptor alpha, and CCR7 ligands in lymph node development. *J. Exp. Med.* **2003**, *197*, 1191–1198. [CrossRef]
9. Gunn, M.D.; Ngo, V.N.; Ansel, K.M.; Ekland, E.H.; Cyster, J.G.; Williams, L.T. A B-cell-homing chemokine made in lymphoid follicles activates Burkitt's lymphoma receptor-1. *Nature* **1998**, *391*, 799–803. [CrossRef] [PubMed]
10. El-Haibi, C.P.; Singh, R.; Gupta, P.; Sharma, P.K.; Greenleaf, K.N.; Singh, S.; Lillard, J.W., Jr. Antibody Microarray Analysis of Signaling Networks Regulated by Cxcl13 and Cxcr5 in Prostate Cancer. *J. Proteom. Bioinform.* **2012**, *5*, 177–184. [CrossRef]
11. Chen, D.; Zhang, J.; Peng, W.; Weng, C.; Chen, J. Urinary CXC motif chemokine 13 is a noninvasive biomarker of antibodymediated renal allograft rejection. *Mol. Med. Rep.* **2018**, *18*, 2399–2406. [CrossRef]
12. Halloran, P.F.; Famulski, K.; Reeve, J. The molecular phenotypes of rejection in kidney transplant biopsies. *Curr. Opin. Organ Transpl.* **2015**, *20*, 359–367. [CrossRef]
13. Einecke, G.; Reeve, J.; Mengel, M.; Sis, B.; Bunnag, S.; Mueller, T.F.; Halloran, P.F. Expression of B cell and immunoglobulin transcripts is a feature of inflammation in late allografts. *Am. J. Transpl.* **2008**, *8*, 1434–1443. [CrossRef] [PubMed]
14. Carpio, V.N.; Noronha Ide, L.; Martins, H.L.; Jobim, L.F.; Gil, B.C.; Kulzer, A.S.; Loreto Mda, S.; Goncalves, L.F.; Manfro, R.C.; Veronese, F.V. Expression patterns of B cells in acute kidney transplant rejection. *Exp. Clin. Transpl.* **2014**, *12*, 405–414.
15. Firl, D.J.; Benichou, G.; Kim, J.I.; Yeh, H. A Paradigm Shift on the Question of B Cells in Transplantation? Recent Insights on Regulating the Alloresponse. *Front Immunol.* **2017**, *8*, 80. [CrossRef] [PubMed]
16. Hippen, B.E.; DeMattos, A.; Cook, W.J.; Kew, C.E., 2nd; Gaston, R.S. Association of CD20+ infiltrates with poorer clinical outcomes in acute cellular rejection of renal allografts. *Am. J. Transpl.* **2005**, *5*, 2248–2252. [CrossRef]
17. Tsai, E.W.; Rianthavorn, P.; Gjertson, D.W.; Wallace, W.D.; Reed, E.F.; Ettenger, R.B. CD20+ lymphocytes in renal allografts are associated with poor graft survival in pediatric patients. *Transplantation* **2006**, *82*, 1769–1773. [CrossRef]
18. Steinmetz, O.M.; Panzer, U.; Kneissler, U.; Harendza, S.; Lipp, M.; Helmchen, U.; Stahl, R.A. BCA-1/CXCL13 expression is associated with CXCR5-positive B-cell cluster formation in acute renal transplant rejection. *Kidney Int.* **2005**, *67*, 1616–1621. [CrossRef] [PubMed]
19. Loupy, A.; Haas, M.; Solez, K.; Racusen, L.; Glotz, D.; Seron, D.; Nankivell, B.J.; Colvin, R.B.; Afrouzian, M.; Akalin, E.; et al. The Banff 2015 Kidney Meeting Report: Current Challenges in Rejection Classification and Prospects for Adopting Molecular Pathology. *Am. J. Transpl.* **2017**, *17*, 28–41. [CrossRef]
20. Schiffer, L.; Henke-Gendo, C.; Wilsdorf, N.; Hussein, K.; Pape, L.; Schmitt, C.; Haller, H.; Schiffer, M.; Klein, C.; Kreipe, H.; et al. CXCL13 as a novel marker for diagnosis and disease monitoring in pediatric PTLD. *Am. J. Transpl.* **2012**, *12*, 1610–1617. [CrossRef]
21. Worthmann, K.; Gueler, F.; von Vietinghoff, S.; Davalos-Misslitz, A.; Wiehler, F.; Davidson, A.; Witte, T.; Haller, H.; Schiffer, M.; Falk, C.S.; et al. Pathogenetic role of glomerular CXCL13 expression in lupus nephritis. *Clin. Exp. Immunol.* **2014**, *178*, 20–27. [CrossRef] [PubMed]
22. Gueler, F.; Rong, S.; Gwinner, W.; Mengel, M.; Brocker, V.; Schon, S.; Greten, T.F.; Hawlisch, H.; Polakowski, T.; Schnatbaum, K.; et al. Complement 5a receptor inhibition improves renal allograft survival. *J. Am. Soc. Nephrol.* **2008**, *19*, 2302–2312. [CrossRef] [PubMed]
23. Ishikawa, S.; Nagai, S.; Sato, T.; Akadegawa, K.; Yoneyama, H.; Zhang, Y.Y.; Onai, N.; Matsushima, K. Increased circulating CD11b+CD11c+ dendritic cells (DC) in aged BWF1 mice which can be matured by TNF-alpha into BLC/CXCL13-producing DC. *Eur. J. Immunol.* **2002**, *32*, 1881–1887. [CrossRef]
24. Xu, X.; Han, Y.; Wang, Q.; Cai, M.; Qian, Y.; Wang, X.; Huang, H.; Xu, L.; Xiao, L.; Shi, B. Characterisation of Tertiary Lymphoid Organs in Explanted Rejected Donor Kidneys. *Immunol. Invest.* **2016**, *45*, 38–51. [CrossRef]
25. Rong, S.; Lewis, A.G.; Kunter, U.; Haller, H.; Gueler, F. A knotless technique for kidney transplantation in the mouse. *J. Transpl.* **2012**, *2012*, 127215. [CrossRef]
26. Gueler, F.; Shushakova, N.; Mengel, M.; Hueper, K.; Chen, R.; Liu, X.; Park, J.K.; Haller, H.; Wensvoort, G.; Rong, S. A novel therapy to attenuate acute kidney injury and ischemic allograft damage after allogenic

kidney transplantation in mice. *PLoS ONE* **2015**, *10*, e0115709. [CrossRef]

27. Hueper, K.; Gutberlet, M.; Brasen, J.H.; Jang, M.S.; Thorenz, A.; Chen, R.; Hertel, B.; Barrmeyer, A.; Schmidbauer, M.; Meier, M.; et al. Multiparametric Functional MRI: Non-Invasive Imaging of Inflammation and Edema Formation after Kidney Transplantation in Mice. *PLoS ONE* **2016**, *11*, e0162705. [CrossRef] [PubMed]
28. Haas, M.; Sis, B.; Racusen, L.C.; Solez, K.; Glotz, D.; Colvin, R.B.; Castro, M.C.; David, D.S.; David-Neto, E.; Bagnasco, S.M.; et al. Banff 2013 meeting report: Inclusion of c4d-negative antibody-mediated rejection and antibody-associated arterial lesions. *Am. J. Transpl.* **2014**, *14*, 272–283. [CrossRef] [PubMed]
29. Team, R.C. *A Language and Environment for Statistical Computing*; R Foundation for Statistical Computing: Vienna, Austria; Available online: https://www.R-project.org (accessed on 1 May 2018).
30. Touloumis, A. R Package multgee: A Generalized Estimating Equations Solver for Multinomial Responses. *J. Stat. Softw.* **2015**, *64*, 1–14. [CrossRef]

12

Renal Chemerin Expression is Induced in Models of Hypertensive Nephropathy and Glomerulonephritis and Correlates with Markers of Inflammation and Fibrosis

Alexander Mocker [1], Karl F. Hilgers [2], Nada Cordasic [2], Rainer Wachtveitl [2], Carlos Menendez-Castro [1], Joachim Woelfle [1], Andrea Hartner [1,†] and Fabian B. Fahlbusch [1,*,†]

1 Department of Pediatrics and Adolescent Medicine, University Hospital of Erlangen, 91054 Erlangen, Germany; alexmocker@t-online.de (A.M.); Carlos.Menendez-Castro@uk-erlangen.de (C.M.-C.); joachim.woelfle@uk-erlangen.de (J.W.); andrea.hartner@uk-erlangen.de (A.H.)

2 Department of Nephrology and Hypertension, University Hospital of Erlangen, 91054 Erlangen, Germany; karl.hilgers@uk-erlangen.de (K.F.H.); Nada.Cordasic@uk-erlangen.de (N.C.); Rainer.Wachtveitl@uk-erlangen.de (R.W.)

* Correspondence: fabian.fahlbusch@uk-erlangen.de

† These authors contributed equally to this work.

Abstract: Chemerin and its receptor, chemokine-like receptor 1 (CmklR1), are associated with chemotaxis, inflammation, and endothelial function, especially in metabolic syndrome, coronary heart disease, and hypertension. In humans, circulating chemerin levels and renal function show an inverse relation. So far, little is known about the potential role of chemerin in hypertensive nephropathy and renal inflammation. Therefore, we determined systemic and renal chemerin levels in 2-kidney-1-clip (2k1c) hypertensive and Thy1.1 nephritic rats, respectively, to explore the correlation between chemerin and markers of renal inflammation and fibrosis. Immunohistochemistry revealed a model-specific induction of chemerin expression at the corresponding site of renal damage (tubular vs. glomerular). In both models, renal expression of chemerin (RT-PCR, Western blot) was increased and correlated positively with markers of inflammation and fibrosis. In contrast, circulating chemerin levels remained unchanged. Taken together, these findings demonstrate that renal chemerin expression is associated with processes of inflammation and fibrosis-related to renal damage. However, its use as circulating biomarker of renal inflammation seems to be limited in our rat models.

Keywords: chemerin; CmklR1; 2-kidney-1-clip; 2k1c; Thy1.1 nephritis; renovascular hypertension; renal inflammation; renal injury; renal fibrosis

---

1. Introduction

The significance of end-stage renal disease (ESRD) remains clinically relevant due to its high mortality and morbidity, as well as the lack of effective preventive therapeutic interventions [1]. ESRD results from different forms of renal injury, e.g., arterial hypertension or glomerulonephritis [2,3]. Alterations in the renal microenvironment trigger pathologic immune cell responses with a subsequent acceleration of progressive renal failure, in the setting of loss of glomeruli, tubular atrophy and fibrosis, with reduced glomerular filtration rate (GFR) [2,4]. Unfortunately, the molecular pathways driving persistent renal inflammation are only partly understood to date. Therefore, further research is warranted regarding the regulatory components of inflammation-induced kidney damage in order to develop targeted therapeutics to prevent ESRD effectively. Chemokines and cytokines are both important regulatory mediators of kidney inflammation and potential therapeutic targets [5,6]. They are produced by resident kidney cells, particularly by podocytes, tubular and mesangial cells, as well as by microvascular endothelial cells [6]. Certain mediator combinations determine the recruitment of specific leukocyte subtypes to sites of renal inflammation [2].

Recently, the adipokine chemerin, also known as tazarotene-induced gene 2 protein (TIG2) or retinoic acid receptor responder protein 2 (RARRES2), was introduced as a novel chemoattractant protein [7]. It acts as a ligand for the G protein-coupled receptor CmklR1, also known as ChemR23, and was found to stimulate chemotaxis of dendritic cells and macrophages to sites of inflammation [7,8]. Beyond its classical role in adipogenesis and adipocyte metabolism [9,10], the potential involvement of chemerin in cardiovascular and renal dysfunction has recently been acknowledged [11]. Chemerin appears to form an integral link in metabolic syndrome, connecting obesity, the related dysfunctional cardiometabolic state, and the associated chronic inflammation of adipose tissue [12].

Several investigations have addressed circulating chemerin levels and their pathophysiologic relevance in cohorts with chronic kidney disease [11]. Unrelated to the method of determination [11], serum creatinine is significantly and independently associated with serum chemerin [13,14]. The level of circulating chemerin has been shown to be dependent on GFR and inversely correlated with renal function. A two-fold increase of serum chemerin has been reported in patients on hemodialysis [15]. These results were strengthened by an investigation of ESRD-patients undergoing kidney transplantation [14], whose elevated serum chemerin levels returned to baseline values observed in healthy controls three months after transplant. Furthermore, elevated chemerin levels persisted in ESRD patients on hemodialysis compared to healthy controls or kidney transplanted patients. Nonetheless, hemodialysis reduced high serum chemerin levels to some extent [16]. With adipose tissue as the main source of circulating chemerin [9], it remains to be determined whether elevated serum chemerin levels are due to the increase of fat mass in metabolic phenotypes or to the related renal damage leading to impaired renal elimination. The latter seems more likely [11], as patients with chronic kidney disease showed no difference in subcutaneous adipose tissue chemerin production at the mRNA level [16]. However, the role of visceral adipose tissue cannot be completely ruled out [11]. Also, beyond its role in chemerin elimination, the kidney itself may influence serum chemerin concentrations via its synthesis, as chemerin expression can be found in animal kidneys [9]. In order to investigate the role of renal chemerin and its potential use as a diagnostic marker of kidney disease, our current study characterized its systemic and local expression in established animal models of hypertensive nephropathy and glomerulonephritis using 2-kidney-1-clip (2k1c) hypertensive and Thy1.1 nephritic rats, respectively.

2. Results

2.1. *Chemerin is Induced in Kidneys Exposed to High Blood Pressure*

Five weeks after clipping of the left renal artery, the weights of the contralateral right kidneys exposed to high blood pressure were significantly higher than the right kidneys of the sham-operated controls (Table 1). Blood pressure and left ventricular weights of 2k1c rats were increased compared to controls (Table 1). Serum urea and creatinine, as markers of renal damage, were elevated in 2k1c rats compared to controls (Table 1). The expression levels of chemerin were significantly higher in the right kidneys of 2k1c hypertensive animals compared to the kidneys of controls (Figure 1A). Immunohistochemical evaluation of chemerin in kidneys revealed some discrete vascular and distal tubular staining for chemerin in control kidneys, with a prominent increase in chemerin immunoreactivity in the tubulo-interstitium of hypertensive kidneys (Figure 1B). The expression of the chemerin receptor CmklR1 was also induced in hypertensive kidneys (Figure 1C). Moreover, a Western blot analysis revealed an increase in chemerin protein in hypertensive kidneys (Figure 2).

Table 1. Physiological parameters of 2k1c experimental groups.

Physiological Parameter	Sham	2k1c	p-Value
Rel. right kidney weight (mg/g body weight)	3.21 ± 0.06	4.87 ± 0.25	<0.001
Serum urea (mg/dL)	37.74 ± 1.13	80.92 ± 11.26	<0.001
Serum creatinine (mg/dL)	0.195 ± 0.007	0.335 ± 0.038	<0.001
Rel. left ventricular weight (mg/g body weight)	2.05 ± 0.04	3.03 ± 0.21	0.003
Mean arterial blood pressure (mm Hg)	113.2 ± 2.6	203.7 ± 5.0	0.014

Sham, sham-operated control group; 2k1c, hypertensive group. Data are means ± standard error of the mean. $p < 0.05$ 2k1c versus sham was considered significant.

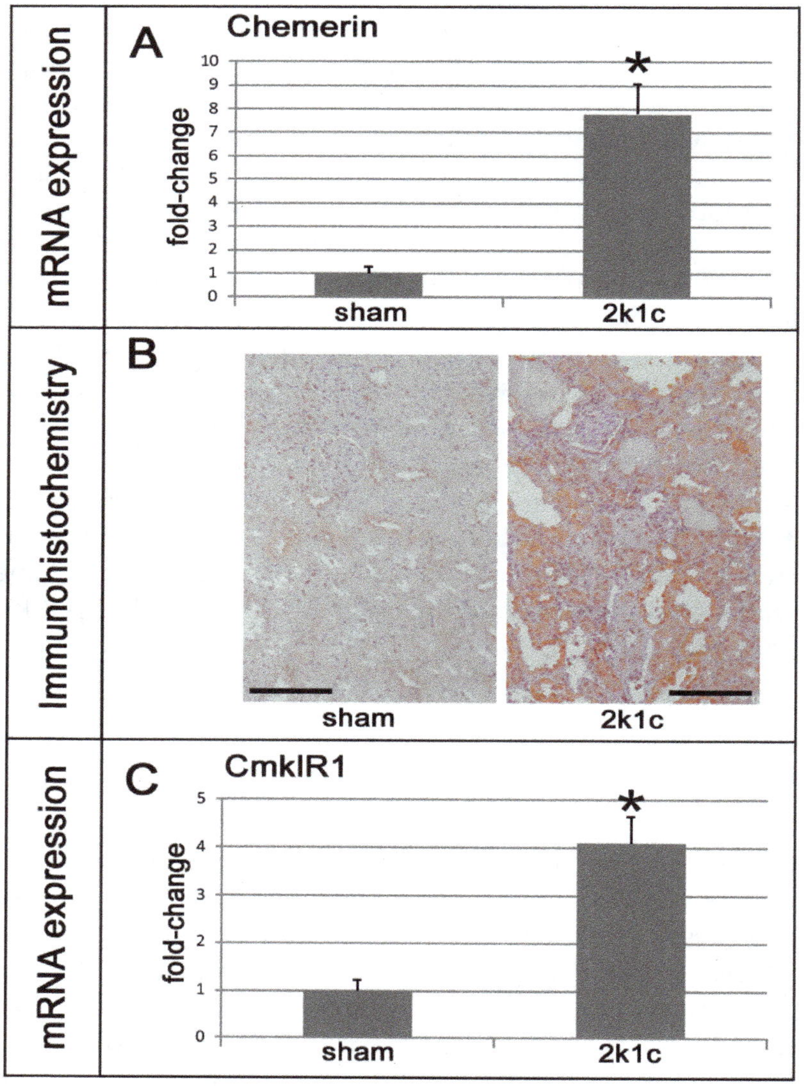

Figure 1. Chemerin and CmklR1 in 2k1c hypertensive nephropathy. (**A**) Chemerin mRNA expression levels in the kidneys of 2k1c hypertensive (2k1c) and control (sham) rats. (**B**) Exemplary photomicrographs of renal tissue from hypertensive (2k1c) and control (sham) rats stained for chemerin. Black bar represents 100 μm. (**C**) CmklR1 mRNA expression levels in the kidneys of 2k1c hypertensive (2k1c) and control (sham) rats. * $p < 0.05$ vs. sham control kidneys.

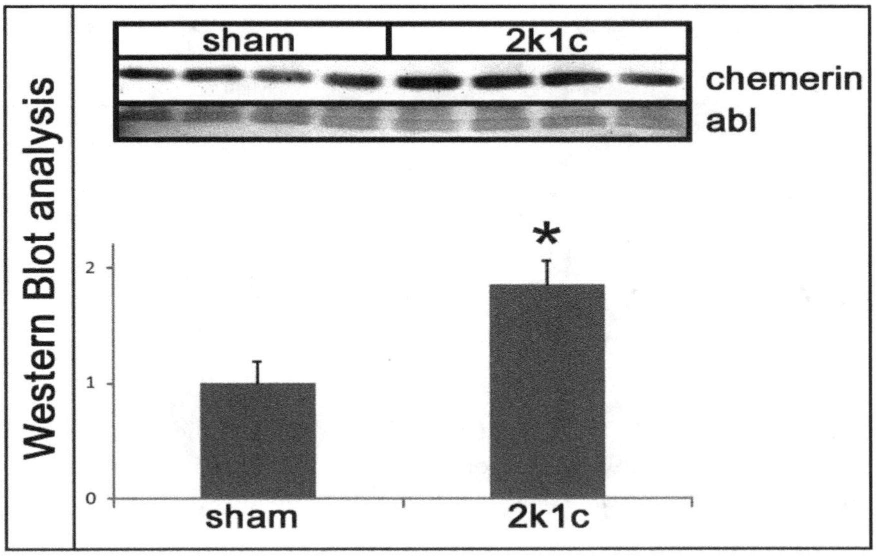

Figure 2. Western blot analysis of chemerin protein expression in the hypertensive kidneys of 2k1c rats. Amido black staining (abl) of the blot served as a loading control. Bar graph: densitometric analysis of Western Blot. * $p < 0.05$ vs. sham control kidneys.

2.2. In Kidneys Exposed to High Blood Pressure, Chemerin Expression Correlates with Markers of Renal Damage, Inflammation, and Fibrosis

Increased infiltration of M1 and M2 macrophages, neutrophil granulocytes, as well as total and helper T-cells, but not of cytotoxic T-cells into the right kidneys of 2k1c rats was observed (Table 2 and Figure 3). Exemplary photomicrographs are shown in Supplementary Figures S1–S3. The expression of TGFβ-1, a central mediator of tissue fibrosis [17], was upregulated in the kidneys of 2k1c rats (Table 3). Moreover, increased smooth muscle actin expression and the presence of more smooth muscle actin positive interstitial cells indicate pronounced fibroblast activation [18] in the right kidney of hypertensive rats (Table 3). Consequently, the expression of the matrix components fibronectin and collagens I, III, and IV was augmented in the right kidneys of these rats (Table 3). The expression of collagens I and IV in right kidney tissue was more prominent in 2k1c rats than in the right kidneys of control rats (Table 3 and Figure 3). Exemplary photomicrographs are shown in Supplementary Figure S4.

Table 2. Inflammatory cell infiltration in the kidneys of 2k1c.

Cell Type	Sham	2k1c	*p*-Value
M2 macrophages (CD163 pos. cells/cortical view)	0.09 ± 0.04	0.86 ± 0.20	<0.001
Neutrophil granulocytes (myeloperoxidase pos. cells/cortical view)	0.53 ± 0.15	1.49 ± 0.30	0.039
Total T-cells (CD3 pos. cells/cortical view)	1.23 ± 0.47	4.88 ± 1.81	0.046
Helper T-cells (CD4 pos. cells/cortical view)	11.56 ± 3.37	75.45 ± 14.60	0.002
Cytotoxic T-cells (CD8a pos. cells/cortical view)	3.12 ± 0.38	4.76 ± 0.35	0.456

Sham, sham-operated control group; 2k1c, hypertensive group. Data are means ± standard error of the mean. $p < 0.05$ 2k1c versus sham was considered significant.

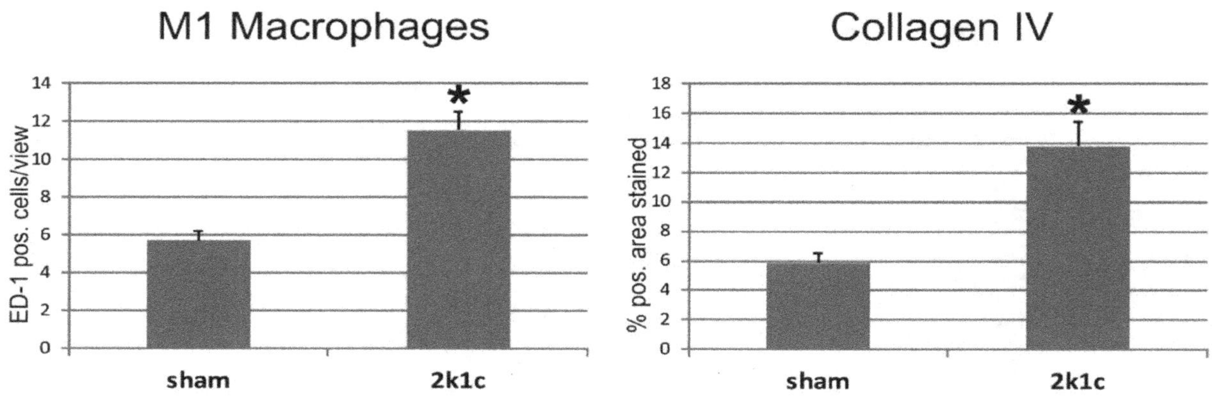

Figure 3. M1 macrophage infiltration and expansion of collagen IV in the tubulointerstitial area of rats with 2k1c hypertensive nephropathy. Sham, control sham operation; ED-1, M1 macrophage marker; * $p < 0.05$ vs. sham control kidneys, data are means ± error of the mean.

Table 3. Markers of renal fibrosis in 2k1c.

Fibrotic Marker	Sham	2k1c	p-Value
TGFβ-1 expression (fold change)	1.00 ± 0.25	3.69 ± 0.44	0.001
Smooth muscle actin expression (fold change)	1.00 ± 0.21	5.89 ± 0.96	0.014
Activated fibroblasts (smooth muscle actin pos. cells/cortical view)	0.26 ± 0.04	5.74 ± 1.50	0.002
Fibronectin expression (fold change)	1.00 ± 0.24	8.81 ± 1.55	0.003
Collagen I expression (fold change)	1.00 ± 0.32	4.42 ± 0.78	0.024
Collagen I stain (% pos. cells/cortical view)	4.66 ± 0.44	7.98 ± 1.14	0.001
Collagen III expression (fold change)	1.00 ± 0.49	18.25 ± 5.32	0.004
Collagen IV expression (fold change)	1.00 ± 0.22	6.03 ± 0.83	0.001

Sham, sham-operated control group; 2k1c, hypertensive group. Data are means ± standard error of the mean. $p < 0.05$ 2k1c versus sham was considered significant.

The expression of chemerin in the right kidney of hypertensive rats correlated with serum levels of urea and creatinine, but not with blood pressure levels (Table 4). There was a correlation between chemerin expression and M1 macrophage and neutrophil granulocyte infiltration into the right kidneys (Figure 4). Chemerin expression also correlated with fibroblast activation, TGFβ-1 expression and the expression of several matrix molecules (Table 4 and Figure 4). Furthermore, there was a high correlation of chemerin expression with the expression of its receptor CmklR1 (Table 4).

2.3. Chemerin is Induced in Glomeruli Afflicted with Thy1.1 Nephritis and Correlates with Markers of Renal Damage, Inflammation, and Fibrosis

Two weeks after the induction of a Thy1.1 glomerulonephritis, an increase in serum creatinine and albuminuria were observed (Table 5). Glomerular M1 macrophage infiltration and renal collagen IV expression were increased in nephritic kidneys (Figure 5 and Figure S5). Blood pressure was not altered in Thy1.1 nephritic rats (Table 5). Chemerin expression was increased in the renal tissue of Thy1.1 nephritic rats (Figure 6A). Staining for chemerin revealed prominent glomerular immunoreactivity in nephritic glomeruli, while in control glomeruli, only some podocytes stained positive (Figure 6B). The expression of the chemerin receptor CmklR1 was also somewhat increased (Figure 6C).

Table 4. Correlation of markers of renal damage, inflammation, and fibrosis with chemerin expression in 2k1c.

Chemerin (mRNA Expression)	r	*p*-Value
Serum creatinine (mg/dL)	0.62	**0.009**
Serum urea (mg/dL)	0.77	**<0.001**
Mean arterial blood pressure (mm Hg)	0.42	0.12
M1 macrophages (ED-1 pos. cells/view)	0.71	**0.001**
M2 macrophages (CD163 pos. cells/view)	0.51	0.16
Total T-cells (CD3 pos. cells/view)	0.27	0.40
Cytotoxic T-cells (CD8a pos. cells/view)	0.47	0.11
Helper T-cells (CD4 pos. cells/view)	−0.14	0.63
Neutrophil granulocytes (MPO pos. cells/view)	0.83	**<0.001**
Activated myofibroblasts (SMA-pos. cells/view)	0.74	**0.003**
Smooth muscle actin (mRNA expression)	0.65	**0.005**
Fibronectin (mRNA expression)	0.86	**<0.001**
Collagen I (% pos. area stained)	0.65	**0.043**
Collagen I (mRNA expression)	0.83	**<0.001**
Collagen III (mRNA expression)	0.84	**<0.001**
Collagen IV (% pos. area stained)	0.64	**0.014**
Collagen IV (mRNA expression)	0.90	**<0.001**
TGFβ-1 (mRNA expression)	0.73	**0.001**
CmklR1 (mRNA expression)	0.89	**<0.001**

r = Spearman–Rho correlation coefficient r, statistical significance was defined as *p*-value < 0.05.

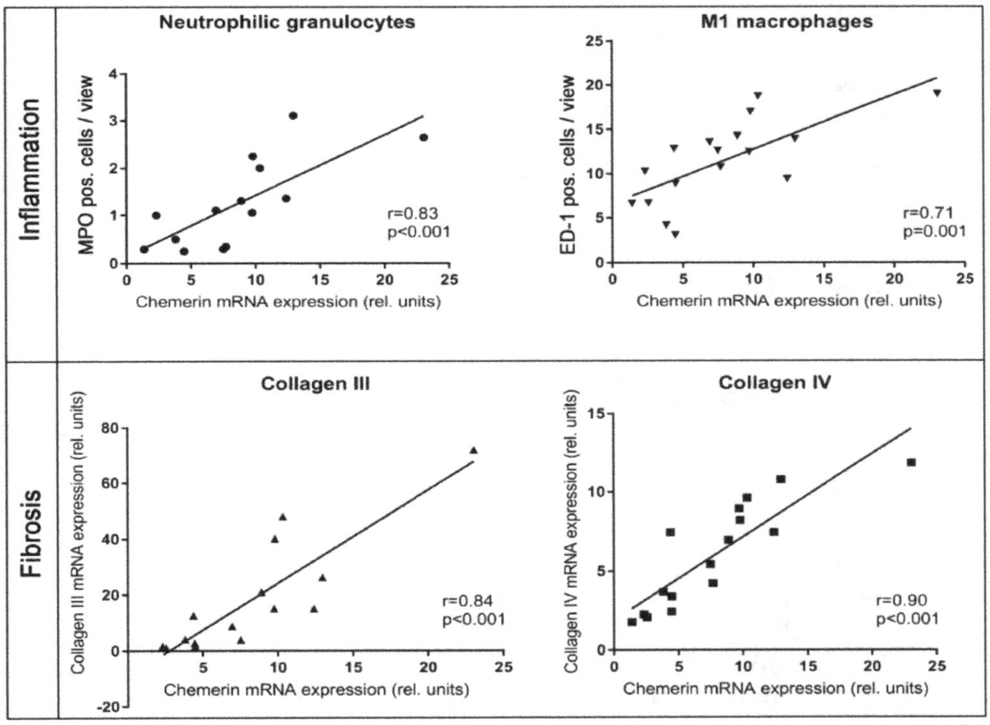

Figure 4. Correlation of chemerin expression with infiltration of neutrophilic granulocytes and M1 macrophages and the expression of collagens III and IV. MPO, myeloperoxidase (marker for neutrophil granulocytes), ED-1, marker for rat M1 macrophages.

Table 5. Markers of renal damage and blood pressure in Thy1 glomerulonephritis.

Damage Marker	NaCl	Thy1	p-Value
Rel. right kidney weight (mg/g body weight)	4.30 ± 0.15	8.57 ± 0.18	<0.01
Albuminuria (mg/24 h)	0.80 ± 0.19	725.79 ± 303.13	<0.01
Serum creatinine (mg/dL)	0.19 ± 0.01	0.34 ± 0.03	<0.01
Cytotoxic T-cells (CD8a pos. cells/cortical view)	3.51 ± 0.56	5.72 ± 0.41	n.s.
Helper T-cells (CD4 pos. cells/cortical view)	3.05 ± 0.61	6.23 ± 2.39	n.s.
Mean arterial blood pressure (mm Hg)	118.5 ± 1.5	123.7 ± 6.3	n.s.
Rel. left ventricular weight (mg/g body weight)	2.23 ± 0.11	2.49 ± 0.09	n.s.

NaCl, NaCl infused control group; Thy1, glomerulonephritic group. Data are means ± standard error of the mean. $p < 0.05$ 2k1c versus sham was considered significant.

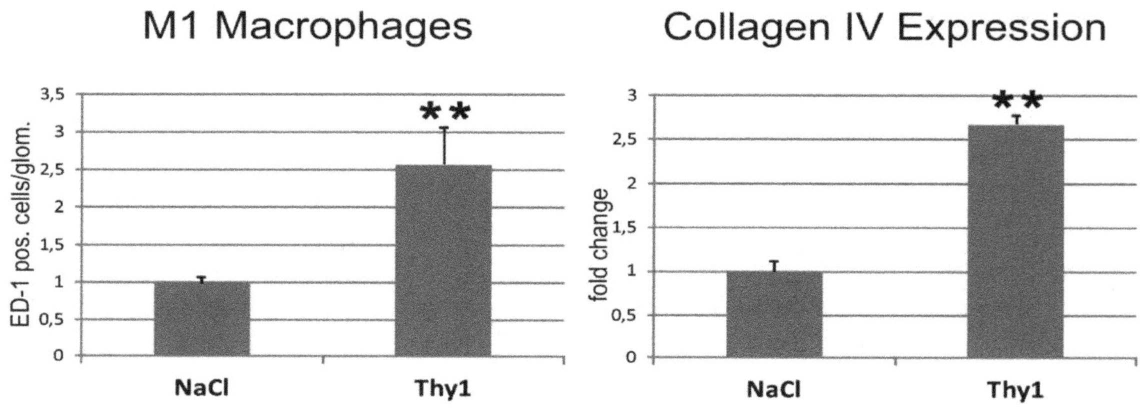

Figure 5. Glomerular M1 macrophage infiltration and collagen IV expression in the renal cortex of rats with anti-Thy1.1 mesangioproliferative glomerulonephritis. NaCl, control vehicle-injected; ED-1, M1 macrophage marker; ** $p < 0.01$; data are means ± error of the mean.

The expression of chemerin in kidneys with Thy1.1 glomerulonephritis correlated with serum creatinine levels, albuminuria, glomerular infiltration of M1 macrophages, and renal collagen IV expression (Table 6). A correlation between chemerin expression and CmklR1 expression was also detected (Table 6).

Table 6. Correlation of markers of renal damage, inflammation and fibrosis with chemerin expression in Thy1 glomerulonephritis.

Chemerin (mRNA Expression)	r	p-Value
CmklR1 (mRNA expression)	0.89	**0.001**
Serum creatinine (mg/dL)	0.73	**0.017**
Albuminuria (mg/24h)	0.73	**0.016**
Mean arterial blood pressure (mm Hg)	0.42	0.262
M1 macrophages (ED-1 pos. cells/view)	0.72	**0.019**
Cytotoxic T-cells (CD8a pos. cells/view)	0.58	0.082
Helper T-cells (CD4 pos. cells/view)	0.39	0.266
Collagen IV (mRNA expression)	0.83	**0.005**

r = Spearman–Rho correlation coefficient r, statistical significance was defined as p-value < 0.05.

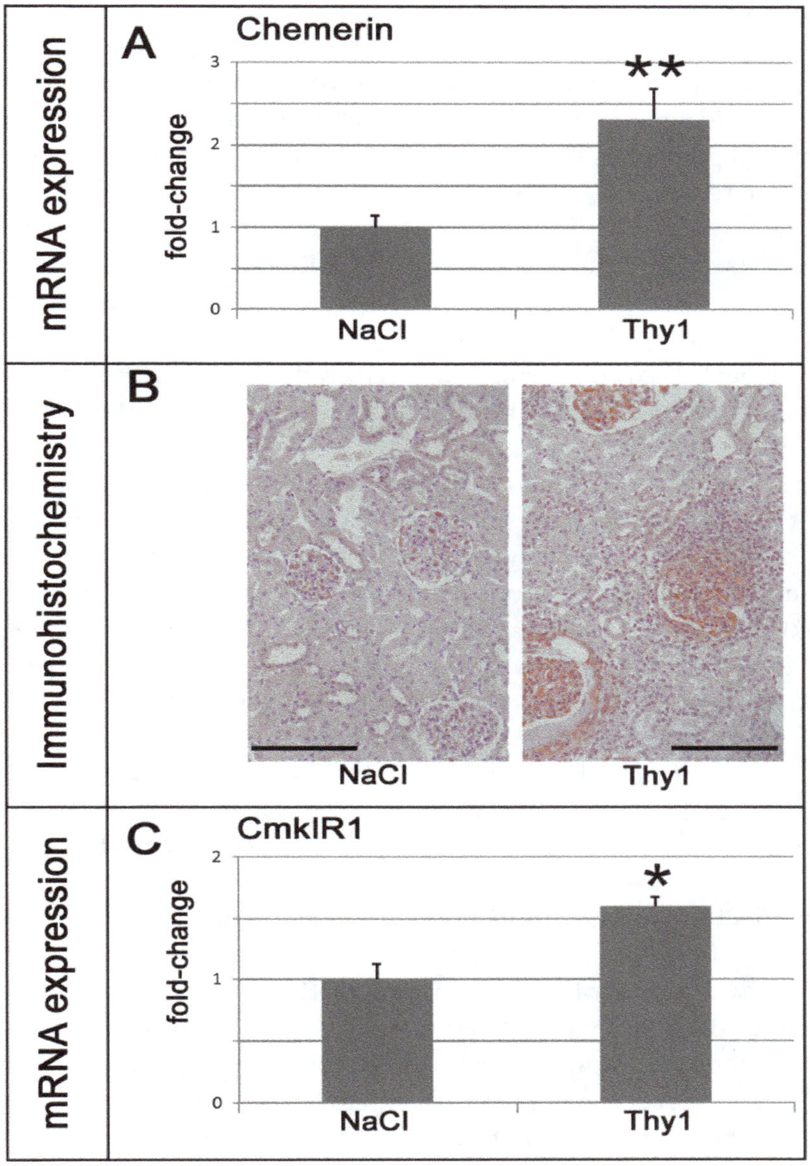

Figure 6. Chemerin and CmklR1 in anti-Thy1.1 glomerulonephritis: (**A**) mRNA expression of chemerin levels in the kidneys of Thy1.1 nephritic (Thy1) and control (NaCl) rats. (**B**) Localization of chemerin protein in renal sections of Thy1.1 nephritic and control rats. Black bar represents 100 μm. (**C**) mRNA expression of the chemerin receptor CmklR1 levels in the kidneys of Thy1.1 nephritic (Thy1) and control (NaCl) rats. NaCl, NaCl infused controls. Thy1, anti-Thy1.1 infused glomerulonephritic animals. ** $p < 0.01$, * $p < 0.05$ vs. control kidneys.

2.4. *Chemerin Plasma Levels are Not Increased in Rat Models of Renal Injury*

To clarify whether increases of renal tissue chemerin are also reflected by increases in plasma chemerin, ELISA assays were performed. In 2k1c hypertensive rats, plasma chemerin was not increased compared to sham-operated controls (1.15 ± 0.06 ng/mL in hypertensive rats versus 1.29 ± 0.11 ng/mL in controls). Likewise, in Thy1.1 glomerulonephritic rats, plasma chemerin levels were similar to the plasma levels of control rats (1.13 ± 0.19 ng/mL in nephritic rats versus 1.22 ± 0.10 ng/mL in controls).

3. Discussion

We have demonstrated specific induction of local expression patterns of chemerin related to the underlying model of renal injury, i.e., tubular-interstitial (2k1c, in kidneys exposed to high blood pressure) and glomerular damage (Thy1.1 nephritis). In our study, renal chemerin expression positively correlated with markers of renal damage and inflammation in 2k1c hypertensive animals and Thy1.1 nephritic rats, indicating a possible involvement of chemerin in these processes, as seen in adipose tissue [19]. Concomitantly, the expression of the chemerin receptor CmklR1 was also found to be induced in hypertensive kidneys, while somewhat increased in anti-Thy1.1 treated animals. Of the three known chemerin receptors (i.e., chemokine-like receptor 1 (CmklR1), G-protein-coupled receptor (GPR) 1, and C-C motif receptor-like (CCRL) 2, only CmklR1 sufficiently mediates intracellular signaling functions (reviewed by [12]). Besides its expression in hematopoietic tissues, CmklR1 is strongly expressed in cells of the immune system (e.g., blood monocytes, monocyte-derived human macrophages, immature dendritic cells, CD4+ T lymphocytes) [7,20]. CmklR1 directs the migration of immune cells to lymphoid organs and inflamed tissues [21]. Thus, the observed renal damage in our models might have partly resulted from chemerin-induced, CmklR1-mediated chemoattraction of immune cells to the respective sites of renal damage (i.e., tubulo-interstitium in 2k1c model and glomerulus in Thy1.1 nephritic rats).

Interestingly, CmklR1 expression was additionally observed in human microvascular endothelial cells (ECs) by Kaur et al. [22]. Thus, para-/autocrine effects of chemerin on renal vasculature in our model are also possible. Kaur et al. showed that the expression of the receptor was significantly up-regulated by pro-inflammatory cytokines in human ECs and had strong angiogenic potential via activation of PI3K/Akt and MAPK pathways in these cells [22]. The involvement of an imbalance of angiogenesis-related factors in the progression of CKD and the therapeutic potential of modulating these factors in CKD has been acknowledged (reviewed by [23]). Furthermore, Kaur et al. showed that chemerin was able to induce the activity of members of the matrix metalloproteinase (MMP) family in ECs [22], which play an important role in the degradation of the extracellular matrix (ECM) [24]. This effect is also crucial in the development and progression of CKD; however, non-proteolytic functions of MMPs might also play a role [24]. In line with these observations, we found chemerin to correlate with markers of renal fibrosis.

So far, the exact mechanisms of renal chemerin induction in our animals remain unknown. However, a potential role of angiotensin 2 (Ang II) in the regulation of chemerin expression has been proposed by others. Using a model of diabetic nephropathy, Yu et al. [25] were able to show that the expression of chemerin in the kidney of diabetic rats was significantly elevated compared to control animals, suggesting that chemerin might be relevant to the model-specific renal pathology. Treatment with irbesartan (Ang II type 1 receptor antagonist) appeared to reduce the renal chemerin expression in these diabetic animals secondary to a reduction in renin–angiotensin system (RAS) components [25].

The Goldblatt 2k1c rat hypertension model is a long-established and widely employed model in the study of renal artery stenosis and renovascular hypertension [26,27]. We have observed that the RAS, including Ang II, is closely related with the 2k1c model [28] since their levels are elevated in the development and maintenance of hypertension in these animals: Early on, hypertension in 2k1c animals is characterized by increased plasma renin levels in response to low renal arterial pressure and subsequently by an increase in circulating Ang II. Later, hypertension is maintained by a continuously activated RAS, as contralateral pressure diuresis of the unaffected kidney prevents hypervolemia [29,30]. Persistent elevation of Ang II also triggers an inflammatory response, characterized by the infiltration of macrophages (ED-1), tubular overexpression of macrophage chemotactic and adhesion molecules, such as osteopontin (OPN), MCP-1 and the expression of inflammatory cytokines, ultimately aggravating renal damage induced by hypertension [3,31,32].

A potential interaction of Ang II with chemerin in the 2k1c model remains to be determined. Ang II is a key mediator of CKD. A blockade of the Ang II type 1 receptor prevents lethal malignant hypertension [28]. It is also understood that Ang II mediates renal fibrosis by stimulating the endogenous synthesis of transforming growth factor-β (TGF-β) [33] in damaged kidney cells, thereby stimulating the synthesis of the extracellular matrix (ECM), and inhibiting the action of MMPs [34]. TGF-β induces the transformation of fibroblasts into myofibroblasts (α-smooth muscle actin-positive cells, α-SMA) and stimulates the expression of fibronectin (FN) and collagen type III (Col III).

This induces the development of renal fibrosis, leads to functional deterioration and increases kidney damage [34–36]. Notably, we have found that renal chemerin levels correlated positively with these Ang II-dependent markers of inflammation and fibrosis in both our models of renal injury. Moreover, other RAS-associated factors, such as aldosterone/mineralocorticoid receptor [37] or the activity of the angiotensin-converting enzyme (ACE) [38], might be relevant in the function of renal chemerin.

Similar to 2k1c animals, RAS activation also plays a pivotal role in the progression of glomerulonephritis (GN) in Thy1.1 nephritic rats [39]. Thus, potential cross-talk of chemerin and Ang II [25] at the glomerular level might be conceivable. The immunohistochemically observed glomerular expression of chemerin in our Thy1.1 nephritic rats closely resembled glomerular cyto/chemokine expression patterns typically found in nephritic renal damage [40], thereby underscoring the potential role of chemerin as a damage-site specific chemoattractant. The most commonly used model of selective mesangial cell damage [41–43], anti-Thy1.1-induced glomerulonephritis, resembles some human forms of GN [44], where the renal damage is characterized by the continued accumulation of ECM, related to the overproduction of glomerular TGF-β.

As a limitation, the role of Ang II in our 2k1c animals and Thy1.1. nephritic rats remains speculative due to the lack of functional data regarding RAS signaling. Future studies are needed to uncover the mechanistic insights of chemerin signaling transduction pathways in the kidney, with a special focus on the exploration of potential therapeutic targets for renal fibrosis and inflammation.

Despite the association of increased chemerin with (renal) inflammation and fibrosis, Yamamoto et al. found an association of elevated chemerin levels with a survival advantage in dialysis patients [45]. This seems controversial, as CKD induces premature vascular aging with vascular calcification and increased arterial stiffness [46]. In addition, previous studies had indicated a role of CmklR1 for the vascular smooth muscle cell (VSMC) atherosclerotic phenotype [47], characterized by vascular inflammation and intimal hyperplasia [48,49]. Surprisingly, chemerin seemed to inhibit atherogenesis through CmklR1 [48,50]. Carracedo et al. [51] were able to show that chemerin treatment of isolated wild-type mouse VSMCs significantly reduced phosphate-induced calcification and increased expression of the calcification inhibitor matrix-gla-protein (MGP). In contrast, VSMCs of CmklR1 knock-out mice were devoid of these effects. This suggests that elevated chemerin might, in fact, exert a direct protective vascular role in CKD, while negatively altering the local microenvironment via attraction of immune cells at the same time.

In contrast to findings in humans [11], we did not observe an induction of circulating chemerin. So far, the majority of existing human reports focus on elevated circulating levels of chemerin in CKD patients, while little is known about the local renal expression of the protein. Based on our finding of increased chemerin expression in ESRD, one could speculate that this may contribute to the reported increase of circulating chemerin levels in ESRD, apart from the postulated reduced chemerin renal elimination capacity associated with ESRD [14]. However, as we were unable to detect an increase of circulating chemerin levels in both animal models of our study, it remains uncertain to what extent such local changes in our rodent models might translate into a significant increase of circulating chemerin levels observed in human ESRD.

The lack of increased circulating chemerin seemed unrelated to an inoperative experimental design. Clipping of the left renal artery and anti-Thy1.1 treatment both sufficiently reduced kidney function, as determined by a ~2-fold increase in serum urea and creatinine. Also, renal weight was significantly increased in both rodent models. These results match findings previously obtained by our group in 2k1c rats [52]. It is possible that despite the detectable renal affliction of our animals and its correlation with local chemerin expression, the functional renal restriction might not have been relevant enough to fully resemble the level of kidney failure seen in human ESRD [14]. Thus, the renal capacity to eliminate increasing levels of circulating chemerin might still have been sufficient in the examined animal models.

A current methodological limitation in the field of chemerin research is the lack of analysis of the multitude of existing chemerin pre-cursors [12,19]. Chemerin is proteolytically processed (e.g., by cathepsin G, elastase, plasmin, and tryptase) into different active and inactive chemerin peptides, such as pre-prochemerin and mature prochemerin, which might exert specific functions on their own.

In summary, our findings provide novel evidence that renal chemerin expression in 2k1c and Thy1.1 nephritic rats are associated with markers of kidney inflammation and fibrosis. However, we did not find elevated levels of circulating chemerin in these animals. Thus, chemerin might not serve as a biomarker in these models.

4. Materials and Methods

4.1. Experimental Procedures

All animal experiments were performed in compliance with the DIRECTIVE 2010/63/EU of the European Parliament and were approved by the local government authorities (Regierung of Mittelfranken, AZ 54-2532.1-51/12, 22 October 2013 and AZ 55.2.2532-2-526, 18 October 2017). All efforts were made to minimize suffering in the animal cohort. Rats were housed in a room maintained at 22 ± 2 °C, exposed to a 12-h dark/light cycle. The animals had unlimited access to standard rodent nutrition and tap water.

Induction of hypertensive nephropathy: Two-kidney, one-clip renovascular hypertension (2k1c) was induced in male Sprague–Dawley rats (Charles River, Sulzfeld, Germany) weighing 150–170 g by placing a silver clip of 0.2 mm internal diameter around the left renal artery through a flank incision under isoflurane anesthesia as previously described (n = 25) [53]. Control animals underwent a sham operation without placement of the clip (n = 10). Analgesia was provided post-operatively in all animals, and as needed later on. Five weeks after the clipping of the renal artery, the experiment was terminated, and renal tissue was collected.

Induction of acute glomerulonephritis: Male Sprague-Dawley rats (150 to 200 g) were obtained from Charles River Deutschland. Anti-Thy1.1 nephritis was induced in uninephrectomized rats by a single intravenous injection of 1 mg/kg body weight anti-Thy1.1 antibody into the tail vein in light isoflurane anesthesia. Controls received solvent only (n = 5 per group). The monoclonal antibody against Thy1.1 (ER4) was from Antibody Solutions (Santa Clara, CA, USA). Anti-Thy1.1 nephritis is an acute mesangioproliferative glomerulonephritis with mesangial expansion and glomerulosclerosis peaking at days 7 to 14 of disease [42,54]. On day 13, animals were housed in metabolic cages for 24 h to collect urine. Five animals per group were sacrificed on day 14 after induction of nephritis and renal tissue was obtained for further evaluation.

4.2. Blood Pressure Measurements

At the end of the experiment, rats were weighed and instrumented with femoral artery catheters for intraarterial blood pressure measurements in anesthesia, as described previously [55]. Measurements were performed on the same day after termination of anesthesia and a recovery phase of 2 h in conscious animals via transducers connected to a polygraph (Hellige, Freiburg, Germany).

4.3. Measurement of Serum and Urine Parameters

For urine collection, anti-Thy1.1 nephritic animals were put in metabolic cages for 24 h on the day before sacrifice. Albumin excretion was assessed by enzyme-linked immunosorbent assay (Bethyl Laboratories, Biomol, Hamburg, Germany). For serum analysis, blood was collected from catheters. Thereafter, rats were euthanized by bleeding in deep anesthesia. Plasma creatinine and plasma urea were analyzed using an automatic analyzer Integra 1000 (Roche Diagnostics, Mannheim, Germany). Plasma chemerin was determined using a commercially available ELISA kit (MyBiosource, Biozol, Eching, Germany) according to the manufacturer's protocol.

4.4. *Tissue Sampling*

After organ weighing, kidneys were decapsulated. Both poles of each kidney and the apical tip of the left ventricle were immediately snap-frozen on liquid nitrogen for protein or RNA extraction. One 6 mm slice of the kidney was put in paraformaldehyde solution (for detection of chemerin), while another 6 mm slice of the remaining kidney was put in methyl-Carnoy solution (60% methanol, 30% chloroform and 10% glacial acetic acid) for fixation. After overnight fixation, tissues were dehydrated by bathing in increasing concentrations of alcohol and embedded in paraffin. Three μm sections were cut with a Leitz SM 2000 R microtome (Leica Instruments, Nussloch, Germany).

4.5. *Immunohistochemistry*

Tissue was processed as described [56]. Immunohistochemical detection of chemerin, collagen I, collagen IV, α-smooth muscle actin (SMA), ED-1, myeloperoxidase (MPO), CD3, CD4, CD8a, and CD163 was performed in methyl Carnoy-fixed tissue sections. Antibodies used are described in Supplementary Table S1. The specificity of the chemerin antibody was confirmed by staining in control tissue: rat skin, lung and testes (see Supplementary Figure S6). Interstitial collagens I and IV were quantified in 30 medium-power views (magnification x200) by means of an 11 × 11-point grid or by densitometric analysis using MetaVue software (Molecular Devices, Sunnyvale, CA, USA). The percentage of grid points corresponding with a stained area or the percentage of stained area in relation to the total area was calculated. SMA, ED-1, MPO, CD3, CD4, CD8a, and CD163 positive cells were counted in 20 medium-power cortical views. All histological evaluations were done by a single investigator blinded to the group assignment.

4.6. *Western Blot Analysis*

Frozen renal tissue was homogenized, protein samples were prepared as described [57] and separated on a denaturing SDS-PAGE gel [58]. After electrophoresis, the gels were electroblotted onto PVDF membranes (Hybond-P, GE Amersham, Munich, Germany), blocked with Rotiblock (Roth, Karlsruhe, Germany) for 1 h and incubated overnight with a primary antibody to chemerin. Protein bands were visualized with secondary horseradish peroxidase-conjugated IgG antibodies (Santa Cruz Biotechnology, 1:50,000), using the Pierce ECL+ system (Thermo Fisher Scientific, Waltham, MA, USA). Blots were quantified using a luminescent imager (LAS-1000, Fujifilm, Berlin, Germany) and Aida 2.1 image analysis software (Raytest, Berlin, Germany). Loading of the blot was quantified by Amido Black staining solution (Sigma, Taufkirchen, Germany).

4.7. *Real-Time Polymerase Chain Reaction (PCR) Analyses*

Renal tissue was homogenized in RLT buffer reagent (Qiagen, Hilden, Germany) with an ultraturrax for 30 s, total RNA was extracted from homogenates by RNeasy Mini columns (Qiagen) according to the manufacturer's protocol, and real-time RT-PCR was performed [59]. First-strand cDNA was synthesized with TaqMan reverse transcription reagents (Applied Biosystems, Darmstadt, Germany) using random hexamers as primers. Reactions without Multiscribe reverse transcriptase were used as negative controls for genomic DNA contamination. PCR was performed with a StepOnePlus™ sequence detector system (Applied Biosystems, Darmstadt, Germany) and TaqMan or SYBR Green Universal PCR master mix (Applied Biosystems), as described previously [57]. All samples were run in duplicates. Specific mRNA levels in hypertensive animals relative to sham-operated controls were calculated and normalized to a housekeeping gene (18S) with the ΔΔCt method as specified by the manufacturer (Applied Biosystems). Primer pairs used for experiments are shown in Supplementary Table S2.

4.8. *Statistical Analysis*

Data are expressed as mean ± standard error of the mean (SEM). After testing for normality distribution using Shapiro–Wilk's test, we performed Student's *t*-test or the Mann–Whitney U-test, where appropriate. A p-value < 0.05 was considered significant. To assess correlations between chemerin and markers of inflammation and fibrosis, Spearman's correlation coefficients (Spearman's rho) were calculated. Calculations were carried out using the SPSS 19 software (IBM, Ehningen, Germany) and GraphPad Prism 7.00 (GraphPad Software, La Jolla, CA, USA).

Supplementary Materials:
Figure S1: Exemplary photomicrographs of kidneys with 2k1c nephropathy and control kidneys (sham) stained for the M1 macrophage marker ED1 and the M2 macrophage marker CD163. Figure S2: Exemplary photomicrographs of kidneys with 2k1c nephropathy and control kidneys (sham) stained for the neutrophil marker myeloperoxidase and the T-cell marker CD3. Figure S3: Exemplary photomicrographs of kidneys with 2k1c nephropathy and control kidneys (sham) stained for the T-helper cell marker CD4 and the cytotoxic T-cell marker CD8a. Figure S4: Exemplary photomicrographs of kidneys with 2k1c nephropathy and control kidneys (sham) stained for collagen I and collagen IV. Figure S5: Exemplary photomicrographs of kidneys with Thy1 induced glomerulonephritis and control kidneys (NaCl) stained for the M1 macrophage marker ED1. Figure S6. Specificity testing of the chemerin antibody. The antibody stained skin (Luangsay S et al. 2009, J Immunol 183; Vermi W et al. 2005, J Exp Med 201), lung (Luangsay S et al. 2009, J Immunol 183) and testes (Li L et al. 2014, J Endocrinol 220), as described before. Black arrowheads point to the chemerin positive keratinocyte layer in a skin sample, to the chemerin positive ciliated epithelium of the lung bronchioles and to chemerin positive Leydig cells in testes. Table S1. Antibodies used for immunohistochemistry. Table S2. Primer sequences.

Author Contributions: A.M. acquired data, interpreted the results and drafted the manuscript. R.W., C.M.-C. and N.C. acquired data, interpreted the results and revised the manuscript. A.H. and F.B.F. designed the work, interpreted the data and drafted the manuscript. K.F.H. designed the work and revised the manuscript. J.W. critically revised the manuscript. All authors gave final approval of the manuscript to be published.

Acknowledgments: We thank Miroslava Kupraszewicz-Hutzler and Astrid Ziegler for their excellent technical assistance. A large part of the experimental procedures and respective data acquisition was performed by Alexander Mocker in fulfillment of the requirements for obtaining the degree "Dr. med." at the Friedrich-Alexander-University of Erlangen-Nürnberg, Dept. of Pediatrics and Adolescent Medicine, Germany. The authors thank J. A. Bello MD, FACR, Professor of Clinical Radiology and Neurosurgery, Director of Neuroradiology, Albert Einstein College of Medicine, Montefiore Medical Center, New York, NY, USA for language editing.

References

1. Breyer, M.D.; Susztak, K. Developing Treatments for Chronic Kidney Disease in the 21st Century. *Semin. Nephrol.* **2016**, *36*, 436–447. [CrossRef] [PubMed]
2. Ernandez, T.; Mayadas, T.N. The Changing Landscape of Renal Inflammation. *Trends Mol. Med.* **2016**, *22*, 151–163. [CrossRef] [PubMed]
3. Hilgers, K.F.; Hartner, A.; Porst, M.; Mai, M.; Wittmann, M.; Hugo, C.; Ganten, D.; Geiger, H.; Veelken, R.; Mann, J.F. Monocyte chemoattractant protein-1 and macrophage infiltration in hypertensive kidney injury. *Kidney Int.* **2000**, *58*, 2408–2419. [CrossRef] [PubMed]
4. Shafi, T.; Coresh, J. 1 - Chronic Kidney Disease: Definition, Epidemiology, Cost, and Outcomes. In *Chronic Kidney Disease, Dialysis, and Transplantation (Fourth Edition), Himmelfarb, J.*; Ikizler, T.A., Ed.; Eds. Elsevier: Philadelphia, PA, USA, 2019.
5. Wada, T.; Matsushima, K.; Kaneko, S. The role of chemokines in glomerulonephritis. *Front. Biosci.* **2008**, *13*, 3966–3974. [CrossRef] [PubMed]
6. Chung, A.C.; Lan, H.Y. Chemokines in renal injury. *J. Am. Soc. Nephrol.* **2011**, *22*, 802–809. [CrossRef] [PubMed]
7. Wittamer, V.; Franssen, J.D.; Vulcano, M.; Mirjolet, J.F.; Le Poul, E.; Migeotte, I.; Brezillon, S.; Tyldesley, R.; Blanpain, C.; Detheux, M.; et al. Specific recruitment of antigen-presenting cells by chemerin, a novel processed ligand from human inflammatory fluids. *J. Exp. Med.* **2003**, *198*, 977–985. [CrossRef] [PubMed]
8. Xu, H.; Barnes, G.T.; Yang, Q.; Tan, G.; Yang, D.; Chou, C.J.; Sole, J.; Nichols, A.; Ross, J.S.; Tartaglia, L.A.; et al. Chronic inflammation in fat plays a crucial role in the development of obesity-related insulin resistance. *J. Clin. Investig.* **2003**, *112*, 1821–1830. [CrossRef]
9. Bozaoglu, K.; Bolton, K.; McMillan, J.; Zimmet, P.; Jowett, J.; Collier, G.; Walder, K.; Segal, D. Chemerin is a novel adipokine associated with obesity and metabolic syndrome. *Endocrinology* **2007**, *148*, 4687–4694. [CrossRef]

10. Goralski, K.B.; McCarthy, T.C.; Hanniman, E.A.; Zabel, B.A.; Butcher, E.C.; Parlee, S.D.; Muruganandan, S.; Sinal, C.J. Chemerin, a novel adipokine that regulates adipogenesis and adipocyte metabolism. *J. Biol. Chem.* **2007**, *282*, 28175–28188. [CrossRef]
11. Bonomini, M.; Pandolfi, A. Chemerin in renal dysfunction and cardiovascular disease. *Vascul. Pharmacol.* **2016**, *77*, 28–34. [CrossRef]
12. Kaur, J.; Mattu, H.S.; Chatha, K.; Randeva, H.S. Chemerin in human cardiovascular disease. *Vascul. Pharmacol.* **2018**, *110*, 1–6. [CrossRef] [PubMed]
13. Hu, W.; Feng, P. Elevated serum chemerin concentrations are associated with renal dysfunction in type 2 diabetic patients. *Diabetes Res. Clin. Pract.* **2011**, *91*, 159–163. [CrossRef] [PubMed]
14. Rutkowski, P.; Sledzinski, T.; Zielinska, H.; Lizakowski, S.; Goyke, E.; Szrok-Wojtkiewicz, S.; Swierczynski, J.; Rutkowski, B. Decrease of serum chemerin concentration in patients with end stage renal disease after successful kidney transplantation. *Regul. Pept.* **2012**, *173*, 55–59. [CrossRef] [PubMed]
15. Pfau, D.; Bachmann, A.; Lossner, U.; Kratzsch, J.; Bluher, M.; Stumvoll, M.; Fasshauer, M. Serum levels of the adipokine chemerin in relation to renal function. *Diabetes Care* **2010**, *33*, 171–173. [CrossRef] [PubMed]
16. Blaszak, J.; Szolkiewicz, M.; Sucajtys-Szulc, E.; Konarzewski, M.; Lizakowski, S.; Swierczynski, J.; Rutkowski, B. High serum chemerin level in CKD patients is related to kidney function, but not to its adipose tissue overproduction. *Ren Fail.* **2015**, *37*, 1033–1038. [CrossRef] [PubMed]
17. Meng, X.M.; Tang, P.M.; Li, J.; Lan, H.Y. TGF-beta/Smad signaling in renal fibrosis. *Front. Physiol.* **2015**, *6*, 82. [CrossRef]
18. Meran, S.; Steadman, R. Fibroblasts and myofibroblasts in renal fibrosis. *Int. J. Exp. Pathol.* **2011**, *92*, 158–167. [CrossRef]
19. Ernst, M.C.; Sinal, C.J. Chemerin: At the crossroads of inflammation and obesity. *Trends Endocrinol. Metab.* **2010**, *21*, 660–667. [CrossRef]
20. Arita, M.; Ohira, T.; Sun, Y.P.; Elangovan, S.; Chiang, N.; Serhan, C.N. Resolvin E1 selectively interacts with leukotriene B4 receptor BLT1 and ChemR23 to regulate inflammation. *J. Immunol.* **2007**, *178*, 3912–3917. [CrossRef]
21. Vermi, W.; Riboldi, E.; Wittamer, V.; Gentili, F.; Luini, W.; Marrelli, S.; Vecchi, A.; Franssen, J.D.; Communi, D.; Massardi, L.; et al. Role of ChemR23 in directing the migration of myeloid and plasmacytoid dendritic cells to lymphoid organs and inflamed skin. *J. Exp. Med.* **2005**, *201*, 509–515. [CrossRef]
22. Kaur, J.; Adya, R.; Tan, B.K.; Chen, J.; Randeva, H.S. Identification of chemerin receptor (ChemR23) in human endothelial cells: Chemerin-induced endothelial angiogenesis. *Biochem. Biophys. Res. Commun.* **2010**, *391*, 1762–1768. [CrossRef] [PubMed]
23. Maeshima, Y.; Makino, H. Angiogenesis and chronic kidney disease. *Fibrogenesis Tissue Repair* **2010**, *3*, 13. [CrossRef] [PubMed]
24. Cheng, Z.; Limbu, M.H.; Wang, Z.; Liu, J.; Liu, L.; Zhang, X.; Chen, P.; Liu, B. MMP-2 and 9 in Chronic Kidney Disease. *Int. J. Mol. Sci.* **2017**, *18*. [CrossRef] [PubMed]
25. Yu, Q.X.; Zhang, H.; Xu, W.H.; Hao, F.; Liu, S.L.; Bai, M.M.; Mu, J.W.; Zhang, H.J. Effect of Irbesartan on Chemerin in the Renal Tissues of Diabetic Rats. *Kidney Blood Press Res.* **2015**, *40*, 467–477. [CrossRef] [PubMed]
26. Goldblatt, H.; Lynch, J.; Hanzal, R.F.; Summerville, W.W. Studies on Experimental Hypertension : I. The Production of Persistent Elevation of Systolic Blood Pressure by Means of Renal Ischemia. *J. Exp. Med.* **1934**, *59*, 347–379. [CrossRef]
27. Goldblatt, H.; Kahn, J.R.; Hanzal, R.F. Studies on Experimental Hypertension : Ix. The Effect on Blood Pressure of Constriction of the Abdominal Aorta above and Below the Site of Origin of Both Main Renal Arteries. *J. Exp. Med.* **1939**, *69*, 649–674. [CrossRef]
28. Hilgers, K.F.; Hartner, A.; Porst, M.; Veelken, R.; Mann, J.F. Angiotensin II type 1 receptor blockade prevents lethal malignant hypertension: Relation to kidney inflammation. *Circulation* **2001**, *104*, 1436–1440. [CrossRef]
29. Wiesel, P.; Mazzolai, L.; Nussberger, J.; Pedrazzini, T. Two-kidney, one clip and one-kidney, one clip hypertension in mice. *Hypertension* **1997**, *29*, 1025–1030. [CrossRef]
30. Corbier, A.; Lecaque, D.; Secchi, J.; Depouez, B.; Hamon, G. Effects of 4 weeks of treatment with trandolapril on renal hypertension and cardiac and vascular hypertrophy in the rat. *J. Cardiovasc. Pharmacol.* **1994**, *23*, S26–S29. [CrossRef]
31. Ozawa, Y.; Kobori, H.; Suzaki, Y.; Navar, L.G. Sustained renal interstitial macrophage infiltration following chronic angiotensin II infusions. *Am. J. Physiol. Renal Physiol.* **2007**, *292*, F330–F339. [CrossRef]

32. Mezzano, S.A.; Aros, C.A.; Droguett, A.; Burgos, M.E.; Ardiles, L.G.; Flores, C.A.; Carpio, D.; Vio, C.P.; Ruiz-Ortega, M.; Egido, J. Renal angiotensin II up-regulation and myofibroblast activation in human membranous nephropathy. *Kidney Int.* **2003**, *64*, S39–S45. [CrossRef] [PubMed]
33. Yang, F.; Chung, A.C.; Huang, X.R.; Lan, H.Y. Angiotensin II induces connective tissue growth factor and collagen I expression via transforming growth factor-beta-dependent and -independent Smad pathways: The role of Smad3. *Hypertension* **2009**, *54*, 877–884. [CrossRef] [PubMed]
34. Border, W.A.; Noble, N.A. Interactions of transforming growth factor-beta and angiotensin II in renal fibrosis. *Hypertension* **1998**, *31*, 181–188. [CrossRef] [PubMed]
35. Mezzano, S.A.; Ruiz-Ortega, M.; Egido, J. Angiotensin II and renal fibrosis. *Hypertension* **2001**, *38*, 635–638. [CrossRef] [PubMed]
36. Wolf, G.; Schneider, A.; Wenzel, U.; Helmchen, U.; Stahl, R.A. Regulation of glomerular TGF-beta expression in the contralateral kidney of two-kidney, one-clip hypertensive rats. *J. Am. Soc. Nephrol.* **1998**, *9*, 763–772. [PubMed]
37. Hoppmann, J.; Perwitz, N.; Meier, B.; Fasshauer, M.; Hadaschik, D.; Lehnert, H.; Klein, J. The balance between gluco- and mineralo-corticoid action critically determines inflammatory adipocyte responses. *J. Endocrinol.* **2010**, *204*, 153–164. [CrossRef] [PubMed]
38. John, H.; Hierer, J.; Haas, O.; Forssmann, W.G. Quantification of angiotensin-converting-enzyme-mediated degradation of human chemerin 145-154 in plasma by matrix-assisted laser desorption/ionization-time-of-flight mass spectrometry. *Anal. Biochem.* **2007**, *362*, 117–125. [CrossRef]
39. Urushihara, M.; Kinoshita, Y.; Kondo, S.; Kagami, S. Involvement of the intrarenal renin-angiotensin system in experimental models of glomerulonephritis. *J. Biomed. Biotechnol.* **2012**, *2012*, 601786. [CrossRef]
40. Anders, H.J.; Vielhauer, V.; Schlondorff, D. Chemokines and chemokine receptors are involved in the resolution or progression of renal disease. *Kidney Int.* **2003**, *63*, 401–415. [CrossRef]
41. Ishizaki, M.; Masuda, Y.; Fukuda, Y.; Sugisaki, Y.; Yamanaka, N.; Masugi, Y. Experimental mesangioproliferative glomerulonephritis in rats induced by intravenous administration of anti-thymocyte serum. *Acta Pathol. Jpn.* **1986**, *36*, 1191–1203. [CrossRef]
42. Hartner, A.; Schocklmann, H.; Prols, F.; Muller, U.; Sterzel, R.B. Alpha8 integrin in glomerular mesangial cells and in experimental glomerulonephritis. *Kidney Int.* **1999**, *56*, 1468–1480. [CrossRef] [PubMed]
43. Sakai, N.; Iseki, K.; Suzuki, S.; Mori, T.; Hagino, S.; Zhang, Y.; Yokoya, S.; Kawasaki, Y.; Suzuki, J.; Isome, M.; et al. Uninephrectomy induces progressive glomerulosclerosis and apoptosis in anti-Thy1 glomerulonephritis. *Pathol. Int.* **2005**, *55*, 19–26. [CrossRef] [PubMed]
44. Kawachi, H.; Iwanaga, T.; Toyabe, S.; Oite, T.; Shimizu, F. Mesangial sclerotic change with persistent proteinuria in rats after two consecutive injections of monoclonal antibody 1-22-3. *Clin. Exp. Immunol.* **1992**, *90*, 129–134. [CrossRef] [PubMed]
45. Yamamoto, T.; Qureshi, A.R.; Anderstam, B.; Heimburger, O.; Barany, P.; Lindholm, B.; Stenvinkel, P.; Axelsson, J. Clinical importance of an elevated circulating chemerin level in incident dialysis patients. *Nephrol. Dial. Transplant.* **2010**, *25*, 4017–4023. [CrossRef] [PubMed]
46. Mukai, H.; Dai, L.; Chen, Z.; Lindholm, B.; Ripsweden, J.; Brismar, T.B.; Heimburger, O.; Barany, P.; Qureshi, A.R.; Soderberg, M.; et al. Inverse J-shaped relation between coronary arterial calcium density and mortality in advanced chronic kidney disease. *Nephrol. Dial. Transplant.* **2018**. [CrossRef] [PubMed]
47. Carracedo, M.; Artiach, G.; Witasp, A.; Claria, J.; Carlstrom, M.; Laguna-Fernandez, A.; Stenvinkel, P.; Back, M. The G-protein coupled receptor ChemR23 determines smooth muscle cell phenotypic switching to enhance high phosphate-induced vascular calcification. *Cardiovasc Res.* **2019**, *115*, 1557–1566. [CrossRef] [PubMed]
48. Artiach, G.; Carracedo, M.; Claria, J.; Laguna-Fernandez, A.; Back, M. Opposing Effects on Vascular Smooth Muscle Cell Proliferation and Macrophage-induced Inflammation Reveal a Protective Role for the Proresolving Lipid Mediator Receptor ChemR23 in Intimal Hyperplasia. *Front. Pharmacol.* **2018**, *9*, 1327. [CrossRef]
49. Laguna-Fernandez, A.; Checa, A.; Carracedo, M.; Artiach, G.; Petri, M.H.; Baumgartner, R.; Forteza, M.J.; Jiang, X.; Andonova, T.; Walker, M.E.; et al. ERV1/ChemR23 Signaling Protects Against Atherosclerosis by Modifying Oxidized Low-Density Lipoprotein Uptake and Phagocytosis in Macrophages. *Circulation* **2018**, *138*, 1693–1705. [CrossRef]
50. Sato, K.; Yoshizawa, H.; Seki, T.; Shirai, R.; Yamashita, T.; Okano, T.; Shibata, K.; Wakamatsu, M.J.; Mori, Y.; Morita, T.; et al. Chemerin-9, a potent agonist of chemerin receptor (ChemR23), prevents atherogenesis.

Clin. Sci. (Lond) **2019**, *133*, 1779–1796. [CrossRef]

51. Carracedo, M.; Witasp, A.; Qureshi, A.R.; Laguna-Fernandez, A.; Brismar, T.; Stenvinkel, P.; Back, M. Chemerin inhibits vascular calcification through ChemR23 and is associated with lower coronary calcium in chronic kidney disease. *J. Int. Med.* **2019**, *286*, 449–457. [CrossRef]
52. Hartner, A.; Jagusch, L.; Cordasic, N.; Amann, K.; Veelken, R.; Jacobi, J.; Hilgers, K.F. Impaired Neovascularization and Reduced Capillary Supply in the Malignant vs. Non-malignant Course of Experimental Renovascular Hypertension. *Front. Physiol.* **2016**, *7*, 370. [CrossRef] [PubMed]
53. Mai, M.; Hilgers, K.F.; Wagner, J.; Mann, J.F.; Geiger, H. Expression of angiotensin-converting enzyme in renovascular hypertensive rat kidney. *Hypertension* **1995**, *25*, 674–678. [CrossRef] [PubMed]
54. Baker, A.J.; Mooney, A.; Hughes, J.; Lombardi, D.; Johnson, R.J.; Savill, J. Mesangial cell apoptosis: The major mechanism for resolution of glomerular hypercellularity in experimental mesangial proliferative nephritis. *J. Clin. Investig.* **1994**, *94*, 2105–2116. [CrossRef] [PubMed]
55. Menendez-Castro, C.; Fahlbusch, F.; Cordasic, N.; Amann, K.; Munzel, K.; Plank, C.; Wachtveitl, R.; Rascher, W.; Hilgers, K.F.; Hartner, A. Early and late postnatal myocardial and vascular changes in a protein restriction rat model of intrauterine growth restriction. *PLoS ONE* **2011**, *6*, e20369. [CrossRef]
56. Menendez-Castro, C.; Hilgers, K.F.; Amann, K.; Daniel, C.; Cordasic, N.; Wachtveitl, R.; Fahlbusch, F.; Plank, C.; Dotsch, J.; Rascher, W.; et al. Intrauterine growth restriction leads to a dysregulation of Wilms' tumour supressor gene 1 (WT1) and to early podocyte alterations. *Nephrol Dial. Transplant.* **2013**, *28*, 1407–1417. [CrossRef]
57. Menendez-Castro, C.; Toka, O.; Fahlbusch, F.; Cordasic, N.; Wachtveitl, R.; Hilgers, K.F.; Rascher, W.; Hartner, A. Impaired myocardial performance in a normotensive rat model of intrauterine growth restriction. *Pediatr. Res.* **2014**, *75*, 697–706. [CrossRef]
58. Laemmli, U.K. Cleavage of structural proteins during the assembly of the head of bacteriophage T4. *Nature* **1970**, *227*, 680–685. [CrossRef]
59. Gibson, U.E.; Heid, C.A.; Williams, P.M. A novel method for real time quantitative RT-PCR. *Genome Res.* **1996**, *6*, 995–1001. [CrossRef]

13

Kidney Cells Regeneration: Dedifferentiation of Tubular Epithelium, Resident Stem Cells and Possible Niches for Renal Progenitors

Nadezda V. Andrianova [1,2], Marina I. Buyan [1], Ljubava D. Zorova [2,3], Irina B. Pevzner [2,3], Vasily A. Popkov [2,3], Valentina A. Babenko [2,3], Denis N. Silachev [2,3], Egor Y. Plotnikov [2,3,4,*] and Dmitry B. Zorov [2,3,*]

1 Faculty of Bioengineering and Bioinformatics, Lomonosov Moscow State University, 119992 Moscow, Russia; andnadya12@gmail.com (N.V.A.); marinanenart@gmail.com (M.I.B.)

2 A.N. Belozersky Institute of Physico-Chemical Biology, Lomonosov Moscow State University, 119992 Moscow, Russia; lju_2003@list.ru (L.D.Z.); irinapevzner@mail.ru (I.B.P.); popkov.vas@gmail.com (V.A.P.); nucleus-90@yandex.ru (V.A.B.); silachevdn@belozersky.msu.ru (D.N.S.)

3 V.I. Kulakov National Medical Research Center of Obstetrics, Gynecology and Perinatology, 117997 Moscow, Russia

4 Sechenov First Moscow State Medical University, Institute of Molecular Medicine, 119991 Moscow, Russia

* Correspondence: plotnikov@belozersky.msu.ru (E.Y.P.); zorov@belozersky.msu.ru (D.B.Z.)

Abstract: A kidney is an organ with relatively low basal cellular regenerative potential. However, renal cells have a pronounced ability to proliferate after injury, which undermines that the kidney cells are able to regenerate under induced conditions. The majority of studies explain yielded regeneration either by the dedifferentiation of the mature tubular epithelium or by the presence of a resident pool of progenitor cells in the kidney tissue. Whether cells responsible for the regeneration of the kidney initially have progenitor properties or if they obtain a "progenitor phenotype" during dedifferentiation after an injury, still stays the open question. The major stumbling block in resolving the issue is the lack of specific methods for distinguishing between dedifferentiated cells and resident progenitor cells. Transgenic animals, single-cell transcriptomics, and other recent approaches could be powerful tools to solve this problem. This review examines the main mechanisms of kidney regeneration: dedifferentiation of epithelial cells and activation of progenitor cells with special attention to potential niches of kidney progenitor cells. We attempted to give a detailed description of the most controversial topics in this field and ways to resolve these issues.

Keywords: renal stem cells; differentiation; scattered tubular cells; papilla; niches

1. Introduction

Despite the fact that the kidney has relatively low basal cellular regenerative potential, tubular epithelial cells have a pronounced ability to proliferate after injury [1]. However, the complexity of the renal tissue in mammals and the low rate of cell renewal makes it difficult to study kidney regeneration mechanisms. In this regard, there is still no consensus on what cells are responsible for the recovery of tubular epithelium after injury [2]. A number of hypotheses have been proposed about the nature of regenerative potential in the kidney tissue. The majority of studies assign the basis of such regenerative potential either to the dedifferentiation of the mature tubular epithelium or to the presence of a resident pool of progenitor cells in the kidney tissue [3,4].

The hypothesis of dedifferentiation as a mechanism of renal tissue restoration was based on the analysis of proliferation after ischemia/reperfusion (I/R) or exposure to damaging agents showing that more than half of all tubular epithelium becomes positively stained for proliferation markers (PCNA, Ki-67, BrdU) [5–8]. In addition, some morphological changes were observed in the tubular epithelial cells, which together with the aforementioned data was interpreted as dedifferentiation of these cells [9]. Furthermore, cells indicated the appearance of markers of an embryonic kidney, which could be assumed as a return to a less differentiated state [10–12]. Since then, a lot of evidence has been accumulated about the dominant role of dedifferentiation in the restoration of renal tissue after injury, including data obtained in transgenic animals.

Subsequently, there was additional evidence indicating the possible existence of a population of progenitor cells (so-called scattered tubular cells, STCs) in the adult kidney which had a more pronounced regenerative potential than differentiated tubular epithelium [13–15]. These cells were initially found in the kidneys of rodents [13] and then they were also described in humans [16,17]. Human kidneys have become a very convenient object for progenitor cells studying due to the presence of specific marker CD133 with glycosylated epitope being a "gold standard" to consider these cells as progenitor cells in humans [16,18], as well as in some other mammals [19,20]. Lack of this marker in rodents forces to use other markers for identification of the progenitor population there and determines the need for experiments with transgenic animals expressing fluorescent markers in progenitor cells [21]. A large number of such markers have been proposed (Tables 1 and 2), which apparently characterize the population of progenitor cells in both human and rodent kidneys [22–24].

Table 1. Conventional markers used for the detection of progenitor cells or the dedifferentiation of tubular epithelial cells. Markers, which are used for progenitor cells detection, are partially different for human and rodent kidneys. Foxm1 is the only marker specific for dedifferentiation. Other markers are used both for dedifferentiated cells and progenitor cells and not selective. Empty fields indicate that the marker was not reported for specified conditions.

	Marker	**Progenitor Cells**		**Dedifferentiation**
		Human	***Rodents***	
Markers of progenitor cells	ALDH1	[18,25]	-	-
	BrdU retention	Not applicable	[13,26–28]	-
	CD24	[16–18,25,29–31]	[15]	-
	CD44	[30,32]	[33]	-
	CD73	[30,32]	-	-
	CD133	[16–18,29–32,34]	Not applicable	-
	C-kit	-	[14,35]	-
	Musculin	-	[36]	-
	NCAM1	[37]	-	-
	NFATc1	-	[38]	-
	S100A6	[16,18,25]	-	-
	Sall1	[25,37]	[39]	-
	Sca-1	-	[14,15,35,36,40]	-
	SIX2	[37,41]	-	-
Marker of dedifferentiation	Foxm1	-	-	[42,43]
Non-selective markers	Nestin	[44]	[35]	[45]
	Pax-2	[25,30,32,34,37,44]	[14,33,35,46]	[8,11,47–49]
	Sox9	-	[50]	[42,51]
	Vimentin	[16–18,25,30,31,44]	[13,14,26,33,35]	[9,42,47,48,52,53]

Table 2. Markers of progenitor cells located in the papilla of human or rodent kidney.

Marker	The Papilla of Human Kidney	The Papilla of Rodent Kidney
BrdU retention	Not applicable	[27,54–59]
CD133	[60,61]	Not applicable
mTert	-	[59]
Nestin	[60,61]	[55,62]
Oct4	[60,61]	-
Pax-2	[61]	-
Sca-1	-	[63]
Troy/TNFRSF19	-	[64]
Vimentin	[61]	-
Zfyve27	-	[65]

The identification of cells responsible for the restoration of tubular epithelium is in the scope of regenerative medicine [66,67]. This review examines the main mechanisms of kidney regeneration: dedifferentiation of the epithelium and activation of progenitor cells with special attention to potential niches of kidney progenitor cells. We attempted to give a detailed description of the most controversial issues in this area. In particular, we considered issues based on defects of techniques involved in the detection of progenitor cells and on the inability of discrimination of tubular epithelium proliferation from progenitor cells preexistence.

2. Dedifferentiation or Recruitment of Progenitor Cells?

2.1. Dedifferentiation

In the kidneys of adult organisms, a renewal rate the cell population is very slow, however, it dramatically enhances after injury [5]. Staining for various proliferative markers, for example, proliferating cell nuclear antigen (PCNA), Ki-67, and evaluating the accumulation of probes such as bromodeoxyuridine (BrdU) showed that injury-induced cell proliferation in the kidney tissue is not associated with some specific regeneration centers, but goes stochastically [7,8]. In this regard, the first hypothesis explaining the restoration of lost renal cells was the dedifferentiation of the tubular epithelium [5,68]. For a long time, it was believed that any renal epithelial cell has a regenerative potency in response to injury [9,69,70].

After exposure to a damaging factor, a peak of proliferation in the kidney tissue was observed usually occurring on the 2nd day, whereas normal epithelial morphology is normally restored within 5–7 days after challenge [1]. Histological analysis of the kidney tissue distinguishes 4 stages of the regeneration process. At the first stage, the death of tubular epithelium is observed, occurring by apoptosis, necrosis, or another death mode, and it is usually accompanied by an inflammatory reaction. In the second stage, survived tubular cells exhibit changes in normal differentiated epithelial phenotypes, such as a loss of brush border, tubular flattening, and rapid loss of cell polarity [71,72]. During this stage, cells undergo epithelial-mesenchymal transition, detected by overexpression of vimentin, which is a marker of mesenchymal cells [9,52]. The third phase is associated with increased levels of growth factors, such as IGF1, HGF, FGFs, and enhanced proliferation of a majority of kidney cells [73]. Growth factors stimulate cells in the G_0 phase and promote their entry into the cell cycle [74]. The regeneration process is terminated after the recovery of the normal morphology of epithelial cells and restoration of nephron function [75]. Thus, regeneration through dedifferentiation refers to the sequence of histological changes including loss of mature epithelium morphology, epithelial-mesenchymal transition, proliferation to replace lost cells, and re-differentiation [5].

S3 segment of the proximal tubule located near the cortico-medullary junction is known as the most vulnerable part of the nephron [76,77]. Remarkably, the S3 segment also exhibits the most pronounced proliferation after injury compared to other segments of the nephron [78]. Therefore, the majority of studies investigating mechanisms of kidney regeneration are focused on this particular area. Double staining with chlorodeoxyuridine (CldU) and antibodies against Ki-67 revealed that within 48 h after I/R more than 55% of the cells, mainly in the S3 segment, reentered the cell cycle or even passed the S phase [8].

There is a direct histological confirmation of the dedifferentiation of tubular epithelium. In the injured tubules, dividing cells were detected revealing both epithelial and proliferative markers [52,69]. Particularly, dividing cells in the S3 segment of proximal tubules and in the distal tubules had a basolateral expression of Na-K-ATPase (a marker of terminal epithelial differentiation) at the same level as neighboring non-proliferating cells [69], and cells survived after injury carrying intact nuclei actively proliferated and expressed vimentin. Paradoxically, actively proliferating cells continued the expression of Kim-1 [79], a well-known marker of the injured proximal tubular epithelium [80]. Usually, around 35–50% of survived kidney cells begin to express this protein in response to injury [81]. In a strange way, the co-expression of an alarming damaging factor Kim-1 with proliferative factor vimentin in tubular cells after an injury has been currently interpreted as evidence for the proliferation of injured epithelium [8]. It is unclear, whether it reflects the compensatory mechanism for replenishment renal loss of functionality, although it seems dangerous for the organism to reproduce damaged cells.

In addition to vimentin, during kidney regeneration markers specific to kidney development appeared, i.g., Pax-2, and neural cell adhesion molecule 1 (NCAM1). Transcription factor Pax-2 is almost not expressed in adult kidneys, except the collecting ducts and papilla [11]. However, after ischemic or nephrotoxic kidney injury, Pax-2 expression is significantly increased in the survived tubular epithelium, indicating the appearance of cells with immature phenotype [11,49]. NCAM1 is widely represented during nephrogenesis, but it is not detected in the differentiated tubular epithelium [49]. However, upon injury or isolation of kidney cells for culturing, epithelium starts to express NCAM1 again [37]. NCAM1-positive cells exhibit features of epithelial-mesenchymal transformation and possess robust clonal capacity, adopting a progenitor phenotype [82].

Similarly to Pax-2 and NCAM1, another marker of dedifferentiation, Sox9, is actively involved in embryogenesis [51], but is not presented in the kidney tissue of adult organisms [83]. Sox9 expression increases by more than 20-fold 24 h after I/R and its elevated level persists up to 30 days after injury [51]. Over 40% of Sox9-positive cells also express Ki-67 and locate in a scattered-like manner, mainly in the proximal tubules. Sox9+ cells co-express injury markers, neutrophil gelatinase-associated lipocalin (NGAL) and Kim-1, which may indicate that these cells represent injured epithelium. In addition, experiments were performed using lineage tracing showed that Sox9+ cells really contributed to kidney regeneration [51].

In addition, nestin, the protein belonging to intermediate filaments, was recently proposed as a marker of dedifferentiation. After subtotal nephrectomy, the expression of nestin was increased in epithelial cells bordering the injured area [45]. These cells actively proliferated, so the expression of nestin was suggested as a dedifferentiation-associated feature.

2.2. *Progenitor Cells*

2.2.1. Progenitor Cells in Rodent Kidneys

The first assumption of the presence of progenitor cells in the kidneys arose in the study of Maeshima et al. [13]. In this study, adult intact rats were treated with BrdU, which accumulated in cells in the S-phase [84]. Analysis of kidney cells was conducted 2 weeks after the end of the 7-days BrdU administration and allowed to identify cells with the slow cell cycle. These cells were scattered among other cells of the proximal and distal tubules, so they later became known as scattered tubular cells (STCs), or label-retaining cells (LRCs). To detect possible progenitor properties of LRCs, rats were exposed to I/R, and it was revealed that the number of BrdU+ cells significantly increased 24 h after I/R, most of them were located in 2-cell clusters and expressed PCNA. These cells expressed vimentin as well, and at day 10 began to express E-cadherin (a marker of differentiated epithelium) [85]. Similar data on the presence of LRCs were obtained in newborn mice in which BrdU+ cells were located mainly in the S3 segment and in the papilla [28].

In addition to label retention, these presumably progenitor cells have a more pronounced regenerative potential than non-LRCs. For example, on a three-dimensional gel substrate, they formed tubule-like or tubulocystic structures in response to growth factors treatment [26]. When transplanted into the metanephric kidney, these cells were embedded into epithelial components of a nephron, including proximal tubules, where they demonstrated 3.5–13 times higher proliferative potential [15]. Cells isolated from the S3 segment of adult rat kidneys were able to reconstruct a three-dimensional kidney-like structure in vitro, having all parts of the nephron, including the glomerulus, tubules, and collecting ducts [35]. Moreover, S3-segment cells injected into adult kidney right after ischemia were found in the cortex and medulla confirming their participation in regeneration [14]. However, despite implantation into the kidney tissue, these cells did not cause any significant physiological effects on kidney function estimated by serum creatinine and urea.

A comparative analysis of human and rat renal progenitor cells revealed a population of human scattered tubular cells with a small amount of cytoplasm and mitochondria, without a brush border, which was positive for CD24, CD133 and other progenitors markers [16]. No similar cells with atypical morphology were found in intact rats. The study of renal progenitor cells in rats is complicated by the lack of specific expression of CD24 and glycosylated form of CD133, therefore the search was carried out by the staining for vimentin and CD44 which is another marker for stemness. While absent in intact tissue, vimentin-positive cells with atypical morphology appeared de novo after unilateral ureteral obstruction. The cells (appeared in areas with severe tubules damage) were located singly or in chains of cells and did not have a brush border [16]. However, the emergence of progenitor cells de novo may be only the result of the dedifferentiation.

A similar situation was observed for transcription factor Sox9, which sometimes is used as a marker of progenitor STCs in mice [50]. For a number of tissues, Sox9 is considered to characterize the population of progenitor cells, for example, in hair follicles, retina, and nerve tissue [12,86,87]. However, in renal tissue, cells begin to actively express Sox9 only after injury. Therefore, although they possess many features of progenitor cells (expression of CD133 and Lgr4, the ability to differentiate into adipogenic, osteogenic and chondrogenic cultures), their appearance can be attributed only to dedifferentiation of some renal cells [50].

Sall1, CD24, Sca-1, and nestin have also been proposed as markers of renal progenitor cells. Sall1 is a transcription factor involved in nephrogenesis [88]. Analysis of its expression in the adult kidney revealed that about 0.5% of all cells contained Sall1 located mainly in the cortico-medullary junction [39]. After I/R, 90% of Sall1-positive cells started to proliferate and 5% of these cells showed asymmetric cell division with one of the two adjacent Sall1-positive cells. CD24 is a glycoprotein that is selectively expressed in immature cells of different tissues and it is almost absent in differentiated cells [89]. The presence of this marker was shown in the population of progenitor cells in rodent kidneys [15], however, it is not always possible to obtain its specific staining [16]. Another important marker is Sca-1, which was initially detected as a marker of hematopoietic stem cells until its association with renal progenitor cells was shown [14,15,36,40]. Finally, the aforementioned nestin, intermediate filaments protein, unambiguously associated with progenitor cells in nervous tissue [90], was also found in the cells of some kidney compartments, which are considered as niches for progenitor cells, particularly, the papilla and cortico-medullary junction [62].

In a recent study, the analysis of kidney progenitor cells was performed using transgenic mice with doxycycline-induced random labeling of all tubular epithelial cells by permanent recombination of a single-color-encoding gene [46]. Analysis carried out 30 days after an acute kidney injury (AKI) showed that tubules consisted of clones of cells with the same color and mainly located in the S3 segment of the kidney. Calculations based on the percentage of differently colored clones demonstrated that only a small number of epithelial cells underwent mitosis after I/R, most of them were Pax-2-positive. During regeneration, these cells formed single-colored clones of more than 10 cells. Only Pax-2+ cells fully passed the mitotic cycle, whereas the rest of the tubular epithelium has undergone an endoreplication cycle [46].

Further evidence for the presence of progenitor cells pool in rodent kidneys came from the study of Rinchevich et al. using the so-called rainbow mice [91]. These mice express multicolored reporter constructs allowing to detect cells with segment-specific clonogenic and proliferative potential. One month after the induction of reporter protein expression in intact mice, the clones were observed as small groups of 2–3 cells with the same color. After a longer period, the clones increased to groups consisting of more than 8 cells and they were located both in the cortical substance and in the medulla, in particular, the papilla. The findings showed that tubulogenesis exists in the adult kidney and only a subset of adult epithelial cells was responsible for it. The number of clones of the same color increased after I/R, and most of them (60%) were found in the cortical substance. Thus, this study proved the presence of a functional population of renal progenitor cells [91]. However, it still remains unclear whether these cells belong to a separate pool or they originate from the epithelium transiently acquiring a progenitor phenotype [92].

2.2.2. Progenitor Cells in Human Kidneys

After the discovery of progenitor cells in rodent kidneys, there were studies demonstrating the existence of such cells in human kidneys [27,32]. A population of cells with morphology and progenitor properties different from normal epithelial cells was isolated in the proximal tubules. The main markers of this population were CD24, CD133, and vimentin, and cells were scattered throughout the proximal tubule in the normal human kidney [16]. If compared to conventional epithelial cells, these cells contained less cytoplasm, fewer mitochondria, and had no brush border [16]. The average number of progenitor cells in the cortical substance of the human kidney was estimated at 0.5–4% [17,32] or slightly more (3%–12%) [31]. Most CD133+ cells in the human kidney are located in the S3 segment of the proximal tubules [27,93]. It is noteworthy that this region is most susceptible to damaging factors, but at the same time, it has a remarkable capacity to rerestore its structure and function [77,94].

A convenient feature of human kidney progenitor cells, absent in similar rodent cells, is the presence of CD133, a specific marker of undifferentiated cells. Although CD133 is abundant in both immature and differentiated cells, specific glycosylated epitopes (CD133/1 and CD133/2) have been found only on immature cells in humans [95,96], such as hematopoietic stem/progenitor cells and tissue-specific progenitor cells [97]. The glycosylated form of CD133 has been shown to be expressed in S-shaped bodies in the fetal kidney and co-expressed with Ki-67 [93]. Thus, CD133 is a widely used marker of progenitor cells, however, when staining for this antigen, it is very important to monitor the specificity of antibodies, to exclusively recognize the epitope related to undifferentiated cells only [98]. For confirmation of the results of CD133 detection, cells often are examined for CD24, which usually co-expresses with CD133 [99].

It has been shown that cells positive for CD24/CD133 in various parts of the nephron can be considered as a population of resident progenitor cells. They have the ability to expansion, self-renewal, and epithelial differentiation both in vitro and in vivo [16,17,31,32]. In culture, they are able to differentiate into tubular, osteogenic, neuronal, adipose cells and to repair tubular structures [100]. In vitro, they have the ability to form spheres, which is a specific feature of stem cells [18] and to proliferate for a long time without signs of cell senescence [25]. These cells contain fewer mitochondria than conventional epithelial cells [16], which was confirmed by electron microscopy using gold-conjugated vimentin antibodies, as well as by double immunofluorescence staining for CD133 and mitochondrial markers [31]. However, despite the reduced mitochondrial content, CD133+ cells demonstrate increased Bcl-2 expression [16,18]. CD133 itself is known to participate in glucose uptake [101], and stem cells, in general, are prone to anaerobic metabolism [102]. Probably, the combination of these factors explains the increased resistance of these cells to apoptosis [17].

In addition, cells expressing CD24 and CD133 have a pronounced regenerative potential when administered to mice with severe combined immunodeficiency (SCID) exposed to I/R [100]. A population of human CD133+ papillary cells also possesses a profound nephroprotective potential when administered to rats subjected to glycerol-induced acute tubular damage. It provides restoration of kidney function, preventing tubular necrosis and stimulating proliferation of their own resident cells [30]. CD133+ cells also show signs of proliferation in the renal biopsy material from patients suffering renal insults [17,31]. Despite the fact that the high proliferative activity of putative progenitor cells has been widely shown, it should be kept in mind that cells can behave in vitro in a completely different way than in the organism [48]. For example, human CD133+ cells injected after kidney injury have been shown to be implanted into the tubules of embryonic kidneys, but not in adult rat kidneys [103].

It was found that, apart from CD24 and CD133, another 49 proteins were expressed in the kidney in the same scattered pattern [16]. Among them, there are already mentioned Pax-2 and Sox9, however, colocalization with CD24 or CD133 was shown only for vimentin, S100A6 and several other proteins, e.g., aldehyde dehydrogenase 1 [18]. Recently, a transcriptional profile of CD133+ cells was obtained by RNA sequencing [25]. Overexpression of CD24, PAX-2, vimentin, aldehyde dehydrogenase 1, S100A6, as well as of some other markers were detected.

The existence of progenitor cells distributed in the kidney in a scattered-like manner raises the question of their origin in the process of nephrogenesis [17]. CD133 and CD24 are expressed under kidney development, with the main cluster located in the urinal pole of Bowman's capsule, and a small portion located in the distal tubules in the junction with the glomerulus. It is assumed that during the growth of the kidney, the cells spread and formed the STCs observed in the adult kidney [104]. This once again proves the indissoluble connection of STCs of tubules with the population of glomerular parietal cells, which are recognized as a pool of progenitor cells for podocytes and contain the same markers as STCs [105].

2.3. State of the Art

Thus, there is still a discussion about the genuine nature of the regenerating mechanisms in the adult kidneys of humans and other mammals [1]. The main problem is the lack of specific methods and unique markers for distinguishing between dedifferentiation and progenitor cells' preexistence [2]. For instance, vimentin, which in some studies used as a marker of dedifferentiation and epithelial-mesenchymal transition [9], is also overexpressed in the population of cells defined as progenitors [5].

A similar discussion is going around Kim-1 [106], which is a common marker of the injured proximal tubular epithelium [79,80]. For a long time, the coexpression of vimentin and Kim-1 in the same cells was considered as strict evidence of the dedifferentiation of the injured epithelium as a regenerative mechanism [79]. However, several studies showed that progenitor cells also express Kim-1 after injury [16,18]. To resolve the issue, transgenic mice were created expressing a fluorescent construct under the Kim-1 promoter [42]. The study revealed that Kim-1 was not expressed in renal cells of intact animals. Therefore Kim-1 could not be a marker of the resident progenitor cells. After I/R, in the kidney tissue, clones of cells were found expressing Kim-1, vimentin, Sox9, and Ki67, that was interpreted as a return to the dedifferentiated state rather than a proliferation of resident tubular progenitors. In addition, in this study transcription factor, Foxm1 was described as a new potential marker of dedifferentiated kidney cells [42]. Foxm1 was overexpressed in the injured proximal tubular epithelium, especially in the S3 segment.

The identification of embryonic kidney markers does not resolve the existing contradictions. On the one hand, markers that take part in the process of nephrogenesis should presumably appear during dedifferentiation [1]. On the other hand, a population of progenitor cells, if exists, may also express neonatal kidney markers [23]. For instance, Pax-2 overexpression has been suggested as an argument in favor of the dedifferentiation of mature tubular epithelium after injury [11]. However, in the intact kidney, a population of Pax-2+ cells was also found, which constituted about 10% of cells in the S3 segment [46].

A similar situation occurs around Sox9 [1], initially proposed as a marker of dedifferentiated epithelium due to its expression during nephrogenesis [51]. After an injury, Sox9 colocalized with markers of injured tubular epithelium, such as NGAL and Kim-1 [51]. However, in the intact adult kidney, Sox9-positive cells were found representing a small population of scattered cells that started to proliferate after injury [50], suggesting Sox9 more likely associated with progenitors.

It still remains unclear whether the population of progenitor cells differs from mature tubular epithelium by the number of mitochondria. On the one hand, in adult rat kidney, STCs were characterized by a large number of mitochondria [107]. On the other, in human kidneys, it was found that STCs had a small amount of these organelles [16,31]. Since the content of mitochondria has a very strong effect on cell metabolism, accurate information about the number of these organelles in progenitor cells could help in the development of methods for affecting these cells.

There is a serious limitation in studying renal progenitor cells due to using CD133 as a key marker of undifferentiated cells in human kidneys [108]. Firstly, the glycosylated epitope of CD133 is present in the kidneys of humans, primates, and pigs, but it is absent in rodents [109], which are the main experimental animals. Secondly, the level of glycosylation depends on the stage of cell differentiation [98]. Therefore, the usage of antibodies recognizing CD133 outside the glycosylated epitope can lead to incorrect results [96]. So it is crucial to monitor the specificity of antibodies to the glycosylated epitope in order to selectively determine the pool of progenitor cells. Finally, CD133 antigenic specificity may not only be a limitation of the technique but also indicates differences in the mechanism for kidney regeneration in humans and rodents [2]. For instance, it has been suggested that in humans, progenitor cells could preexist in the tubules, while, in rodents, dedifferentiation might predominate as the main regeneration mechanism [16]. However, this hypothesis was questioned by the detection of progenitor cells in rodent kidneys using other markers [38,50,64].

Thus, the majority of studies support the idea that after injury, the adult kidneys acquire a population of cells with pronounced regenerative potential. However, it remains unclear whether these cells arose from dedifferentiated epithelial cells or from the preexisting population of progenitor cells. The current views on these mechanisms are summarized in Figure 1.

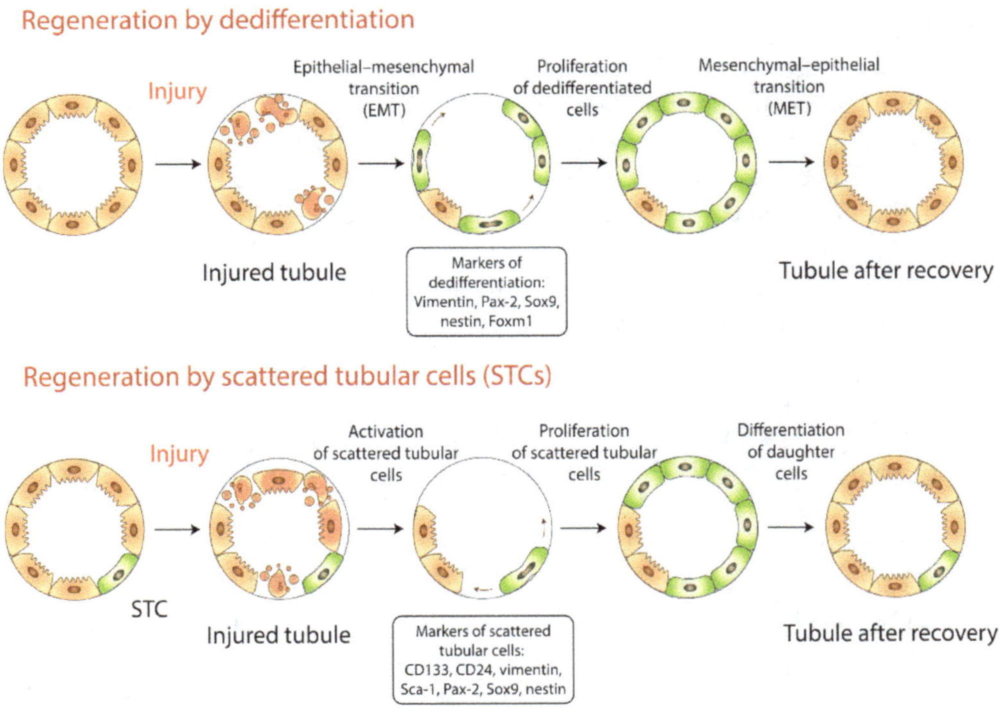

Figure 1. Two major putative mechanisms of kidney tissue regeneration: dedifferentiation of tubular epithelial cells and proliferation of resident renal progenitors with subsequent differentiation.

3. Renal Papilla as a Niche for Progenitor Cells

Morphologically, papilla belongs to the inner layer of renal medulla and plays a crucial role in urine concentration due to residing Henle's loop of juxtamedullary nephrons [110]. Some studies suggest papilla as a putative niche for progenitor cells [55,62,111]. This hypothesis is based on the presence of a large number of cells with the slow cell cycle in the papilla and those cells carrying markers of progenitor cells [2]. Moreover, the papilla is a place with unique conditions that are simultaneously hyperosmotic and hypoxic [112]. The hypoxic microenvironment is a distinguishing feature for stem cell niches in the other organs, such as bone marrow and brain [113]. Papilla cells along with STCs in proximal tubules express progenitor cell markers, for instance, glycated CD133 in human kidneys or nestin in rodent kidneys, and these cells change their properties during tissue regeneration [30,61,62]. Furthermore, papilla cells are positive for embryonic kidney markers, for instance, Pax-2 [11] and TNFRSF19 [64], even in intact adult kidneys.

Papilla as a niche for progenitor cells was suggested in 2004 by Oliver et al., who tried to discover renal resident progenitor cells and outline their properties [55]. The research was based on the observation that organ-specific adult stem cells in a number of tissues have a slow cell cycle that can be detected by retention of BrdU, which integrates into DNA molecule during replication [84]. The study was performed on neonatal rats and mice, which are characterized by the ongoing process of nephrogenesis for a few days after birth. Newborn rodents were injected with BrdU solution, and label retention was estimated 2 months later in the kidney tissue. As a result, in papilla, a population of LRCs was found, with a slow cell cycle, which resided mostly in interstitium although some of them were colocalized with markers of tubular epithelial cells. These LRCs were not bone marrow-derived or belong to endothelial cells. However, after I/R, BrdU-positive cells were absent in the cortex and medulla, which refuted the hypothesis about LRCs migration towards injured areas of the kidney [55].

However, the BrdU labeling assay has several restrictions. The assay mechanism bases on the ability of bromodeoxyuridine to replace thymidine during replication with such replacements being detected by specific antibodies [84]. Label levels slowly decrease in the daughter cells when cells divide after label withdraw. Due to the slow cycle, stem and progenitor cells contain the label for a longer time [114]. However, all cells in S-phase accumulate BrdU during its administration that is the main limitation of the assay [7].

As a result of limitations with BrdU labeling assay, there were attempts to detect progenitor cells in the papilla using lineage tracing in transgenic mice expressing green fluorescent protein (GFP)-fused histone protein (H2B-GFP) under tetracycline-sensitive promotor [115]. The assay was based on the high stability of H2B-GFP protein in the cells with a slow cycle. Consequently, stimulation of its expression before the mice's birth resulted in the detection of cells with a slow cycle even within months after birth [58]. This assay confirmed that cells with slow cycles were located mainly in the papilla, but not in the outer medulla or cortex. Moreover, GFP-positive cells migrated toward the upper part of the papilla where these cells formed chain-like structures of proliferating cells positive for Ki-67 [58].

The population of papilla stem cells was also found in transgenic mice expressing GFP under the nestin promoter [90]. Nestin is considered to be a marker of progenitor cells, including the kidney [60,116]. Those mice had GFP-positive cells mainly in the papilla, and only a small amount was located in the cortico-medullary junction [62]. In the study, evidence was found that GFP-positive cells migrate from the papilla to cortex [90]. The main limitation of the model was a constitutive nestin expression in the adult podocytes and in some endotheliocytes [117,118]. Furthermore, nestin expression in podocytes has been shown to rise during some pathological conditions [119,120].

One more approach for detecting cells with a slow cell cycle is in using mTert-GFP as a reporter system, thus labeling telomerase-expressing embryonic stem cells [59]. On the one hand, such a reporter was chosen because telomerase is a biomarker of stem cells. On the other hand, knockout of mTert leads to the increased severity of AKI, which is believed to be associated with inhibiting of mTert-expressing renal progenitor cell population [121]. The majority of GFP+ cells were observed in the papilla (about 10% of all papillary cells); a small amount was detected in the outer medulla, but not in the cortex. Colocalization with the other cell type-specific proteins showed that mTert was expressed primarily in epithelial cells [59].

Based on the suggestion that papillary progenitor cells have the same cell markers as other tissues progenitor cells GFP-positive cells from H2B-GFP transgenic mice were obtained by fluorescence-activated cell sorting (FACS), and their specific markers were defined. Only protrudin (Zfyve27) demonstrated selective expression in the papilla and it was absent in the other kidney areas [65]. Protrudin-positive cells appeared not to contribute to normal kidney maintenance, however, after severe kidney injury, cells started to proliferate and generate long tubular segments located preferentially in the kidney medulla [65]. Additionally, these cells had many morphological characteristics specific to migratory cells [122].

Considering this data, it was suggested that different kidney areas might have different progenitor cell pools [65] (Figure 2). For instance, papillary LRCs could be activated only in response to severe injury and they restore mainly epithelium in the medulla. This suggestion correlates with the experiments performed on the other epithelial tissues which showed the existence of progenitor cell pools responding to damaging factors being responsible for restoring anatomically various parts of an organ [123,124].

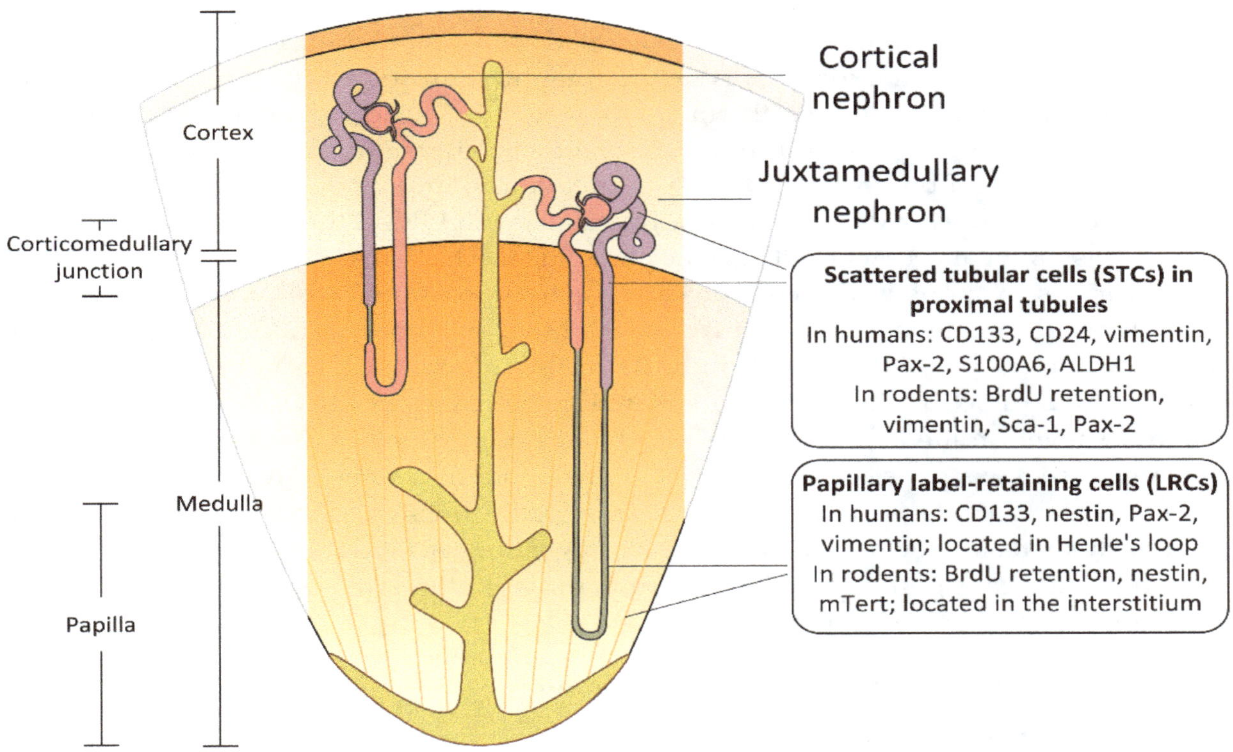

Figure 2. Major suggested niches of renal progenitor cells based on the immunophenotyping with specific surface markers and label retention approach. There are two putative niches for progenitor cells: proximal tubules (especially their S3-segments) and papilla. Progenitor cells in human and rodents kidneys are characterized by slightly different markers listed in Table 2. It is worth noting some differences in the location of progenitor cells: in the papilla of rodent kidney, label-retaining cells (LRCs) reside in the interstitium, while in human kidneys these progenitors constitute the Henle's loop among differentiated cells of the nephron.

Interestingly, papillary progenitor cells were found both in rodents [55,62] and human kidneys [60,61], but with some differences in the localization of the cells. In rodents, a preferential interstitial localization of progenitor cells was observed [55,58,62], while human progenitors were found primarily inside Henle's loops [60]. Both in rodents and humans, these cells were colocalized with the conventional progenitor cell markers. It was shown that CD133+ and nestin+ cells in Henle's loop were located both in the papilla and cortex of the human kidneys. CD133+ cells obtained from the human papilla actively proliferated; after injection into mice embryonic kidney, they integrated into tubules and were involved in tubulogenesis [60]. Similarly, rodent papilla contained cells expressing nestin and telomerase [59,62,125], and papillary cells from pig kidneys were positive for progenitor cells markers CD24 and CD133, and they had myogenic, osteogenic, and adipogenic differentiation potential [111].

To date, the involvement of the papillary cells in kidney regeneration is not fully understood. Whether it is achieved through progenitors migration and integration into tubules, or through paracrine mechanisms is not clear. Hypothesis about proliferation and migration of progenitors daughter cells are based on almost 9 fold decrease of LRCs in papilla 3 weeks after I/R injury [55]. However, in GFP-nestin mice such a decrease in LRCs was not shown after I/R [62]. The question is: why so many papillary LRCs lose BrdU label after injury, whereas only a fraction of them proliferate after injury, and apoptosis is not observed in this area [114].

The migration of papillary LRCs was confirmed in the single study using GFP-nestin mice when papillary nestin-GFP+ cells migrated to cortex and medulla after I/R [62]. Other studies with more evidence-based data demonstrated that migration is limited by the medulla [58,65]. Moreover, the mTert-GFP mouse model showed no evidence of the migration of mTert LRCs from the papilla in response to injury [59]. Humphreys et al. reiterated the study with BrdU administration during nephrogenesis; LRCs in their experiments neither migrated during repair from I/R nor selectively proliferated in those conditions [8]. Furthermore, Ki-67 staining in kidneys of mice injected with CldU during infancy showed that LRCs did not demonstrate proliferation after injury in the cortex and medulla [8]. "Chains" of proliferating Ki-67+ cells found in upper papilla did not colocalize with CldU-positive cells. However, despite the negative results with LRCs, Humphreys et al. did not refute that papilla cells might affect other cells via the paracrine mechanisms [54].

Thus, various methods indicated that kidney papilla contains a cell population with a slow cell cycle involved in regeneration processes in the other parts of the kidney [8,28,55]. However, the biological significance of the long-term BrdU-retaining population is not fully understood yet. These cells could be a population that differentiated in the kidney as early as during embryogenesis and then have never proliferated for any reason. On the other hand, LRCs rapidly exit the cell cycle and undergo much fewer divisions than tubular epithelium thus having more significant regenerative capacity after injury [56]. Due to a large number of contradictions in this area, it is difficult to accept unambiguously that a kidney papilla is a niche of progenitor cells. Further experiments are required to clarify the biological significance of this renal papillary cell population and to identify possible mechanisms of its role in regeneration.

4. Potential Approaches Affecting Kidney Regeneration

A discussion around the presence of progenitor cells in the kidneys of adult organisms appears from the requests of regenerative medicine, because if such cells exist, it would be possible to develop approaches selectively enhancing kidney regeneration [66]. The development of such approaches is possible in the case of dedifferentiation as the main mechanism of regeneration, as well. However, the presence of a pool of progenitors with specific markers and their own physiological characteristics increases the chances to find a successful strategy. Therefore, numerous studies are focused on searching and phenotyping these cells [67].

One of the cell therapy approaches is the use of resident progenitor cells obtained from the kidney by isolation, cultivation and subsequent transplantation (autologous or allogeneic) in the injured organ. Such design is frequently described in the experimental works performed on rodents. Recent studies showed that cells could integrate into the tubules of neonatal and adult kidneys, and then either directly or indirectly could influence the regeneration of renal tissue through the paracrine mechanisms [15–17,35]. However, not in all studies the real improvement of the organ functions was achieved [33]. It is known that cell therapy with resident kidney progenitor cells reduces the activation of apoptosis and inflammation [126], improves angiogenesis [127], reduces fibrosis [128,129], and even increases animal survival after kidney injury [130].

On the other hand, attempts are continuing to develop approaches for affecting resident progenitor cells, for example, to increase the activity of glomerular parietal cells, which are known to be progenitors of podocytes. Some compounds, such as glycogen synthase kinases 3-α and -β (GSK3s) inhibitor 6-bromoindirubin-3-oxime (BIO) [131], notch signaling inhibitors [132], interferon [133], steroids [134], and some others enhanced the proliferation of parietal cells and mediated their differentiation into podocytes in vitro [135]. Perhaps, compounds exist that would selectively affect STC or other possible pools of progenitor cells.

However, it should be taken into account that excessive activation of kidney progenitor cells could have unwanted side effects on organ function. For instance, the above-mentioned activation of parietal cells is observed in glomerulonephritis and diabetic nephropathy and does not lead to a positive outcome. Excessive proliferation can generate lesions of cells, extracapillary crescentic glomerulonephritis, collapsing glomerulopathy, tip lesions, and ultimately these processes compromise the normal functioning of the glomerulus [136].

5. Summary

Obviously, a kidney has a pronounced regenerative potential, however, its cellular basis is still not fully understood. No doubt that some renal cells are responsible for the regeneration of the kidney, but whether these cells initially have progenitor properties or they obtain a "progenitor phenotype" during dedifferentiation after an injury, still stays the main question. The major stumbling block in resolving the issue is the lack of specific methods for distinguishing between dedifferentiated cells and resident progenitor cells [2]. The complexity of the morphological structure of the kidney and the evidence of the existence of populations of different progenitor cells led to the suggestion that different parts of the kidney may have various progenitor cell pools. Another hypothesis is that diverse cell populations are activated in response to different damaging stimuli [137]. Finally, it is possible that two mechanisms of regeneration may coexist in the kidney, complement and compensate each other [2,92].

Transgenic animals are a powerful tool to solve this problem, as well as new methods, for example, single-cell transcriptomics, which has already been successfully used to study the kidney recovery after injury [43,138]. It is hoped that the application of these approaches will soon lead to the discovery of the true source of regenerative potential in the kidney and allow regenerative medicine to choose targeted methods for renal tissue regeneration after injury.

Acknowledgments: The authors are very thankful to Anastasia V. Balakireva for her valuable help with the illustrations.

Abbreviations

I/R	Ischemia/reperfusion
AKI	Acute kidney injury
STCs	Scattered tubular cells
LRCs	Label-retaining cells

References

1. Little, M.H.; Kairath, P. Does Renal Repair Recapitulate Kidney Development? *J. Am. Soc. Nephrol.* **2017**, *28*, 34–46. [CrossRef] [PubMed]
2. Huling, J.; Yoo, J.J. Comparing adult renal stem cell identification, characterization and applications. *J. Biomed. Sci.* **2017**, *24*, 32. [CrossRef] [PubMed]

3. Eymael, J.; Smeets, B. Origin and fate of the regenerating cells of the kidney. *Eur. J. Pharmacol.* **2016**, *790*, 62–73. [CrossRef] [PubMed]
4. Kramann, R.; Kusaba, T.; Humphreys, B.D. Who regenerates the kidney tubule? *Nephrol. Dial. Transplant.* **2015**, *30*, 903–910. [CrossRef] [PubMed]
5. Bonventre, J. V Dedifferentiation and proliferation of surviving epithelial cells in acute renal failure. *J. Am. Soc. Nephrol.* **2003**, *14* (Suppl. 1), S55–S61. [CrossRef]
6. Ledda-Columbano, G.M.; Columbano, A.; Coni, P.; Curto, M.; Faa, G.; Pani, P. Cell proliferation in rat kidney induced by 1,2-dibromoethane. *Toxicol. Lett.* **1987**, *37*, 85–90. [CrossRef]
7. Iatropoulos, M.J.; Williams, G.M. Proliferation markers. *Exp. Toxicol. Pathol.* **1996**, *48*, 175–181. [CrossRef]
8. Humphreys, B.D.; Czerniak, S.; DiRocco, D.P.; Hasnain, W.; Cheema, R.; Bonventre, J. V Repair of injured proximal tubule does not involve specialized progenitors. *Proc. Natl. Acad. Sci. USA* **2011**, *108*, 9226–9231. [CrossRef]
9. Witzgall, R.; Brown, D.; Schwarz, C.; Bonventre, J.V. Localization of proliferating cell nuclear antigen, vimentin, c-Fos, and clusterin in the postischemic kidney. Evidence for a heterogenous genetic response among nephron segments, and a large pool of mitotically active and dedifferentiated cells. *J. Clin. Invest.* **1994**, *93*, 2175–2188. [CrossRef]
10. Barker, N.; Rookmaaker, M.B.; Kujala, P.; Ng, A.; Leushacke, M.; Snippert, H.; van de Wetering, M.; Tan, S.; Van Es, J.H.; Huch, M.; et al. Lgr5+ve Stem/Progenitor Cells Contribute to Nephron Formation during Kidney Development. *Cell Rep.* **2012**, *2*, 540–552. [CrossRef]
11. Imgrund, M.; Gröne, E.; Gröne, H.J.; Kretzler, M.; Holzman, L.; Schlöndorff, D.; Rothenpieler, U.W. Re-expression of the developmental gene Pax-2 during experimental acute tubular necrosis in mice. *Kidney Int.* **1999**, *56*, 1423–1431.
12. Poché, R.A.; Furuta, Y.; Chaboissier, M.C.; Schedl, A.; Behringer, R.R. Sox9 is expressed in mouse multipotent retinal progenitor cells and functions in Müller Glial cell development. *J. Comp. Neurol.* **2008**, *510*, 237–250. [CrossRef] [PubMed]
13. Maeshima, A.; Yamashita, S.; Nojima, Y. Identification of renal progenitor-like tubular cells that participate in the regeneration processes of the kidney. *J. Am. Soc. Nephrol.* **2003**, *14*, 3138–3146. [CrossRef] [PubMed]
14. Kitamura, S.; Yamasaki, Y.; Kinomura, M.; Sugaya, T.; Sugiyama, H.; Maeshima, Y.; Makino, H. Establishment and characterization of renal progenitor like cells from S3 segment of nephron in rat adult kidney. *FASEB J.* **2005**, *19*, 1789–1797. [CrossRef] [PubMed]
15. Challen, G.A.; Bertoncello, I.; Deane, J.A.; Ricardo, S.D.; Little, M.H. Kidney Side Population Reveals Multilineage Potential and Renal Functional Capacity but also Cellular Heterogeneity. *J. Am. Soc. Nephrol.* **2006**, *17*, 1896–1912. [CrossRef]
16. Smeets, B.; Boor, P.; Dijkman, H.; Sharma, S.V.; Jirak, P.; Mooren, F.; Berger, K.; Bornemann, J.; Gelman, I.H.; Floege, J.; et al. Proximal tubular cells contain a phenotypically distinct, scattered cell population involved in tubular regeneration. *J. Pathol.* **2013**, *229*, 645–659. [CrossRef]
17. Angelotti, M.L.; Ronconi, E.; Ballerini, L.; Peired, A.; Mazzinghi, B.; Sagrinati, C.; Parente, E.; Gacci, M.; Carini, M.; Rotondi, M.; et al. Characterization of renal progenitors committed toward tubular lineage and their regenerative potential in renal tubular injury. *Stem Cells* **2012**, *30*, 1714–1725. [CrossRef]
18. Lindgren, D.; Boström, A.K.; Nilsson, K.; Hansson, J.; Sjölund, J.; Möller, C.; Jirström, K.; Nilsson, E.; Landberg, G.; Axelson, H.; et al. Isolation and characterization of progenitor-like cells from human renal proximal tubules. *Am. J. Pathol.* **2011**, *178*, 828–837. [CrossRef]
19. Berger, K.; Moeller, M.J. Mechanisms of epithelial repair and regeneration after acute kidney injury. *Semin. Nephrol.* **2014**, *34*, 394–403. [CrossRef]
20. Romagnani, P. Family portrait: Renal progenitor of Bowman's capsule and its tubular brothers. *Am. J. Pathol.* **2011**, *178*, 490–493. [CrossRef]
21. Meyer-Schwesinger, C. The Role of Renal Progenitors in Renal Regeneration. *Nephron* **2016**, *132*, 101–109. [CrossRef]
22. Gupta, S.; Rosenberg, M.E. Do stem cells exist in the adult kidney? *Am. J. Nephrol.* **2008**, *28*, 607–613. [CrossRef] [PubMed]
23. McCampbell, K.K.; Wingert, R.A. Renal stem cells: fact or science fiction? *Biochem. J.* **2012**, *444*, 153–168. [CrossRef] [PubMed]
24. Marcheque, J.; Bussolati, B.; Csete, M.; Perin, L. Concise Reviews: Stem Cells and Kidney Regeneration: An Update. *Stem Cells Transl. Med.* **2019**, *8*, 82–92. [CrossRef] [PubMed]

25. Brossa, A.; Papadimitriou, E.; Collino, F.; Incarnato, D.; Oliviero, S.; Camussi, G.; Bussolati, B. Role of CD133 Molecule in Wnt Response and Renal Repair. *Stem Cells Transl. Med.* **2018**, *7*, 283–294. [CrossRef] [PubMed]
26. Maeshima, A.; Sakurai, H.; Nigam, S.K. Adult kidney tubular cell population showing phenotypic plasticity, tubulogenic capacity, and integration capability into developing kidney. *J. Am. Soc. Nephrol.* **2006**, *17*, 188–198. [CrossRef] [PubMed]
27. Kim, K.; Lee, K.M.; Han, D.J.; Yu, E.; Cho, Y.M. Adult stem cell-like tubular cells reside in the corticomedullary junction of the kidney. *Int. J. Clin. Exp. Pathol.* **2008**, *1*, 232–241.
28. Kim, J.; Kim, J.I.; Na, Y.K.; Park, K.M. Intra-renal slow cell-cycle cells contribute to the restoration of kidney tubules injured by ischemia/reperfusion. *Anat. Cell Biol.* **2011**, *44*, 186. [CrossRef]
29. Sallustio, F.; De Benedictis, L.; Castellano, G.; Zaza, G.; Loverre, A.; Costantino, V.; Grandaliano, G.; Schena, F.P. TLR2 plays a role in the activation of human resident renal stem/progenitor cells. *FASEB J.* **2009**, *24*, 514–525. [CrossRef]
30. Grange, C.; Moggio, A.; Tapparo, M.; Porta, S.; Camussi, G.; Bussolati, B. Protective effect and localization by optical imaging of human renal CD133+ progenitor cells in an acute kidney injury model. *Physiol. Rep.* **2014**, *2*, e12009. [CrossRef]
31. Hansson, J.; Hultenby, K.; Cramnert, C.; Pontén, F.; Jansson, H.; Lindgren, D.; Axelson, H.; Johansson, M.E. Evidence for a morphologically distinct and functionally robust cell type in the proximal tubules of human kidney. *Hum. Pathol.* **2014**, *45*, 382–393. [CrossRef]
32. Bussolati, B.; Bruno, S.; Grange, C.; Buttiglieri, S.; Deregibus, M.C.; Cantino, D.; Camussi, G. Isolation of renal progenitor cells from adult human kidney. *Am. J. Pathol.* **2005**, *166*, 545–555. [CrossRef]
33. Gupta, S.; Verfaillie, C.; Chmielewski, D.; Kren, S.; Eidman, K.; Connaire, J.; Heremans, Y.; Lund, T.; Blackstad, M.; Jiang, Y.; et al. Isolation and characterization of kidney-derived stem cells. *J. Am. Soc. Nephrol.* **2006**, *17*, 3028–3040. [CrossRef] [PubMed]
34. Loverre, A.; Capobianco, C.; Ditonno, P.; Battaglia, M.; Grandaliano, G.; Schena, F.P. Increase of proliferating renal progenitor cells in acute tubular necrosis underlying delayed graft function. *Transplantation* **2008**, *85*, 1112–1119. [CrossRef] [PubMed]
35. Kitamura, S.; Sakurai, H.; Makino, H. Single adult kidney stem/progenitor cells reconstitute three-dimensional nephron structures in vitro. *Stem Cells* **2015**, *33*, 774–784. [CrossRef] [PubMed]
36. Hishikawa, K.; Marumo, T.; Miura, S.; Nakanishi, A.; Matsuzaki, Y.; Shibata, K.; Ichiyanagi, T.; Kohike, H.; Komori, T.; Takahashi, I.; et al. Musculin/MyoR is expressed in kidney side population cells and can regulate their function. *J. Cell Biol.* **2005**, *169*, 921–928. [CrossRef]
37. Buzhor, E.; Omer, D.; Harari-Steinberg, O.; Dotan, Z.; Vax, E.; Pri-Chen, S.; Metsuyanim, S.; Pleniceanu, O.; Goldstein, R.S.; Dekel, B. Reactivation of NCAM1 defines a subpopulation of human adult kidney epithelial cells with clonogenic and stem/progenitor properties. *Am. J. Pathol.* **2013**, *183*, 1621–1633. [CrossRef]
38. Langworthy, M.; Zhou, B.; de Caestecker, M.; Moeckel, G.; Baldwin, H. NFATc1 identifies a population of proximal tubule cell progenitors. *J. Am. Soc. Nephrol.* **2009**, *20*, 311–321. [CrossRef]
39. Abedin, M.J.; Imai, N.; Rosenberg, M.E.; Gupta, S. Identification and characterization of Sall1-expressing cells present in the adult mouse kidney. *Nephron. Exp. Nephrol.* **2011**, *119*, e75–e82. [CrossRef]
40. Iwatani, H.; Ito, T.; Imai, E.; Matsuzaki, Y.; Suzuki, A.; Yamato, M.; Okabe, M.; Hori, M. Hematopoietic and nonhematopoietic potentials of Hoechst low /side population cells isolated from adult rat kidney. *Kidney Int.* **2004**, *65*, 1604–1614.
41. Da Sacco, S.; Thornton, M.E.; Petrosyan, A.; Lavarreda-Pearce, M.; Sedrakyan, S.; Grubbs, B.H.; De Filippo, R.E.; Perin, L. Direct Isolation and Characterization of Human Nephron Progenitors. *Stem Cells Transl. Med.* **2017**, *6*, 419–433. [CrossRef]
42. Chang-Panesso, M.; Kadyrov, F.F.; Lalli, M.; Wu, H.; Ikeda, S.; Kefaloyianni, E.; Abdelmageed, M.M.; Herrlich, A.; Kobayashi, A.; Humphreys, B.D. FOXM1 drives proximal tubule proliferation during repair from acute ischemic kidney injury. *J. Clin. Invest.* **2019**, *129*. [CrossRef]
43. Kirita, Y.; Chang-Panesso, M.; Humphreys, B.D. Recent Insights into Kidney Injury and Repair from Transcriptomic Analyses. *Nephron* **2019**. [CrossRef] [PubMed]
44. Ye, Y.; Wang, B.; Jiang, X.; Hu, W.; Feng, J.; Li, H.; Jin, M.; Ying, Y.; Wang, W.; Mao, X.; et al. Proliferative capacity of stem/progenitor-like cells in the kidney may associate with the outcome of patients with acute tubular necrosis. *Hum. Pathol.* **2011**, *42*, 1132–1141. [CrossRef] [PubMed]
45. Wen, D.; Ni, L.; You, L.; Zhang, L.; Gu, Y.; Hao, C.M.; Chen, J. Upregulation of nestin in proximal tubules may participate in cell migration during renal repair. *Am. J. Physiol. Ren. Physiol.* **2012**, *303*. [CrossRef] [PubMed]

46. Lazzeri, E.; Angelotti, M.L.; Peired, A.; Conte, C.; Marschner, J.A.; Maggi, L.; Mazzinghi, B.; Lombardi, D.; Melica, M.E.; Nardi, S.; et al. Endocycle-related tubular cell hypertrophy and progenitor proliferation recover renal function after acute kidney injury. *Nat. Commun.* **2018**, *9*. [CrossRef] [PubMed]
47. Lin, F.; Moran, A.; Igarashi, P. Intrarenal cells, not bone marrow-derived cells, are the major source for regeneration in postischemic kidney. *J. Clin. Invest.* **2005**, *115*, 1756–1764. [CrossRef] [PubMed]
48. Kusaba, T.; Lalli, M.; Kramann, R.; Kobayashi, A.; Humphreys, B.D. Differentiated kidney epithelial cells repair injured proximal tubule. *Proc. Natl. Acad. Sci. USA* **2014**, *111*, 1527–1532. [CrossRef]
49. Villanueva, S.; Céspedes, C.; Vio, C.P. Ischemic acute renal failure induces the expression of a wide range of nephrogenic proteins. *Am. J. Physiol. Regul. Integr. Comp. Physiol.* **2006**, *290*, R861–R870. [CrossRef]
50. Kang, H.M.; Huang, S.; Reidy, K.; Han, S.H.; Chinga, F.; Susztak, K. Sox9-Positive Progenitor Cells Play a Key Role in Renal Tubule Epithelial Regeneration in Mice. *Cell Rep.* **2016**. [CrossRef]
51. Kumar, S.; Liu, J.; Pang, P.; Krautzberger, A.M.; Reginensi, A.; Akiyama, H.; Schedl, A.; Humphreys, B.D.; McMahon, A.P. Sox9 Activation Highlights a Cellular Pathway of Renal Repair in the Acutely Injured Mammalian Kidney. *Cell Rep.* **2015**, *12*, 1325–1338. [CrossRef]
52. Fujigaki, Y.; Goto, T.; Sakakima, M.; Fukasawa, H.; Miyaji, T.; Yamamoto, T.; Hishida, A. Kinetics and characterization of initially regenerating proximal tubules in S3 segment in response to various degrees of acute tubular injury. *Nephrol. Dial. Transplant.* **2006**, *21*, 41–50. [CrossRef]
53. Gröne, H.J.; Weber, K.; Gröne, E.; Helmchen, U.; Osborn, M. Coexpression of keratin and vimentin in damaged and regenerating tubular epithelia of the kidney. *Am. J. Pathol.* **1987**, *129*, 1–8. [PubMed]
54. Humphreys, B.D.; Valerius, M.T.; Kobayashi, A.; Mugford, J.W.; Soeung, S.; Duffield, J.S.; McMahon, A.P.; Bonventre, J.V. Intrinsic Epithelial Cells Repair the Kidney after Injury. *Cell Stem Cell* **2008**, *2*, 284–291. [CrossRef] [PubMed]
55. Oliver, J.A.; Maarouf, O.; Cheema, F.H.; Martens, T.P.; Al-Awqati, Q. The renal papilla is a niche for adult kidney stem cells. *J. Clin. Invest.* **2004**. [CrossRef] [PubMed]
56. Adams, D.C.; Oxburgh, L. The long-term label retaining population of the renal papilla arises through divergent regional growth of the kidney. *Am. J. Physiol. Physiol.* **2009**, *297*, F809–F815. [CrossRef]
57. Liu, X.; Liu, H.; Sun, L.; Chen, Z.; Nie, H.; Sun, A.; Liu, G.; Guan, G. The role of long-term label-retaining cells in the regeneration of adult mouse kidney after ischemia/reperfusion injury. *Stem Cell Res. Ther.* **2016**, *7*. [CrossRef]
58. Oliver, J.A.; Klinakis, A.; Cheema, F.H.; Friedlander, J.; Sampogna, R.V.; Martens, T.P.; Liu, C.; Efstratiadis, A.; Al-Awqati, Q. Proliferation and migration of label-retaining cells of the kidney papilla. *J. Am. Soc. Nephrol.* **2009**, *20*, 2315–2327. [CrossRef]
59. Song, J.; Czerniak, S.; Wang, T.; Ying, W.; Carlone, D.L.; Breault, D.T.; Humphreys, B.D. Characterization and fate of telomerase-expressing epithelia during kidney repair. *J. Am. Soc. Nephrol.* **2011**, *22*, 2256–2265. [CrossRef]
60. Ward, H.H.; Romero, E.; Welford, A.; Pickett, G.; Bacallao, R.; Gattone, V.H.; Ness, S.A.; Wandinger-Ness, A.; Roitbak, T. Adult human CD133/1(+) kidney cells isolated from papilla integrate into developing kidney tubules. *Biochim. Biophys. Acta* **2011**, *1812*, 1344–1357. [CrossRef]
61. Bussolati, B.; Moggio, A.; Collino, F.; Aghemo, G.; D'Armento, G.; Grange, C.; Camussi, G. Hypoxia modulates the undifferentiated phenotype of human renal inner medullary CD133+ progenitors through Oct4/miR-145 balance. *Am. J. Physiol. Renal Physiol.* **2012**, *302*, F116–F128. [CrossRef]
62. Patschan, D.; Michurina, T.; Shi, H.K.; Dolff, S.; Brodsky, S.V.; Vasilieva, T.; Cohen-Gould, L.; Winaver, J.; Chander, P.N.; Enikolopov, G.; et al. Normal distribution and medullary-to-cortical shift of Nestin-expressing cells in acute renal ischemia. *Kidney Int.* **2007**, *71*, 744–754. [CrossRef]
63. Dekel, B.; Zangi, L.; Shezen, E.; Reich-Zeliger, S.; Eventov-Friedman, S.; Katchman, H.; Jacob-Hirsch, J.; Amariglio, N.; Rechavi, G.; Margalit, R.; et al. Isolation and characterization of nontubular Sca-1+Lin-multipotent stem/progenitor cells from adult mouse kidney. *J. Am. Soc. Nephrol.* **2006** *17*, 3300–3314. [CrossRef] [PubMed]
64. Schutgens, F.; Rookmaaker, M.B.; Blokzijl, F.; Van Boxtel, R.; Vries, R.; Cuppen, E.; Verhaar, M.C.; Clevers, H. Troy/TNFRSF19 marks epithelial progenitor cells during mouse kidney development that continue to contribute to turnover in adult kidney. *Proc. Natl. Acad. Sci. USA* **2017**, *114*, E11190–E11198. [CrossRef [PubMed]
65. Oliver, J.A.; Sampogna, R.V.; Jalal, S.; Zhang, Q.-Y.; Dahan, A.; Wang, W.; Shen, T.H.; Al-Awqati, Q. A Subpopulation of Label-Retaining Cells of the Kidney Papilla Regenerates Injured Kidney Medullary Tubules.

Stem Cell Rep. **2016**, *6*, 757–771. [CrossRef] [PubMed]
66. Aggarwal, S.; Moggio, A.; Bussolati, B. Concise Review: Stem/Progenitor Cells for Renal Tissue Repair: Current Knowledge and Perspectives. *Stem Cells Transl. Med.* **2013**, *2*, 1011–1019. [CrossRef] [PubMed]
67. Pleniceanu, O.; Omer, D.; Harari-Steinberg, O.; Dekel, B. Renal lineage cells as a source for renal regeneration. *Pediatr. Res.* **2018**, *83*, 267–274. [CrossRef] [PubMed]
68. Houghton, D.C.; Hartnett, M.; Campbell-Boswell, M.; Porter, G.; Bennett, W. A light and electron microscopic analysis of gentamicin nephrotoxicity in rats. *Am. J. Pathol.* **1976**, *82*, 589.
69. Vogetseder, A.; Karadeniz, A.; Kaissling, B.; Hir, M. Le Tubular cell proliferation in the healthy rat kidney. *Histochem. Cell Biol.* **2005**, *124*, 97–104. [CrossRef]
70. Vogetseder, A.; Palan, T.; Bacic, D.; Kaissling, B.; Le Hir, M. Proximal tubular epithelial cells are generated by division of differentiated cells in the healthy kidney. *Am. J. Physiol. Cell Physiol.* **2007**, *292*, C807–C813. [CrossRef]
71. Molitoris, B.A.; Hoilien, C.A.; Dahl, R.; Ahnen, D.J.; Wilson, P.D.; Kim, J. Characterization of ischemia-induced loss of epithelial polarity. *J. Membr. Biol.* **1988**, *106*, 233–242. [CrossRef]
72. Solez, K.; Morel-Maroger, L.; Sraer, J.D. The morphology of "acute tubular necrosis" in man: analysis of 57 renal biopsies and a comparison with the glycerol model. *Medicine (Baltimore)* **1979**, *58*, 362–376. [CrossRef]
73. Schena, F.P. Role of growth factors in acute renal failure. *Kidney Int. Suppl.* **1998**, *66*, S11-5. [PubMed]
74. El Sabbahy, M.; Vaidya, V.S. Ischemic kidney injury and mechanisms of tissue repair. *Wiley Interdiscip. Rev. Syst. Biol. Med.* **2011**, *3*, 606–618. [CrossRef] [PubMed]
75. Devarajan, P.; Mishra, J.; Supavekin, S.; Patterson, L.T.; Steven Potter, S. Gene expression in early ischemic renal injury: clues towards pathogenesis, biomarker discovery, and novel therapeutics. *Mol. Genet. Metab.* **2003**, *80*, 365–376. [CrossRef] [PubMed]
76. Spiegel, D.M.; Shanley, P.F.; Molitoris, B.A. Mild ischemia predisposes the S3 segment to gentamicin toxicity. *Kidney Int.* **1990**, *38*, 459–464. [CrossRef] [PubMed]
77. Sekine, M.; Monkawa, T.; Morizane, R.; Matsuoka, K.; Taya, C.; Akita, Y.; Joh, K.; Itoh, H.; Hayashi, M.; Kikkawa, Y.; et al. Selective depletion of mouse kidney proximal straight tubule cells causes acute kidney injury. *Transgenic Res.* **2012**, *21*, 51–62. [CrossRef] [PubMed]
78. Vogetseder, A.; Picard, N.; Gaspert, A.; Walch, M.; Kaissling, B.; Le Hir, M. Proliferation capacity of the renal proximal tubule involves the bulk of differentiated epithelial cells. *Am. J. Physiol. Physiol.* **2008**, *294*, C22–C28. [CrossRef]
79. Ichimura, T.; Hung, C.C.; Yang, S.A.; Stevens, J.L.; Bonventre, J.V. Kidney injury molecule-1: a tissue and urinary biomarker for nephrotoxicant-induced renal injury. *Am. J. Physiol. Physiol.* **2004**, *286*, F552–F563. [CrossRef]
80. Ichimura, T.; Bonventre, J.V.; Bailly, V.; Wei, H.; Hession, C.A.; Cate, R.L.; Sanicola, M. Kidney injury molecule-1 (KIM-1), a putative epithelial cell adhesion molecule containing a novel immunoglobulin domain, is up-regulated in renal cells after injury. *J. Biol. Chem.* **1998**, *273*, 4135–4142. [CrossRef]
81. Berger, K.; Bangen, J.-M.; Hammerich, L.; Liedtke, C.; Floege, J.; Smeets, B.; Moeller, M.J. Origin of regenerating tubular cells after acute kidney injury. *Proc. Natl. Acad. Sci. USA* **2014**, *111*, 1533–1538. [CrossRef]
82. Romagnani, P.; Rinkevich, Y.; Dekel, B. The use of lineage tracing to study kidney injury and regeneration. *Nat. Rev. Nephrol.* **2015**, *11*, 420–431. [CrossRef]
83. Chaboissier, M.C.; Kobayashi, A.; Vidal, V.I.P.; Lützkendorf, S.; van de Kant, H.J.G.; Wegner, M.; de Rooij, D.G.; Behringer, R.R.; Schedl, A. Functional analysis os Sox8 and Sox9 during sex determination in the mouse. *Development* **2004**, *131*, 1891–1901. [CrossRef] [PubMed]
84. Cavanagh, B.L.; Walker, T.; Norazit, A.; Meedeniya, A.C.B. Thymidine analogues for tracking DNA synthesis. *Molecules* **2011**, *16*, 7980–7993. [CrossRef] [PubMed]
85. Piepenhagen, P.A.; Peters, L.L.; Lux, S.E.; Nelson, W.J. Differential expression of Na+-K+-ATPase, ankyrin, fodrin, and E- cadherin along the kidney nephron. *Am. J. Physiol. Cell Physiol.* **1995**, *269*, C1417–C1432. [CrossRef] [PubMed]
86. Nowak, J.A.; Polak, L.; Pasolli, H.A.; Fuchs, E. Hair follicle stem cells are specified and function in early skin morphogenesis. *Cell Stem Cell* **2008**, *3*, 33–43. [CrossRef] [PubMed]
87. Cheung, M.; Briscoe, J. Neural crest development is regulated by the transcription factor Sox9. *Development* **2003**, *130*, 5681–5693. [CrossRef] [PubMed]
88. Yamashita, K.; Sato, A.; Asashima, M.; Wang, P.C.; Nishinakamura, R. Mouse homolog of SALL1, a causative gene for Townes-Brocks syndrome, binds to A/T-rich sequences in pericentric heterochromatin via its

C-terminal zinc finger domains. *Genes Cells* **2007**, *12*, 171–182. [CrossRef] [PubMed]
89. Shirasawa, T.; Akashi, T.; Sakamoto, K.; Takahashi, H.; Maruyama, N.; Hirokawa, K. Gene expression of CD24 core peptide molecule in developing brain and developing non-neural tissues. *Dev. Dyn.* **1993**, *198*, 1–13. [CrossRef]
90. Mignone, J.L.; Kukekov, V.; Chiang, A.S.; Steindler, D.; Enikolopov, G. Neural Stem and Progenitor Cells in Nestin-GFP Transgenic Mice. *J. Comp. Neurol.* **2004**, *469*, 311–324. [CrossRef]
91. Rinkevich, Y.; Montoro, D.T.; Contreras-Trujillo, H.; Harari-Steinberg, O.; Newman, A.M.; Tsai, J.M.; Lim, X.; Van-Amerongen, R.; Bowman, A.; Januszyk, M.; et al. In vivo clonal analysis reveals lineage-restricted progenitor characteristics in mammalian kidney development, maintenance, and regeneration. *Cell Rep.* **2014**. [CrossRef]
92. Chang-Panesso, M.; Humphreys, B.D. Cellular plasticity in kidney injury and repair. *Nat. Rev. Nephrol.* **2017**, *13*, 39–46. [CrossRef]
93. Kim, K.; Park, B.-H.; Ihm, H.; Kim, K.M.; Jeong, J.; Chang, J.W.; Cho, Y.M. Expression of stem cell marker CD133 in fetal and adult human kidneys and pauci-immune crescentic glomerulonephritis. *Histol. Histopathol.* **2011**, *26*, 223–232. [PubMed]
94. Lieberthal, W.; Nigam, S.K. Acute renal failure. I. Relative importance of proximal vs. distal tubular injury. *Am. J. Physiol.* **1998**, *275*, F623–F632. [CrossRef] [PubMed]
95. Kemper, K.; Sprick, M.R.; De Bree, M.; Scopelliti, A.; Vermeulen, L.; Hoek, M.; Zeilstra, J.; Pals, S.T.; Mehmet, H.; Stassi, G.; et al. The AC133 epitope, but not the CD133 protein, is lost upon cancer stem cell differentiation. *Cancer Res.* **2010**, *70*, 719–729. [CrossRef] [PubMed]
96. Angelotti, M.L.; Lazzeri, E.; Lasagni, L.; Romagnani, P. Only anti-CD133 antibodies recognizing the CD133/1 or the CD133/2 epitopes can identify human renal progenitors. *Kidney Int.* **2010**, *78*, 620–621. [CrossRef] [PubMed]
97. Corbeil, D.; Röper, K.; Hellwig, A.; Tavian, M.; Miraglia, S.; Watt, S.M.; Simmons, P.J.; Peault, B.; Buck, D.W.; Huttner, W.B. The human AC133 hematopoietic stem cell antigen is also expressed in epithelial cells and targeted to plasma membrane protrusions. *J. Biol. Chem.* **2000**, *275*, 5512–5520. [CrossRef]
98. Mizrak, D.; Brittan, M.; Alison, M.R. CD 133: Molecule of the moment. *J. Pathol.* **2008**, *214*, 3–9. [CrossRef]
99. Romagnani, P.; Remuzzi, G. CD133+ renal stem cells always co-express CD24 in adult human kidney tissue. *Stem Cell Res.* **2014**, *12*, 828–829. [CrossRef]
100. Sagrinati, C.; Netti, G.S.; Mazzinghi, B.; Lazzeri, E.; Liotta, F.; Frosali, F.; Ronconi, E.; Meini, C.; Gacci, M.; Squecco, R.; et al. Isolation and characterization of multipotent progenitor cells from the Bowman's capsule of adult human kidneys. *J. Am. Soc. Nephrol.* **2006**, *17*, 2443–2456. [CrossRef]
101. Chen, H.; Luo, Z.; Dong, L.; Tan, Y.; Yang, J.; Feng, G.; Wu, M.; Li, Z.; Wang, H. CD133/prominin-1-mediated autophagy and glucose uptake beneficial for hepatoma cell survival. *PLoS ONE* **2013**, *8*, e56878. [CrossRef]
102. Rehman, J. Empowering self-renewal and differentiation: The role of mitochondria in stem cells. *J. Mol. Med.* **2010**, *88*, 981–986. [CrossRef]
103. Santeramo, I.; Perez, Z.H.; Illera, A.; Taylor, A.; Kenny, S.; Murray, P.; Wilm, B.; Gretz, N. Human kidney-derived cells ameliorate acute kidney injury without engrafting into renal tissue. *Stem Cells Transl. Med.* **2017**. [CrossRef] [PubMed]
104. Romagnani, P.; Lasagni, L.; Remuzzi, G. Renal progenitors: An evolutionary conserved strategy for kidney regeneration. *Nat. Rev. Nephrol.* **2013**, *9*, 137–146. [CrossRef] [PubMed]
105. Shankland, S.J.; Freedman, B.S.; Pippin, J.W. Can podocytes be regenerated in adults? *Curr. Opin. Nephrol. Hypertens.* **2017**, *26*, 154–164. [CrossRef] [PubMed]
106. Humphreys, B.D. Kidney injury, stem cells and regeneration. *Curr. Opin. Nephrol. Hypertens.* **2014**, *23*, 25–31. [CrossRef]
107. Forbes, M.S.; Thornhill, B.A.; Galarreta, C.I.; Chevalier, R.L. A population of mitochondrion-rich cells in the pars recta of mouse kidney. *Cell Tissue Res.* **2016**, *363*, 791–803. [CrossRef]
108. Bussolati, B.; Camussi, G. Therapeutic use of human renal progenitor cells for kidney regeneration. *Nat. Rev. Nephrol.* **2015**. [CrossRef]
109. Romagnani, P. Of mice and men: The riddle of tubular regeneration. *J. Pathol.* **2013**, *229*, 641–644. [CrossRef]
110. Vanslambrouck, J.; Li, J.; Little, M.H. The renal papilla: An enigma in damage and repair. *J. Am. Soc. Nephrol.* **2011**, *22*, 2145–2147. [CrossRef]
111. Burmeister, D.M.; McIntyre, M.K.; Montgomery, R.K.; Gómez, B.I.; Dubick, M.A. Isolation and Characterization of Multipotent CD24+ Cells From the Renal Papilla of Swine. *Front. Med.* **2018**, *5*.

[CrossRef]
112. Pannabecker, T.L.; Layton, A.T. Targeted delivery of solutes and oxygen in the renal medulla: role of microvessel architecture. *Am. J. Physiol. Renal Physiol.* **2014**, *307*, F649–F655. [CrossRef]
113. Mohyeldin, A.; Garzón-Muvdi, T.; Quiñones-Hinojosa, A. Oxygen in stem cell biology: A critical component of the stem cell niche. *Cell Stem Cell* **2010**, *7*, 150–161. [CrossRef] [PubMed]
114. Humphreys, B.D. Slow-Cycling Cells in Renal Papilla: Stem Cells Awaken? *J. Am. Soc. Nephrol.* **2009**. [CrossRef] [PubMed]
115. Tumbar, T.; Guasch, G.; Greco, V.; Blanpain, C.; Lowry, W.E.; Rendl, M.; Fuchs, E. Defining the epithelial stem cell niche in skin. *Science* **2004**, *303*, 359–363. [CrossRef] [PubMed]
116. Wiese, C.; Rolletschek, A.; Kania, G.; Blyszczuk, P.; Tarasov, K.V.; Tarasova, Y.; Wersto, R.P.; Boheler, K.R.; Wobus, A.M. Nestin expression-A property of multi-lineage progenitor cells? *Cell. Mol. Life Sci.* **2004**. [CrossRef] [PubMed]
117. Chen, J.; Boyle, S.; Zhao, M.; Su, W.; Takahashi, K.; Davis, L.; DeCaestecker, M.; Takahashi, T.; Brever, M.D.; Hao, C.M. Differential expression of the intermediate filament protein nestin during renal development and its localization in adult podocytes. *J. Am. Soc. Nephrol.* **2006**, *17*, 1283–1291. [CrossRef]
118. Kirik, O.V.; Korzhevskii, D.E. Expression of neural stem cell marker nestin in the kidney of rats and humans. *Bull. Exp. Biol. Med.* **2009**, *147*, 539–541. [CrossRef]
119. Zou, J.; Yaoita, E.; Watanabe, Y.; Yoshida, Y.; Nameta, M.; Li, H.; Qu, Z.; Yamamoto, T. Upregulation of nestin, vimentin, and desmin in rat podocytes in response to injury. *Virchows Arch.* **2006**, *448*, 485–492. [CrossRef]
120. Perry, J.; Ho, M.; Viero, S.; Zheng, K.; Jacobs, R.; Thorner, P.S. The intermediate filament nestin is highly expressed in normal human podocytes and podocytes in glomerular disease. *Pediatr. Dev. Pathol.* **2007**, *10*, 369–382. [CrossRef]
121. Westhoff, J.H.; Schildhorn, C.; Jacobi, C.; Hömme, M.; Hartner, A.; Braun, H.; Kryzer, C.; Wang, C.; Von Zglinicki, T.; Kränzlin, B.; et al. Telomere shortening reduces regenerative capacity after acute kidney injury. *J. Am. Soc. Nephrol.* **2010**, *21*, 327–336. [CrossRef]
122. Ridley, A.J.; Schwartz, M.A.; Burridge, K.; Firtel, R.A.; Ginsberg, M.H.; Borisy, G.; Parsons, J.T.; Horwitz, A.R. Cell Migration: Integrating Signals from Front to Back. *Science* **2003**, *302*, 1704–1709. [CrossRef]
123. Solanas, G.; Benitah, S.A. Architecture of the Interfolliculer epidermis. *Nat. Rev. Mol. Cell Biol.* **2013**, *14*, 737–748. [CrossRef] [PubMed]
124. Yousefi, M.; Li, L.; Lengner, C.J. Hierarchy and Plasticity in the Intestinal Stem Cell Compartment. *Trends Cell Biol.* **2017**, *27*, 753–764. [CrossRef] [PubMed]
125. Wang, J.; Lin, G.; Alwaal, A.; Zhang, X.; Wang, G.; Jia, X.; Banie, L.; Villalta, J.; Lin, C.S.; Lue, T.F. Kinetics of Label Retaining Cells in the Developing Rat Kidneys. *PLoS ONE* **2015**. [CrossRef] [PubMed]
126. Gupta, A.K.; Jadhav, S.H.; Tripathy, N.K.; Nityanand, S. Fetal kidney cells can ameliorate ischemic acute renal failure in rats through their anti-inflammatory, anti-apoptotic and anti-oxidative effects. *PLoS ONE* **2015**, *10*. [CrossRef] [PubMed]
127. Gupta, A.K. Fetal kidney stem cells ameliorate cisplatin induced acute renal failure and promote renal angiogenesis. *World J. Stem Cells* **2015**, *7*, 776. [CrossRef] [PubMed]
128. Aggarwal, S.; Grange, C.; Iampietro, C.; Camussi, G.; Bussolati, B. Human CD133 + Renal Progenitor Cells Induce Erythropoietin Production and Limit Fibrosis after Acute Tubular Injury. *Sci. Rep.* **2016**, *6*. [CrossRef]
129. Chen, C.; Chou, K.; Fang, H.; Hsu, C.; Huang, W.; Huang, C.; Huang, C.; Chen, H.; Lee, P. Progenitor-like cells derived from mouse kidney protect against renal fibrosis in a remnant kidney model via decreased endothelial mesenchymal transition. *Stem Cell Res. Ther.* **2015**, *6*. [CrossRef]
130. Lee, P.T.; Lin, H.H.; Jiang, S.T.; Lu, P.J.; Chou, K.J.; Fang, H.C.; Chiou, Y.Y.; Tang, M.J. Mouse kidney progenitor cells accelerate renal regeneration and prolong survival after ischemic injury. *Stem Cells* **2010**, *28*, 573–584. [CrossRef]
131. Lasagni, L.; Angelotti, M.L.; Ronconi, E.; Lombardi, D.; Nardi, S.; Peired, A.; Becherucci, F.; Mazzinghi, B.; Sisti, A.; Romoli, S.; et al. Podocyte Regeneration Driven by Renal Progenitors Determines Glomerular Disease Remission and Can Be Pharmacologically Enhanced. *Stem Cell Rep.* **2015**, *5*, 248–263. [CrossRef]
132. Lasagni, L.; Ballerini, L.; Angelotti, M.L.; Parente, E.; Sagrinati, C.; Mazzinghi, B.; Peired, A.; Ronconi, E.; Becherucci, F.; Bani, D.; et al. Notch activation differentially regulates renal progenitors proliferation and differentiation toward the podocyte lineage in glomerular disorders. *Stem Cells* **2010**, *28*, 1673–1685. [CrossRef]
133. Migliorini, A.; Angelotti, M.L.; Mulay, S.R.; Kulkarni, O.O.; Demleitner, J.; Dietrich, A.; Sagrinati, C.;

Ballerini, L.; Peired, A.; Shankland, S.J.; et al. The antiviral cytokines IFN-α and IFN-β modulate parietal epithelial cells and promote podocyte loss: Implications for IFN toxicity, viral glomerulonephritis, and glomerular regeneration. *Am. J. Pathol.* **2013**, *183*, 431–440. [CrossRef] [PubMed]

134. Zhang, J.; Pippin, J.W.; Krofft, R.D.; Naito, S.; Liu, Z.H.; Shankland, S.J. Podocyte repopulation by renal progenitor cells following glucocorticoids treatment in experimental FSGS. *Am. J. Physiol. Ren. Physiol.* **2013**, *304*, 1375–1389. [CrossRef] [PubMed]
135. Becherucci, F.; Mazzinghi, B.; Allinovi, M.; Angelotti, M.L.; Romagnani, P. Regenerating the kidney using human pluripotent stem cells and renal progenitors. *Expert Opin. Biol. Ther.* **2018**. [CrossRef] [PubMed]
136. Lasagni, L.; Romagnani, P. Glomerular Epithelial Stem Cells: The Good, The Bad, and The Ugly. *J. Am. Soc. Nephrol.* **2010**, *21*, 1612–1619. [CrossRef] [PubMed]
137. Gheisari, Y.; Nassiri, S.M.; Arefian, E.; Ahmadbeigi, N.; Azadmanesh, K.; Jamali, M.; Jahanzad, I.; Zeinali, S.; Vasei, M.; Soleimani, M. Severely damaged kidneys possess multipotent renoprotective stem cells. *Cytotherapy* **2010**, *12*. [CrossRef]
138. Wilson, P.C.; Humphreys, B.D. Kidney and organoid single-cell transcriptomics: the end of the beginning. *Pediatr. Nephrol.* **2019**. [CrossRef]

14

Contribution of Inflammatory Cytokine Interleukin-18 Genotypes to Renal Cell Carcinoma

Wen-Shin Chang [1,†], Te-Chun Shen [1,†], Wei-Lan Yeh [2,†], Chien-Chih Yu [3], Hui-Yi Lin [3], Hsi-Chin Wu [1,4], Chia-Wen Tsai [1,*] and Da-Tian Bau [1,5,6,*]

1. Terry Fox Cancer Research Laboratory, Translational Medicine Research Center, China Medical University Hospital, Taichung 40447, Taiwan; halittlemelon@hotmail.com (W.-S.C.); chestshen@gmail.com (T.-C.S.); wuhc@mail.cmuh.org.tw (H.-C.W.)
2. Institute of New Drug Development, China Medical University, Taichung 40402, Taiwan; wlyeh@mail.cmu.edu.tw
3. School of Pharmacy, China Medical University, Taichung 40402, Taiwan; ccyu@mail.cmu.edu.tw (C.-C.Y.); hylin@mail.cmu.edu.tw (H.-Y.L.)
4. School of Medicine, China Medical University, Taichung 40402, Taiwan
5. Graduate Institute of Biomedical Sciences, China Medical University, Taichung 40402, Taiwan
6. Department of Bioinformatics and Medical Engineering, Asia University, Taichung 41354, Taiwan

* Correspondence: wenwen816@gmail.com (C.-W.T.); artbau2@gmail.com (D.-T.B.)

† These authors contributed equally to this work.

Abstract: Interleukin-18 (*IL-18*) is a multi-functional immuno-mediator in the development and progression of many types of infectious and inflammatory diseases. In this study, we evaluated the contribution of *IL-18* genotypes to renal cell carcinoma (RCC) in Taiwan via the genotyping of *IL-18* -656 (A/C), -607 (A/C), and -137 (G/C). Moreover, we analyzed their interactions with smoking, alcohol drinking, hypertension, and diabetes status. The results showed an association of the AC and CC genotypes of *IL-18* −607 with a significant decrease in the risk of RCC compared with the AA genotype (odds ratio (OR) = 0.44 and 0.35, 95% confidence interval (CI) = 0.27–0.72 and 0.18–0.66, $p = 0.0008$ and 0.0010, respectively). Furthermore, a significantly lower frequency of the C allele at -607 was observed in the RCC group (35.3% vs. 49.8%; OR = 0.53; 95% CI = 0.35–0.71, $p = 0.0003$). However, *IL-18* -656 and -137 did not exhibit a likewise differential distribution of these genotypes between the control and case groups. Stratifying the population according to smoking, alcohol drinking, hypertension, and diabetes status revealed a different distribution of *IL-18* -607 genotypes among non-smokers, non-drinkers, and patients without diabetes, but not among smokers, drinkers, or patients with diabetes. These findings suggest that *IL-18* -607 genotypes may play a role in the etiology and progression of RCC in Taiwan and may serve as a useful biomarker for early detection.

Keywords: genotype; *IL-18*; polymorphism; renal cell carcinoma; Taiwan

---

1. Introduction

Renal cell carcinoma (RCC) is the sixth most frequently diagnosed cancer in men (5%) and the tenth in women (3%) worldwide, thus posing a serious disease burden [1]. From an epidemiological viewpoint, RCC is the most common renal cancer and includes several subtypes that may be distinguished from each other by their histology, genetic background, clinical course, and response to treatment [2,3]. Moreover, there are several potential risk factors for RCC, including physical activity level, obesity, fruit and vegetable intake, cigarette smoking, and alcohol consumption. In addition, there are some common medical comorbidities for RCC, such as hypertension, diabetes, urinary stones, and other forms of chronic kidney diseases [3]. However, to date, no clinically practical genomic biomarker is available for RCC risk prediction. Unfortunately, many RCC patients, even those with advanced-stage tumors, remain asymptomatic [2,4], and the disease proceeds undetected. To make matters worse, up to 30% of RCC patients treated by radical nephrectomy suffer from many adverse effects and will relapse soon after their surgery [5]. Current personal prognostication of RCC is mainly based on histological validation, which may be labor intensive and time consuming, but frequently not useful for establishing a suitable course of treatment. Therefore, genomic molecular markers for early detection of RCC are urgently needed.

Interleukin-18 (IL-18), initially named IFN-γ inducing factor, is a proinflammatory cytokine encoded by the human *IL-18* gene and produced by activated macrophages, epithelial cells, osteoblasts, keratinocytes, and most importantly, cancer cells [6,7]. In syngeneic mice models, supplementary IL-18 administration suppressed the growth of Meth A sarcoma and mouse glioma cells [7–9], suggesting that IL-18 plays an essential role in host mechanisms of defense against tumors. On a molecular level, IL-18 homeostasis is under the control of highly complex machinery involved in chronic inflammation and carcinogenesis, which is of great interest to both immunologists and oncologists. However, the promotive or suppressive effects of IL-18 on carcinogenesis are not yet fully understood. First, IL-18 may exert its tumor-suppressive influences by stimulating IFN-γ production, promoting Th1 differentiation, enhancing the cytotoxic capacities of CD8+ lymphocytes and natural killer cells [7], inducing cancer cells to undergo programmed cell death [10], and suppressing the angiogenesis [7,11]. Second, IL-18 can inhibit the recognition of cancer cells by immune cells, enhancing cancer cell adherence to the vascular wall, increasing the production of angiogenic and growth factors, and providing a pro-metastatic microenvironment [12,13]. Third, the serum levels of IL-18 were found to be higher in cancer patients than in healthy subjects, including bladder cancer [14], ovarian cancer [15], gastrointestinal cancer [16], and non-small cell lung cancer [17]. Fourth, the serum levels of IL-18 were much higher in those from breast cancer patients with metastasis than in those from patients without metastasis and non-cancer healthy subjects, supporting the hypothesis that elevated serum IL-18 levels can be used as non-invasive markers for suspected metastatic potential [18]. All the above findings support the hypothesis that the pleiotropic cytokine IL-18 can biphasically exert both anti-cancerous and pro-cancerous activities [13]. To summarize, the molecular interactions of IL-18 and other molecules are very complex and deeply involved in tumorigenesis.

From a genomic perspective, the expression level of IL-18 appears to be determined by at least two single nucleotide polymorphisms (SNPs) in the promoter at positions -607 (A/C) and -137 (G/C) of the human *IL-18* gene. The former involves an A to C shift that disrupts a potential binding site for the cAMP responsive element binding protein, and the latter involves a G to C shift that abolishes the human histone H4 gene-specific transcription factor-1 (H4TF-1) nuclear factor binding site [19]. The alterations in transcription factor binding capacities determined by these two promoter polymorphisms may affect the overall activity of *IL-18*. Another SNP located in the *IL-18* promoter is -656 (A/C); however, the effects of different genotypes at *IL-18* -656 on cancer risk have not yet been well elucidated. That is to say, the contribution of -656 genotypes in human *IL-18* to autoimmune diseases has started to be examined [15], but their involvement in any type of cancer has not.

As mentioned above, most of the previous genomic studies on human *IL-18* were devoted to examining the association of *IL-18* -607 and -137 polymorphisms with various types of cancer. Some of them revealed positive associations with cancer risk [20–24], while others identified negative ones [25,26]. However, only one such study investigated the association of the -137 and -607 genotypes of *IL-18* with RCC [27]. In that paper, although the authors reported a negative association, they found that the -137 and -607 genotypes of *IL-18* were correlated with more advanced stages of RCC, and the genotype related to a higher production of IL-18 was associated with a larger size and T stage of the tumor [27]. In the present study, the promoter SNPs at positions -656 (A/C, rs1946519), -607 (A/C, rs1946518), and -137 (G/C, rs187238) of the *IL-18* gene were first examined and their genotype distributions analyzed in patients with RCC in Taiwan. In addition, we investigated the interaction of these *IL-18* promoter genotypes with personal behavioral and clinical factors that contribute to RCC susceptibility.

2. Results

2.1. *Comparison of Characteristics Among Patients with Renal Cell Carcinoma (RCC) and Controls*

The frequency distributions in terms of age, gender, and personal behavioral habits for the 92 patients with RCC and the 580 cancer-free controls are summarized and compared in Table 1. Because the control subjects were already matched with patients with RCC for these factors, no difference was observed in terms of age and gender between these groups ($p > 0.05$). Moreover, there was no significant difference between the two groups in the frequency distributions in terms of personal behavioral habits, smoking, alcohol consumption, diabetes status, and family history ($p > 0.05$) (Table 1). An interesting finding was that there was a higher proportion of subjects with hypertension in the RCC group (66.3%) than in the cancer-free group (52.1%) ($p = 0.0130$). The percentage histologically identified as clear cell RCC patients is 77.2%. The percentages of "low" grade and "middle and high grade" are 52.2 and 47.8%, respectively (Table 1).

Table 1. Distributions of the frequencies of selected characteristics among the renal cell carcinoma (RCC) cases and healthy controls.

Characteristics	Cases ($n = 92$)		Controls ($n = 580$)		*p*-Value
	N	%	N	%	
Age (year) (mean ± SD)	58.8 ± 11.7		58.3 ± 11.5		0.8971
≤60	47	51.1%	307	52.9%	0.8223
>60	45	48.9%	273	47.1%	
Gender					
Male	59	64.1%	371	64.0%	1.0000
Female	33	35.9%	209	36.0%	
Smoking status					
Smokers	41	44.6%	220	37.9%	0.2499
Non-smokers	51	55.4%	360	62.1%	
Alcohol drinking status					
Drinkers	37	40.2%	209	36.0%	0.4848
Non-drinkers	55	59.8%	371	64.0%	
Hypertension					
Yes	61	66.3%	302	52.1%	0.0130 *
No	31	33.7%	278	47.9%	
Diabetes					
Yes	21	22.8%	104	17.9%	0.2523
No	71	77.2%	476	82.1%	
Family cancer history					
Yes	6	6.5%	17	2.9%	0.1125
No	86	93.5%	563	97.1%	
Histological types					
Clear cell	71	77.2%			
Non-clear cell	21	22.8%			
Histological grades					
Low	48	52.2%			
Middle and high	44	47.8%			

* Statistically identified as significant based on Chi-square test without Yates' correction.

2.2. *Analysis of the Association of IL-18 Promoter Genotypes and RCC Risk in Taiwan*

The genotype frequencies of *IL-18* -656 (A/C, rs1946519), -607 (A/C, rs1946518), and -137 (G/C, rs187238) for the 92 patients with RCC and the 580 age- and gender-matched healthy control subjects were determined, and the comparative results of codominant, dominant, and recessive models are presented in Table 2. The frequencies of *IL-18* -656 and -137 genotypes in the control group, but not those of *IL-18* -656 ($p = 0.0206$), were in agreement with the Hardy–Weinberg equilibrium.

Table 2. Distribution of *interleukin-18 (IL-18)* genotypes among the renal cell carcinoma patients and non-cancer healthy control subjects.

Genotypes	Controls		Patients		OR (95% CI) [a]	aOR (95% CI) [a]	*p*-Value
	n	%	*n*	%			
***IL-18* -656**							
AA	221	38.1%	32	34.8%	1.00 (Reference)	1.00 (Reference)	
AC	252	43.5%	44	47.8%	1.21 (0.74–1.97)	1.20 (0.69–1.84)	0.4535
CC	107	18.4%	16	17.4%	1.03 (0.54–1.96)	1.04 (0.52–1.93)	0.9218
P_{trend}							0.7311
Carrier comparison							
AA + AC	473	81.6%	76	82.6%	1.00 (Reference)	1.00 (Reference)	
CC	107	18.4%	16	17.4%	0.93 (0.52–1.66)	0.96 (0.56–1.46)	0.8076
AA	221	38.1%	32	34.8%	1.00 (Reference)	1.00 (Reference)	
AC + CC	359	61.9%	60	65.2%	1.15 (0.73–1.83)	1.12 (0.70–1.79)	0.5414
***IL-18* -607**							
AA	144	24.8%	41	44.6%	1.00 (Reference)	1.00 (Reference)	
AC	294	50.7%	37	40.2%	0.44 (0.27–0.72)	0.41 (0.22–0.64)	0.0008 *
CC	142	24.5%	14	15.2%	0.35 (0.18–0.66)	0.33 (0.15–0.58)	0.0010 *
P_{trend}							0.0004 *
Carrier comparison							
AA + AC	438	75.5%	78	84.8%	1.00 (Reference)	1.00 (Reference)	
CC	142	24.5%	14	15.2%	0.55 (0.30-1.00)	0.51 (0.32–0.96)	0.0505
AA	144	24.8%	41	44.6%	1.00 (Reference)	1.00 (Reference)	
AC + CC	436	75.2%	51	55.4%	0.41 (0.26–0.65)	0.39 (0.25–0.66)	0.0001 *
***IL-18* -137**							
GG	463	79.8%	72	78.3%	1.00 (Reference)	1.00 (Reference)	
GC	108	18.6%	18	19.5%	1.07 (0.61-1.87)	1.06 (0.60-1.66)	0.8074
CC	9	1.6%	2	2.2%	1.42 (0.30-6.75)	1.37 (0.35-6.23)	0.6505
P_{trend}							0.8825
Carrier comparison							
GG + GC	571	98.4%	90	97.8%	1.00 (Reference)	1.00 (Reference)	
CC	9	1.6%	2	2.2%	1.41 (0.30-6.63)	1.38 (0.32-5.98)	0.6622
GG	463	79.8%	72	78.3%	1.00 (Reference)	1.00 (Reference)	
GC + CC	117	20.2%	20	21.7%	1.10 (0.64-1.88)	1.10 (0.65-1.85)	0.7289

OR: odds ratio; [a] The ORs were estimated with multivariate logistic regression analysis after being adjusted with age, gender, smoking, alcohol drinking, hypertension, diabetes, and family history status; * Statistically identified as significant based on Chi-square test without Yates' correction.

For the first time, the genotypes at the *IL-18* promoter -607 (A/C) polymorphic site were found to be differentially distributed between RCC cases and control groups (p for trend = 0.0004) (Table 2, middle panel). To explain in detail, the *IL-18* -607 heterozygous AC and homozygous CC genotypes were associated with decreased risks for RCC (OR = 0.44 and 0.35, 95% CI = 0.27–0.72 and 0.18–0.66, p = 0.0008 and 0.0010, respectively) (Table 2, middle panel). After adjusting for the potential confounders, including age, gender, smoking, alcohol consumption, hypertension, diabetes status, and family history status, the significances still existed (Table 2, middle panel). In the dominant and recessive analyzing models, a significant association with the risk for RCC still persisted, as observed for the homozygous CC genotype (Table 2, middle panel). In contrast, none of the genotypes or alleles for *IL-18*, -656, and -137 demonstrated any correlation with RCC risk in any of the subgroups (Table 2).

We further performed allelic frequency analysis for these three *IL-18* genotypes; the results are shown in Table 3. These results demonstrated that the variant allele C comprised only 35.3% in the RCC group, which was significantly less than that (49.8%) in the control group (adjusted OR = 0.53, 95% CI = 0.35–0.71, p = 0.0003), and these results fully confirmed the conclusion derived in Table 2. Consistently, the other two genotypes, *IL-18* -656 and -137, showed no significant association with the risk for RCC (Table 3).

Table 3. Allelic frequency analysis for *interleukin-18 (IL-18)* polymorphisms and renal cell carcinoma.

Allele	Controls *n* (%)	Patients *n* (%)	aOR (95% CI) [a]	*p*-Value
***IL-18* -656**				
G	694 (59.8%)	108 (58.7%)	1.00 (Reference)	
T	466 (40.2%)	76 (41.3%)	1.06 (0.73-1.31)	0.7712
***IL-18* -607**				
A	582 (50.2%)	119 (64.7%)	1.00 (Reference)	
C	578 (49.8%)	65 (35.3%)	0.53 (0.35-0.71)	0.0003 *
***IL-18* -137**				
G	1034 (89.1%)	162 (88.0%)	1.00 (Reference)	
C	126 (10.9%)	22 (12.0%)	1.11 (0.69-1.83)	0.6595

[a] The ORs were estimated with multivariate logistic regression analysis after being adjusted with age, gender, smoking, alcohol drinking, hypertension, diabetes, and family history status. * Statistically identified as significant based on chi-square test without Yates' correction.

2.3. Stratified Analysis of IL-18 Genotypes According to Personal Behavioral and Clinical Factors

We further conducted stratification analysis of the association between *IL-18* -607 genotypes and the risk for RCC based on potential personal behavioral and clinical risk factors among Taiwanese people, including cigarette smoking, alcohol consumption, hypertension, and diabetes status. First, the distributions of the genotype frequencies between the case and control groups among nonsmokers were significantly different, but showed similar proportions for cases and controls among smokers (Figure 1). The adjusted ORs for carriers with genotypes AC and CC at *IL-18* -607 were 0.36 and 0.22 for nonsmokers (95% CI = 0.21–0.63 and 0.11–0.56, respectively) and 0.61 and 0.58 for smokers (95% CI = 0.33–1.31 and 0.24–1.35, respectively), respectively (Figure 1). It appeared that the protective effects of *IL-18* -607 genotypes on the risk for RCC were obvious among nonsmokers, but not among smokers (Figure 1). Second, the distributions of the genotype frequencies between the case and control groups among nondrinkers were significantly different, but showed similar proportions for cases and controls among alcohol drinkers (Figure 2). The adjusted ORs for carriers with genotypes AC and CC at *IL-18* -607 were 0.38 and 0.21 among nondrinkers (95% CI = 0.22–0.70 and 0.09–0.51, respectively) and 0.56 and 0.62 among alcohol drinkers (95% CI = 0.31–1.23 and 0.28–1.41, respectively), respectively (Figure 2). The protective effects of *IL-18* -607 genotypes on the risk for RCC appeared to be obvious among nondrinkers, but not among alcohol drinkers (Figure 2). Third, the distributions of the genotype frequencies between case and control groups among non-hypertensive and hypertensive subjects were both significantly different (Figure 3). The adjusted ORs for carriers with genotypes AC and CC at *IL-18* -607 were 0.39 and 0.24 among subjects without hypertension (95% CI = 0.18–0.81 and 0.11–0.69, respectively) and 0.41 and 0.39 among those with hypertension (95% CI = 0.26–0.84 and 0.18–0.94, respectively), respectively (Figure 3). The protective effects of *IL-18* -607 genotypes on the risk for RCC appeared to be obvious among people with or without hypertension (Figure 3). Finally, the distributions of the genotype frequencies between the case and control groups among subjects without diabetes were significantly different, but presented similar proportions for cases and controls among subjects with diabetes (Figure 4). The adjusted ORs for carriers with genotypes AC and CC at *IL-18* -607 were 0.44 and 0.35 among subjects without diabetes (95% CI = 0.28–0.81 and 0.21–0.68, respectively) and 0.38 and 0.36 among those with diabetes (95% CI = 0.18–1.02 and 0.13–1.58, respectively), respectively (Figure 4). The effects of *IL-18* -607 genotypes on the risk for RCC appeared to be protective among subjects without diabetes, but not among those with diabetes (Figure 4). The sample size of those with a family history of cancer was too small for stratification analysis.

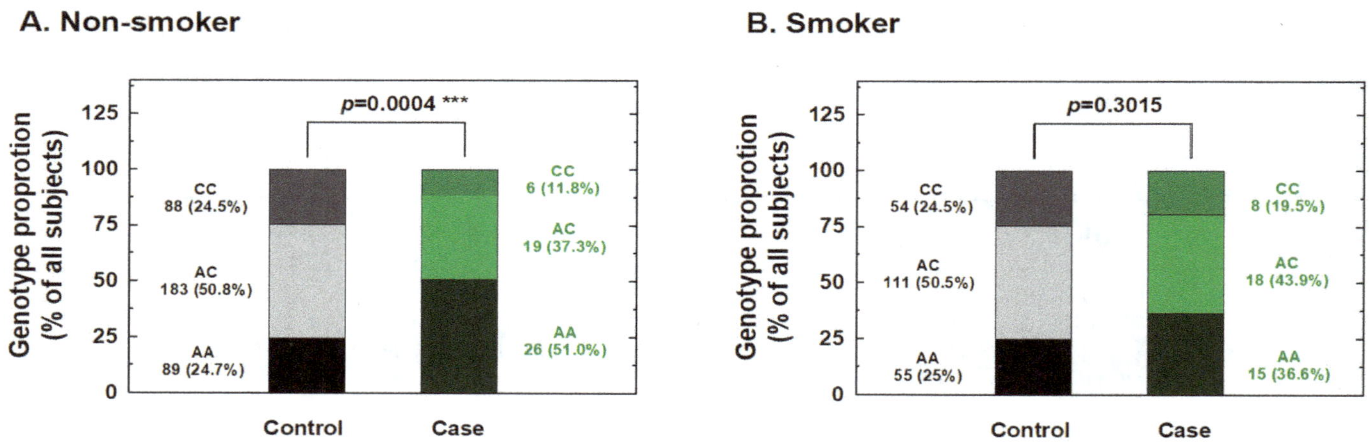

Figure 1. Contribution of *interleukin-18 (IL-18)* promoter -607 genotype to the risk of renal cell carcinoma after stratification by smoking status. The distributions of AA, AC, and CC genotypes at *IL-18* promoter -607 among nonsmokers (**A**) and smokers (**B**). *** Statistically significant between case and control groups.

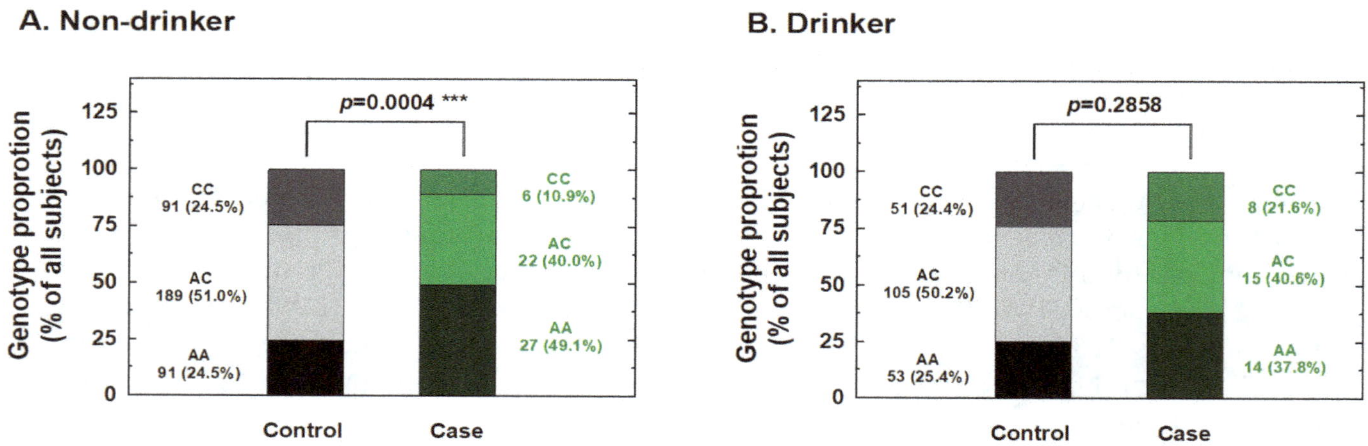

Figure 2. Contribution of *interleukin-18 (IL-18)* promoter -607 genotype to the risk of renal cell carcinoma after stratification by alcohol consumption status. The distributions of AA, AC, and CC genotypes at *IL-18* promoter -607 among nondrinkers (**A**) and drinkers (**B**). *** Statistically significant between case and control groups.

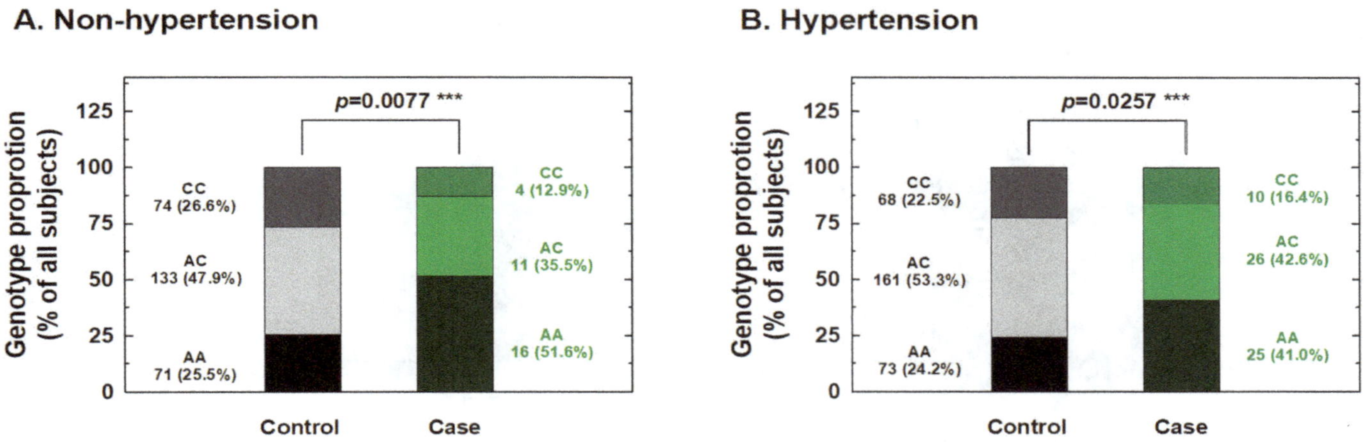

Figure 3. Contribution of *interleukin-18 (IL-18)* promoter -607 genotype to the risk of renal cell carcinoma after stratification by hypertension status. The distributions of AA, AC, and CC genotypes at *IL-18* promoter -607 among non-hypertensive (**A**) and hypertensive subjects (**B**). *** Statistically significant between case and control groups.

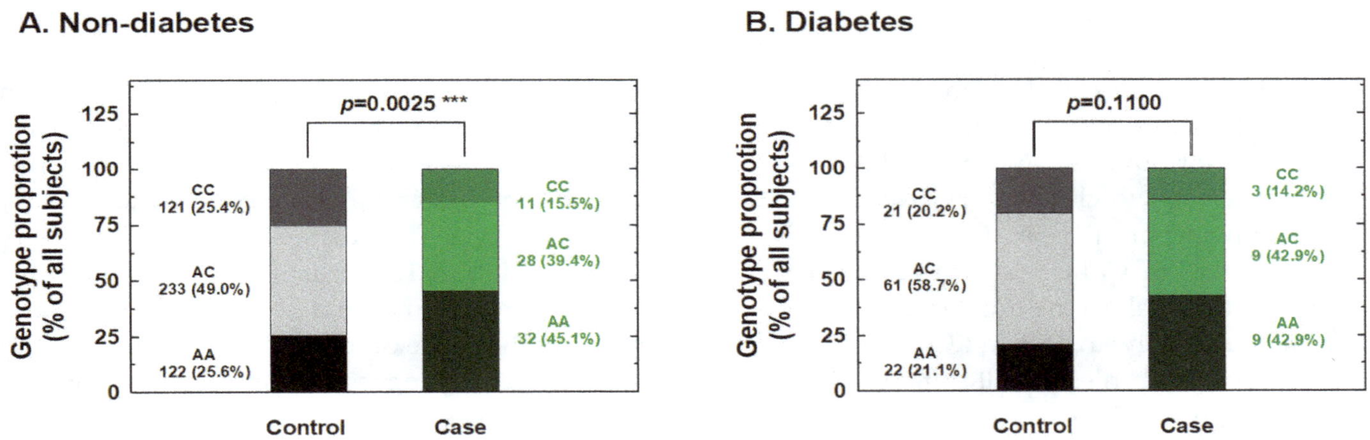

Figure 4. Contribution of *interleukin-18 (IL-18)* promoter -607 genotype to the risk of renal cell carcinoma after stratification by diabetes status. The distributions of AA, AC, and CC genotypes at *IL-18* promoter -607 among subjects without (**A**) and with (**B**) diabetes. *** Statistically significant between case and control groups.

The levels of IL-18 in the serum of 10 RCC patients and 10 healthy controls were determined using ELISA. The results demonstrated that the basal IL-18 levels were significantly higher in RCC patients (212.80 $\pm$ 21.39 pg/mL) than those of control subjects (113.70 $\pm$ 9.94 pg/mL) (p = 0.0001) (Figure 5). According to their *IL-18* -607 genotype distribution, the 10 RCC patients were divided into three subgroups: four patients with the AA genotype (216.25 $\pm$ 12.79 pg/mL), four with AC (206.25 $\pm$ 31.31 pg/mL), and two with CC (219.00 $\pm$ 19.80 pg/mL). There were no significant differences in serum IL-18 levels between different *IL-18* -607 genotypes (AC versus AA: p = 0.5759; CC versus AA: p = 0.8412; and CC versus AC: p = 0.6369).

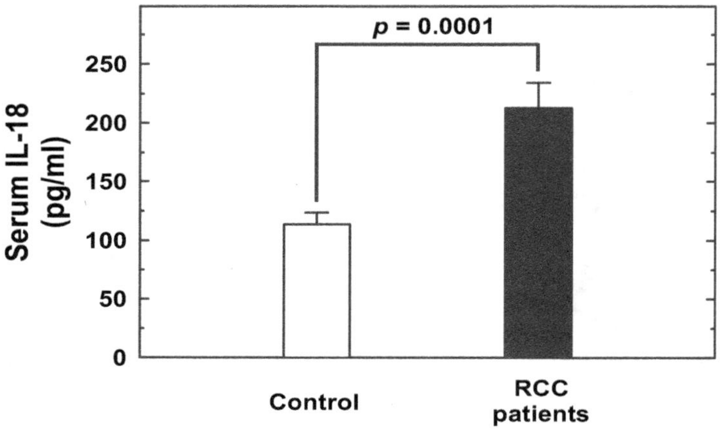

Figure 5. Serum IL-18 levels in 10 RCC patients and 10 healthy control subjects. The serum IL-18 levels were measured by ELISA methodology. The basal levels of serum IL-18 were higher in RCC patients (212.80 ± 21.39 pg/mL) than those of control subjects (113.70 ± 9.94 pg/mL) ($p = 0.0001$). However, no association was found between serum IL-18 levels and specific genotypes. The values are shown as mean ± standard deviation. IL-18, interleukin-18; RCC, renal cell carcinoma; ELISA, enzyme-linked immunosorbent assay.

3. Discussion

The prevalence and death rates of RCC are not ranked as high as those of other cancers in Taiwan. Clinically, surgery is the major course of RCC treatment. However, the symptoms of early-stage RCC are not obvious, and early detection of RCC is not available. Thus, the findings of genomic biomarker(s), which are very useful in rapid and convenient screening, may contribute to early detection and prediction of RCC susceptibility and outcome. For many years, members of the Terry Fox Cancer Fox Cancer Research foundation, including translational scientists and surgeons, have devoted themselves to elucidating specific and practical genomic biomarkers for early detection and prediction in Taiwan, where RCC is a prevalent condition and the cause of many cancer deaths [28–32]. Cytokines play an essential but complex role in the initiation and progression of inflammation and tumorigenesis [33], which is currently still under investigation. The proinflammatory cytokine IL-18 confers protective effects against cancer proliferation, such as that of lung cancer, in several murine models [13,34], and the benefits of recombinant human IL-18 have been shown in preclinical trials for cancer treatment [35]. However, despite the conventional view of IL-18 as an anticancer agent, some studies have also proposed a procancerous behavior for IL-18 under specific conditions [13]. Recently, mounting studies have reported that various cytokine genotypes may influence the serum levels of their counterpart cytokines, which may be closely associated with susceptibility to certain human diseases [19–23,25,26]. Among the numerous SNPs in *IL-18*, three polymorphisms are present in the promoter region of this gene: -656 (G/T), -607 (C/A), and -137 (G/C), and they were reported to cause differences in the transcription factor binding capacity and expression level of IL-18 in serum [19]. The polymorphic genotypes of *IL-18* promoter -607 and -137 were previously found to be associated with the risk of esophageal squamous cell carcinoma [20] and prostate cancer [21] in China, colorectal cancer in Greece [22], ovarian cancer in the USA (Hawaii) [23], and breast cancer in Iran [24]. On the contrary, there were also some negative associations reported between *IL-18* polymorphisms and the risk of head and neck cancers in Iran [26], as well as oral cancer in Greece [25]. Reasonable explanations for these discrepant and diverse findings may involve three possibilities: the dual impact of IL-18 on tumor-immune responses [13], the different types of cancer investigated, and variation among the populations under study [26].

In the current study, the genotypes at polymorphic locations -656 (G/T), -607 (C/A), and -137 (G/C) of the *IL-18* promoter region among RCC patients and healthy individuals in a Taiwan population were first determined and evaluated for their contribution to RCC risk. The results indicated a significantly lower risk for the heterozygous AC and homozygous CC variant genotypes and for the C allele at position -607 of the *IL-18* gene than their counterparts about RCC susceptibility (Tables 2 and 3), even after statistical adjustment for personal behavioral and clinical risk factors. In contrast, no significant association between any genotype or allelic type with RCC risk was found for -656 or -137 of *IL-18* (Tables 2 and 3). The positive findings indicating that genotypes of *IL-18* -607 may be determinants for personal RCC susceptibility were inconsistent with previous findings from the only paper investigating the contribution of *IL-18* genotypes to RCC [27], which returned negative findings. Once again, the inconsistency may be due to the location of Taiwan located in East Asia and the fact that it is an island with a conserved genetic, cultural, and environmental background, much different from the investigated Spanish population [27]. Although the sample size of the current study was similar to theirs (case:control = 92:580 vs. 158:506), we brought forward two novel findings: *IL-18* -607 was a determinant of RCC susceptibility (Tables 2 and 3), and there were positive interactions of this polymorphic site with personal behavioral and clinical factors (Figures 1–4). In the near future, the significant contribution of *IL-18* genotypes to RCC risk evaluation, especially those at *IL-18* -607, should be validated in larger samples and other populations worldwide.

In detail, the stratification of RCC patients and non-cancer subjects according to personal behavior revealed that *IL-18* -607 genotypes may play a significant role in the determination of susceptibility to RCC in non-smokers (Figure 1), non-alcohol drinkers (Figure 2), those with and without hypertension (Figure 3), and those without diabetes (Figure 4), but not in smokers, alcohol drinkers, or those with diabetes (Figures 1, 3 and 4). However, the undermined subtle mechanisms and signaling networks that are responsible for the interaction of IL-18 and other molecules related to the etiology of RCC require further investigation.

The genotype-phenotype association was performed after the measurement of serum levels of IL-18 in 10 RCC patients and 10 healthy controls. The results showed that: (a) the AA genotype at *IL-18* -607 was higher in the RCC patients than the healthy controls (Table 2); (b) the IL-18 levels were higher in the RCC patients than the healthy controls (Figure 5), which is consistent with the previous findings [36]; and (c) there was no difference in the IL-18 levels among RC patients of different *IL-18* -607 genotypes. This finding is consistent with the previous finding in lung cancer [37], but inconsistent with another [38]. The difference and similarity may due to the fact that different populations were investigated. Ours and the former were investigating Taiwanese and Chinese people, respectively, while the latter one was investigating people from Iran.

As for the perspective molecular mechanism, there is literature mentioning that the A to C shift at IL-18 -607 may disrupt the potential binding site for the cAMP responsive element binding protein, thus lowering the expression level of IL-18 [19]. That is to say, the differential genotype at *IL-18* -607 may associate with elevated expression levels of IL-18, as the early detector for RCC, like we showed in Figure 5. The current study does not provide supporting evidence for the hypothesis that any genotype at *IL-18* -607 may associate with elevated expression levels of IL-18, due to the limited samples examined, and confirmation in larger samples is an urgent need. We also have to notice that the alteration of IL-18 may not be the only indicator during RCC carcinogenesis. In 2015, Xu et al. reported that elevated IL-18 together with IL-1b were significantly associated with advanced RCC stages, an elevated recurrence rate, and a shortened survival period among patients with localized RCC [35].

To summarize, this pilot study indicated a significant association between the *IL-18* -607 polymorphism and RCC in Taiwan. Furthermore, to the best of our knowledge, it is also the first to investigate the interaction of *IL-18* genotypes and behavioral and clinical factors in RCC risk. Our results showed a significant association between the *IL-18* -607 polymorphism and RCC, particularly in people without smoking or alcohol drinking behavior, and those without diabetes. However, it should be pointed out that the samples sizes of affected subjects (i.e., smokers, drinkers, and particularly patients with diabetes) were much smaller than those of un-affected subjects, which might be the main reason for the lack of statistically significant associations in the affected subjects. Future larger studies in various populations are needed to validate *IL-18* genotypes as early detective and predictive determinants of RCC.

4. Materials and Methods

4.1. Selected Subjects

This case-control study was performed in the China Medical University Hospital and involved the collection of data from 92 patients with RCC and 580 cancer-free controls matched by age and gender; none of the participants were related to each other by any biological relationship. The diagnosis of RCC, and the grades and types of each patient were histopathologically confirmed by the surgeons and pathologists led by Hsi-Chin Wu. In addition, the age- and gender-matched cancer-free controls were genetically unrelated to any of the recruited participants and had no prior history of any cancer. Originally, we frequency matched seven controls, which were collected in the Health Examination Center of the China Medical University Hospital, for each RCC patient with the same gender and age at ±2 years. After the first-term matching, those with incomplete demographic data about smoking, alcohol drinking status, hypertension, diabetes, or family cancer history, were excluded. A further exclusion criterion for the control subjects was any symptom suggestive of RCC, such as hematuria. Finally, only 580 controls were collected in the study. After obtaining written informed consent, 3–5 mL of venous blood was collected from each participant for genotyping. The study was approved by the Institutional Review Board of China Medical University, and expert members of the Tissue Bank of China Medical University Hospital (DMR98-IRB-209 in 2009) provided their kind assistance. The overall agreement rate among the participants was >85%. Select characteristics of all the participants are summarized and compared in Table 1.

4.2. DNA Preparation and Storage

Genomic DNA from the leukocytes of each study subject was extracted using the QIAamp Blood Mini Kit (Qiagen, Valencia, CA, USA), stored for the long term at −80 °C, simultaneously diluted, and aliquoted and stored for genotyping as a working stock at −20 °C, as we have frequently performed previously [32,39,40].

4.3. *IL-18* Genotype Discrimination Methodology

The genotype discrimination methodology for *IL-18* -137, -607, and -656 genotypes was performed as we described in 2018 [41]. Briefly, -137 (G/C, rs187238) and -607 (A/C, rs1946518) genotyping was performed using the ABI StepOne™ Real-Time PCR System (Applied Biosystems, Foster City, CA, USA) and analyzed using the typical TaqMan assay. Regarding the genotyping of *IL-18* -656 (A/C, rs1946519), the polymerase chain reaction-restriction fragment length polymorphism (PCR-RFLP) methodology was carried out using the primers originally reported in 2005 by Flowaczny et al. [42], with the forward primer being 5′-AGGTCAGTCTTTGCTATCATTCCAGG-3′ and the reverse primer being 5′-CTGCAACAGAAAGTAAGCTTGCGGAGAGG-3′, and a 120-bp fragment nearby the *IL-18* -656 polymorphism was amplified. In detail, approximately 100 ng of genomic DNA of each sample was subjected to PCR, in which the reaction mixture of 25-μL contained 300 mM dNTP, 2 U of Taq DNA polymerase, 1× PCR buffer, 1.5 mM $MgCl_2$, and 0.8 mM of each primer. After mixing up and briefly spinning down, the reaction mixture was heated to 94 °C for 4 min and amplified by 30 cycles using the My Cycler (Biorad, Hercules, CA, USA) with the following steps: denaturation at 94 °C for 60 s, annealing at 60 °C for 60 s, extension at 72 °C for 60 s for each cycle, and a final extension step at 72 °C for 5 min. The volume of the restriction assay was set at 12.5 μL, containing 8 μL of PCR products, 2 U *Mwo* I restriction enzyme, and 1× buffer. The reaction mixture was then incubated for 16 h or overnight at 60 °C. The resultant DNA fragments were subject to electrophoresis in 3.0% agarose gel at 100 V for 30 min. After electrophoresis, ethidium bromide staining was done to observe the DNA fragments under UV (260 nm) light. For the A allele of *IL-18* -656, there was no digestion of the 120-bp PCR fragment, whereas for the C allele of *IL-18* -656, two (96- and 24-bp) fragments were identified.

4.4. Enzyme-linked Immunosorbent Assay (ELISA) for Serum IL-18 Levels

Ten milliliters of blood samples were collected from 10 healthy controls and 10 RCC patients. The blood samples were collected in serum tubes with an accelerating agent for serum separation and kept at a room temperature for 30 min before their further centrifugation for 20 min at 1500× g. Serum was then isolated and stored at −80 °C until IL-18 measurement. The individual level of IL-18 in serum was measured by enzyme-linked immunosorbent assay (ELISA, Newwark, DE, USA) kits.

4.5. Statistical Analysis Methodology

The data of 580 cancer-free healthy controls and 92 patients with RCC who had complete genotypic and clinical details were finally included for statistical analysis, whose results are presented in the form of tables and figures. To ensure that the control subjects in this study were representative of the Taiwanese general population and to exclude the possibility of genotyping error, the deviation of the genotype frequencies of *IL-18* SNPs in the control subjects from those expected under the Hardy–Weinberg equilibrium was assessed using the goodness-of-fit test. Pearson's Chi-square test was used to compare the distribution of *IL-18* genotypes between cases and control groups and in the stratification analysis. The comparison of the continuous factor age was performed and evaluated by the Student's *t*-test. The contribution of *IL-18* genotypes to the risk of developing RCC was estimated by the odds ratios (ORs) and their counterpart 95% confidence intervals (CIs) obtained through logistic regression analysis with adjustment for possible confounders. Any p value < 0.05 was considered to be statistically significant.

Author Contributions: Conceived and designed the experiments: W.-S.C., T.-C.S., and W.-L.Y. Performed the experiments: W.-S.C. and C.-W.T. Analyzed the data: C.-C.Y. and H.-Y.L. Contributed reagents/materials/analysis tools: W.-L.Y. and H.-C.W. Wrote the paper: C.-W.T. and D.-T.B.

Acknowledgments: We thank the Tissuebank and colleagues of the Urinary Department in the China Medical University Hospital for their excellent technical assistance. The genotyping and analyzing work was partially helped by Yun-Chi Wang, Hsin-Ting Li, and Huai-Mei Hsu. The statistical analyses were kindly double checked by Cheng-Li Lin (manpower under MOHW108-TDU-B-212-133004).

References

1. Siegel, R.L.; Miller, K.D.; Jemal, A. Cancer statistics, 2018. *CA Cancer J. Clin.* **2018**, *68*, 7–30. [CrossRef] [PubMed]
2. Ferlay, J.; Shin, H.R.; Bray, F.; Forman, D.; Mathers, C.; Parkin, D.M. Estimates of worldwide burden of cancer in 2008: GLOBOCAN 2008. *Int. J. Cancer* **2010**, *127*, 2893–2917. [CrossRef] [PubMed]
3. Klaassen, Z.; Sayyid, R.K.; Wallis, C.J.D. Lessons learned from the global epidemiology of kidney cancer: A refresher in epidemiology 101. *Eur. Urol.* **2019**, *75*, 85–87. [CrossRef]
4. Niedworok, C.; Dorrenhaus, B.; Vom Dorp, F.; Piotrowski, J.A.; Tschirdewahn, S.; Szarvas, T.; Rubben, H.; Schenck, M. Renal cell carcinoma and tumour thrombus in the inferior vena cava: Clinical outcome of 98 consecutive patients and the prognostic value of preoperative parameters. *World J. Urol.* **2015**, *33*, 1541–1552. [CrossRef]
5. Cohen, H.T.; McGovern, F.J. Renal-cell carcinoma. *N. Engl. J. Med.* **2005**, *353*, 2477–2490. [CrossRef]
6. Okamura, H.; Tsutsi, H.; Komatsu, T.; Yutsudo, M.; Hakura, A.; Tanimoto, T.; Torigoe, K.; Okura, T.; Nukada, Y.; Hattori, K.; et al. Cloning of a new cytokine that induces IFN-gamma production by T cells. *Nature* **1995**, *378*, 88–91. [CrossRef] [PubMed]
7. Nakanishi, K.; Yoshimoto, T.; Tsutsui, H.; Okamura, H. Interleukin-18 is a unique cytokine that stimulates both Th1 and Th2 responses depending on its cytokine milieu. *Cytokine Growth Factor Rev.* **2001**, *12*, 53–72. [CrossRef]
8. Golab, J. Interleukin 18–interferon gamma inducing factor–a novel player in tumour immunotherapy? *Cytokine* **2000**, *12*, 332–338. [CrossRef] [PubMed]

9. Kikuchi, T.; Akasaki, Y.; Joki, T.; Abe, T.; Kurimoto, M.; Ohno, T. Antitumor activity of interleukin-18 on mouse glioma cells. *J. Immunother.* **2000**, *23*, 184–189. [CrossRef] [PubMed]
10. Okano, F.; Yamada, K. Canine interleukin-18 induces apoptosis and enhances Fas ligand mRNA expression in a canine carcinoma cell line. *Anticancer Res.* **2000**, *20*, 3411–3415.
11. Cao, R.; Farnebo, J.; Kurimoto, M.; Cao, Y. Interleukin-18 acts as an angiogenesis and tumor suppressor. *FASEB J.* **1999**, *13*, 2195–2202. [CrossRef] [PubMed]
12. Park, C.C.; Morel, J.C.; Amin, M.A.; Connors, M.A.; Harlow, L.A.; Koch, A.E. Evidence of IL-18 as a novel angiogenic mediator. *J. Immunol.* **2001**, *167*, 1644–1653. [CrossRef] [PubMed]
13. Vidal-Vanaclocha, F.; Mendoza, L.; Telleria, N.; Salado, C.; Valcarcel, M.; Gallot, N.; Carrascal, T.; Egilegor, E.; Beaskoetxea, J.; Dinarello, C.A. Clinical and experimental approaches to the pathophysiology of interleukin-18 in cancer progression. *Cancer Metastasis Rev.* **2006**, *25*, 417–434. [CrossRef] [PubMed]
14. Jaiswal, P.K.; Singh, V.; Srivastava, P.; Mittal, R.D. Association of IL-12, IL-18 variants and serum IL-18 with bladder cancer susceptibility in North Indian population. *Gene* **2013**, *519*, 128–134. [CrossRef]
15. Samsami Dehaghani, A.; Shahriary, K.; Kashef, M.A.; Naeimi, S.; Fattahi, M.J.; Mojtahedi, Z.; Ghaderi, A. Interleukin-18 gene promoter and serum level in women with ovarian cancer. *Mol. Biol. Rep.* **2009**, *36*, 2393–2397. [CrossRef]
16. Haghshenas, M.R.; Hosseini, S.V.; Mahmoudi, M.; Saberi-Firozi, M.; Farjadian, S.; Ghaderi, A. IL-18 serum level and IL-18 promoter gene polymorphism in Iranian patients with gastrointestinal cancers. *J. Gastroenterol. Hepatol.* **2009**, *24*, 1119–1122. [CrossRef]
17. Okamoto, M.; Azuma, K.; Hoshino, T.; Imaoka, H.; Ikeda, J.; Kinoshita, T.; Takamori, S.; Ohshima, K.; Edakuni, N.; Kato, S.; et al. Correlation of decreased survival and IL-18 in bone metastasis. *Intern. Med.* **2009**, *48*, 763–773. [CrossRef]
18. Gunel, N.; Coskun, U.; Sancak, B.; Gunel, U.; Hasdemir, O.; Bozkurt, S. Clinical importance of serum interleukin-18 and nitric oxide activities in breast carcinoma patients. *Cancer* **2002**, *95*, 663–667. [CrossRef]
19. Giedraitis, V.; He, B.; Huang, W.X.; Hillert, J. Cloning and mutation analysis of the human IL-18 promoter: A possible role of polymorphisms in expression regulation. *J. Neuroimmunol.* **2001**, *112*, 146–152. [CrossRef]
20. Wei, Y.S.; Lan, Y.; Liu, Y.G.; Tang, H.; Tang, R.G.; Wang, J.C. Interleukin-18 gene promoter polymorphisms and the risk of esophageal squamous cell carcinoma. *Acta. Oncol.* **2007**, *46*, 1090–1096. [CrossRef]
21. Liu, Y.; Lin, N.; Huang, L.; Xu, Q.; Pang, G. Genetic polymorphisms of the interleukin-18 gene and risk of prostate cancer. *DNA Cell. Biol.* **2007**, *26*, 613–618. [CrossRef] [PubMed]
22. Nikiteas, N.; Yannopoulos, A.; Chatzitheofylaktou, A.; Tsigris, C. Heterozygosity for interleukin-18 -607 A/C polymorphism is associated with risk for colorectal cancer. *Anticancer Res.* **2007**, *27*, 3849–3853. [PubMed]
23. Bushley, A.W.; Ferrell, R.; McDuffie, K.; Terada, K.Y.; Carney, M.E.; Thompson, P.J.; Wilkens, L.R.; Tung, K.H.; Ness, R.B.; Goodman, M.T. Polymorphisms of interleukin (IL)-1alpha, IL-1beta, IL-6, IL-10, and IL-18 and the risk of ovarian cancer. *Gynecol. Oncol.* **2004**, *95*, 672–679. [CrossRef] [PubMed]
24. Khalili-Azad, T.; Razmkhah, M.; Ghiam, A.F.; Doroudchi, M.; Talei, A.R.; Mojtahedi, Z.; Ghaderi, A. Association of interleukin-18 gene promoter polymorphisms with breast cancer. *Neoplasma* **2009**, *56*, 22–25. [CrossRef]
25. Vairaktaris, E.; Serefoglou, Z.C.; Yapijakis, C.; Agapi, C.; Vassiliou, S.; Nkenke, E.; Antonis, V.; Sofia, S.; Neukam, F.W.; Patsouris, E. The interleukin-18 -607A/C polymorphism is not associated with risk for oral cancer. *Anticancer Res.* **2007**, *27*, 4011–4014. [PubMed]
26. Asefi, V.; Mojtahedi, Z.; Khademi, B.; Naeimi, S.; Ghaderi, A. Head and neck squamous cell carcinoma is not associated with interleukin-18 promoter gene polymorphisms: A case-control study. *J. Laryngol. Otol.* **2009**, *123*, 444–448. [CrossRef]
27. Saenz-Lopez, P.; Carretero, R.; Vazquez, F.; Martin, J.; Sanchez, E.; Tallada, M.; Garrido, F.; Cozar, J.M.; Ruiz-Cabello, F. Impact of interleukin-18 polymorphisms-607 and -137 on clinical characteristics of renal cell carcinoma patients. *Hum. Immunol.* **2010**, *71*, 309–313. [CrossRef]
28. Chang, W.S.; Ke, H.L.; Tsai, C.W.; Lien, C.S.; Liao, W.L.; Lin, H.H.; Lee, M.H.; Wu, H.C.; Chang, C.H.; Chen, C.C.; et al. The role of XRCC6 T-991C functional polymorphism in renal cell carcinoma. *Anticancer Res.* **2012**, *32*, 3855–3860.
29. Chang, W.S.; Tsai, C.W.; Wang, S.M.; Wang, S.W.; Wu, H.C.; Ji, H.X.; Lin, C.H.; Wang, Z.H.; Chou, J.C.; Bau, D.T.; et al. Association of caveolin-1 genotypes with renal cell carcinoma risk in Taiwan. *Chin. J. Physiol.* **2014**, *57*, 220–226. [CrossRef]

30. Chang, W.S.; Liao, C.H.; Miao, C.E.; Wu, H.C.; Hou, L.L.; Hsiao, C.L.; Ji, H.X.; Tsai, C.W.; Bau, D.T. The role of functional polymorphisms of cyclooxygenase 2 in renal cell carcinoma. *Anticancer Res.* **2014**, *34*, 5481–5486.
31. Chang, W.S.; Liao, C.H.; Tsai, C.W.; Hu, P.S.; Wu, H.C.; Hsu, S.W.; Ji, H.X.; Hsiao, C.L.; Bau, D.T. The Role of IL-10 Promoter Polymorphisms in Renal Cell Carcinoma. *Anticancer Res.* **2016**, *36*, 2205–2209.
32. Liao, C.H.; Chang, W.S.; Hu, P.S.; Wu, H.C.; Hsu, S.W.; Liu, Y.F.; Liu, S.P.; Hung, H.S.; Bau, D.T.; Tsai, C.W. The Contribution of MMP-7 Promoter Polymorphisms in Renal Cell Carcinoma. *In Vivo* **2017**, *31*, 631–635. [PubMed]
33. Aggarwal, B.B.; Shishodia, S.; Sandur, S.K.; Pandey, M.K.; Sethi, G. Inflammation and cancer: How hot is the link? *Biochem. Pharmacol.* **2006**, *72*, 1605–1621. [CrossRef] [PubMed]
34. Lian, H.; Jin, N.; Li, X.; Mi, Z.; Zhang, J.; Sun, L.; Li, X.; Zheng, H.; Li, P. Induction of an effective anti-tumor immune response and tumor regression by combined administration of IL-18 and Apoptin. *Cancer Immunol. Immunother.* **2007**, *56*, 181–192. [CrossRef] [PubMed]
35. Herzyk, D.J.; Bugelski, P.J.; Hart, T.K.; Wier, P.J. Preclinical safety of recombinant human interleukin-18. *Toxicol. Pathol.* **2003**, *31*, 554–561. [CrossRef] [PubMed]
36. Sozen, S.; Coskun, U.; Sancak, B.; Bukan, N.; Gunel, N.; Tunc, L.; Bozkirli, I. Serum levels of interleukin-18 and nitrite+nitrate in renal cell carcinoma patients with different tumor stage and grade. *Neoplasma* **2004**, *51*, 25–29. [PubMed]
37. Jia, Y.; Zang, A.; Jiao, S.; Chen, S.; Yan, F. The interleukin-18 gene promoter -607 A/C polymorphism contributes to non-small-cell lung cancer risk in a Chinese population. *Onco. Targets. Ther.* **2016**, *9*, 1715–1719. [CrossRef]
38. Xu, L.; Zhu, Y.; An, H.; Liu, Y.; Lin, Z.; Wang, G.; Xu, J. Clinical significance of tumor-derived IL-1β and IL-18 in localized renal cell carcinoma: Associations with recurrence and survival. *Urol. Oncol.* **2015**, *33*, 68.e9–68.e16. [CrossRef]
39. Yueh, T.C.; Wu, C.N.; Hung, Y.W.; Chang, W.S.; Fu, C.K.; Pei, J.S.; Wu, M.H.; Lai, Y.L.; Lee, Y.M.; Yen, S.T.; et al. The Contribution of MMP-7 Genotypes to Colorectal Cancer Susceptibility in Taiwan. *Cancer Genomics Proteomics* **2018**, *15*, 207–212. [CrossRef]
40. Shen, T.C.; Chang, W.S.; Tsai, C.W.; Chao, C.Y.; Lin, Y.T.; Hsiao, C.L.; Hsu, C.L.; Chen, W.C.; Hsia, T.C.; Bau, D.T. The Contribution of Matrix Metalloproteinase-1 Promoter Genotypes in Taiwan Lung Cancer Risk. *Anticancer Res.* **2018**, *38*, 253–257.
41. Huang, C.Y.; Chang, W.S.; Tsai, C.W.; Hsia, T.C.; Shen, T.C.; Bau, D.T.; Shui, H.A. Interleukin-18 promoter genotype is associated with the risk of nasopharyngeal carcinoma in Taiwan. *Cancer Manag. Res.* **2018**, *10*, 5199–5207. [CrossRef] [PubMed]
42. Folwaczny, M.; Glas, J.; Torok, H.P.; Tonenchi, L.; Paschos, E.; Bauer, B.; Limbersky, O.; Folwaczny, C. Polymorphisms of the interleukin-18 gene in periodontitis patients. *J. Clin. Periodontol.* **2005**, *32*, 530–534. [CrossRef] [PubMed]

15

Effects of Farnesiferol B on Ischemia-Reperfusion-Induced Renal Damage, Inflammation and NF-κB Signaling

Lu Zhang [1,2,†], Xianjun Fu [1,†], Ting Gui [1], Tianqi Wang [1], Zhenguo Wang [1], Gerd A. Kullak-Ublick [2,3,*] and Zhibo Gai [1,2,*]

1 College of Traditional Chinese Medicine; Shandong Co-Innovation Center of TCM Formula; Institute for Literature and Culture of Chinese Medicine; Key Laboratory of Traditional Chinese Medicine for Classical Theory, Ministry of Education, Shandong University of Traditional Chinese Medicine, Jinan 250355, China; Lu.zhang@usz.ch (L.Z.); xianxiu@hotmail.com (X.F.); stefina1982@gmail.com (T.G.); wangtianqi9292@gmail.com (T.W.); zhenguo.wang0101@gmail.com (Z.W.)

2 Department of Clinical Pharmacology and Toxicology, University Hospital Zurich, University of Zurich, 8006 Zurich, Switzerland

3 Mechanistic Safety, CMO & Patient Safety, Global Drug Development, Novartis Pharma, 4056 Basel, Switzerland

* Correspondence: gerd.kullak@usz.ch (G.A.K.-U.); gaizhibo@gmail.com (Z.G.)

† These authors contributed equally to this work.

Abstract: Background: G-protein-coupled bile acid receptor (TGR5), a membrane bile acid receptor, regulates macrophage reactivity, and attenuates inflammation in different disease models. However, the regulatory effects of TGR5 in ischemia/reperfusion (I/R)-induced kidney injury and inflammation have not yet been extensively studied. Therefore, we hypothesize that Farnesiferol B, a natural TGR5 agonist, could alleviate renal I/R injury by reducing inflammation and macrophage migration through activating TGR5. Methods: Mice were treated with Farnesiferol B before I/R or sham procedures. Renal function, pathological analysis, and inflammatory mediators were examined. In vitro, the regulatory effects of Farnesiferol B on the Nuclear Factor kappa-light-chain-enhancer of activated B cells (NF-κB) pathway in macrophages were investigated. Results: After I/R, Farnesiferol B-treated mice displayed better renal function and less tubular damage. Farnesiferol B reduced renal oxidative stress and inflammation significantly. In vitro, Farnesiferol B treatment alleviated lipopolysaccharide (LPS)-induced macrophage migration and activation, as well as LPS-induced NF-κB activation through TGR5. Conclusions: Farnesiferol B could protect kidney function from I/R-induced damage by attenuating inflammation though activating TGR5 in macrophages. Farnesiferol B might be a potent TGR5 ligand for the treatment of I/R-induced renal inflammation.

Keywords: inflammation; ischemia/reperfusion injury; Farnesiferol B; Nuclear Factor kappa-light-chain-enhancer of activated B cells (NF-κB); G-protein-coupled bile acid receptor (TGR5)

---

1. Introduction

Ischemia/reperfusion (I/R) is a common complication in patients undergoing major cardiac surgery, kidney transplantation, and those experiencing hemorrhage and dehydration [1]. Ischemia/reperfusion injury (I/RI) after renal transplantation is a well-recognized and prevalent postoperative complication, which has been thought as a risk factor for the loss of tubular epithelial cell function, leading to acute kidney injury (AKI), delayed graft function, as well as acute or chronic organ rejection [2,3]. The process of renal ischemia reperfusion (RIR) is exceedingly complex, including a series of intricate and related events that lead to renal cell injury and ultimately give rise to cell death via apoptosis and necrosis [4]. Even though reperfusion is critically paramount for the repair of ischemic tissue and the survival of patients, the additional cellular damage by itself has provoked much attention, largely due to the production of reactive oxygen species (ROS) and infiltration of neutrophils [5,6].

The mechanism and treatment of I/R on kidney injury is still under exploration. During I/R, toxic products of kidney cells and cytokine release cause damage to renal epithelial tubular cells [7]. Besides, several studies have suggested that I/R leads rise to neutrophil infiltration of kidney tissue and stimulates the oxidative stress processes producing ROS [8]. Oxidative stress directly or indirectly affects all aspects of the kidney damage by the pathway lead to apoptosis, necrosis, fibrosis, tissue damage progression, and renal dysfunction [9]. ROS is considered as both the mediator or a signaling molecule during acute kidney inflammatory diseases [10]. The oxidase activity is elevated soon after ischemic injury, which is may originate from macrophages and/or neutrophils [11]. Moreover, inflammatory cells can also induce post-hypoxic cellular damage by ROS, which in turn gives rise to tubular epithelial cell damage or death by triggering apoptosis and necrosis pathways [12,13].

Early in a classic pharmacopoeia of traditional Chinese medicine book, Ferulae Resina is recorded as widely used for its effects on removing stagnancy (Xiao Ji), dissolving hard mass (Hua Jia), dissipating obstruction (San Pi), and as having anthelmintic properties (Sha Chong). Previous research reported the isolation of Farnesiferol B, a new sesquiterpene that is highly produced in the Apiaceae family, from the roots of Ferula [14,15]. Farnesiferol B has shown anti-plasmodial activity and anti-cytotoxicity effects in rat skeletal fibroblasts, a L6-cell line [16]. In a recent in silico work, Farnesiferol B was confirmed as a TGR5 agonist, also known as a G-protein-coupled bile acid receptor 1 (GPBAR1) activator, which denotes a regulatory effect of Farnesiferol B on inflammation [17].

TGR5 is expressed in several types of cells, including hepatic non-parenchymal cells [18–20]. The renal tubular cells, and immune cells including monocytes and macrophages [21,22]. Recently, it was demonstrated that TGR5 activation could be exploited to confer protection from diabetic nephropathy [23]. Considering that TGR5 activation possesses anti-oxidant and anti-inflammatory roles [23,24] in the kidney, we hypothesized that Farnesiferol B would alleviate renal I/R injury by reducing inflammation and ROS through regulating renal tubular cells and macrophages over TGR5.

In this study, the protective effect of Farnesiferol B was examined in a mouse model of AKI induced by I/R. We investigated the regulatory effects of Farnesiferol B on pro-inflammatory pathways in LPS-treated macrophages.

2. Results

2.1. *Farnesiferol B Protection for Kidney Damage in I/R Kidney*

The overall effect of Farnesiferol B on kidney injury was first explored by histological assessment and creatinine quantification. Haemotoxylin and Eosin (HE) staining and kidney injury marker Kim-1 (kidney injury molecule-1) immunohistochemical staining analysis results show that I/R kidneys are characterized by tubular basal membrane rupture, nuclear infiltration, tubular vacuolization, higher Kim-1 expression, and a higher renal tubular injury score (Figure 1A,B,E). Levels of proximal tubular cell death and cell proliferation were assessed. In the TUNEL assay, the nuclei of TUNEL-positive cells were stained red (Figure 1C), and the levels of cell death were indicated as the percentage of TUNEL-positive cells (Figure 1F). TUNEL-positive cells were observed mainly in the tubular area of the renal cortex. I/R group displayed more TUNEL-positive cells that the sham group (Figure 1C(b) vs. (a)). PCNA expression was observed in proliferating cell nuclei, and was significantly increased in AKI compared with the sham group (Figure 1D,G). Serum creatinine levels in I/R mice were significantly elevated in comparison to sham-operated mice (Figure 1H). The treatment with Farnesiferol B prior to I/R decreased serum creatinine level, attenuating the I/R-induced kidney injury (Figure 1A,C,H). However, Farnesiferol B treatment did not change the I/R-induced cell proliferation (Figure 1D(c) vs. (b)). The above results suggest that, in general, Farnesiferol B treatment protects against the kidney damage caused by I/R.

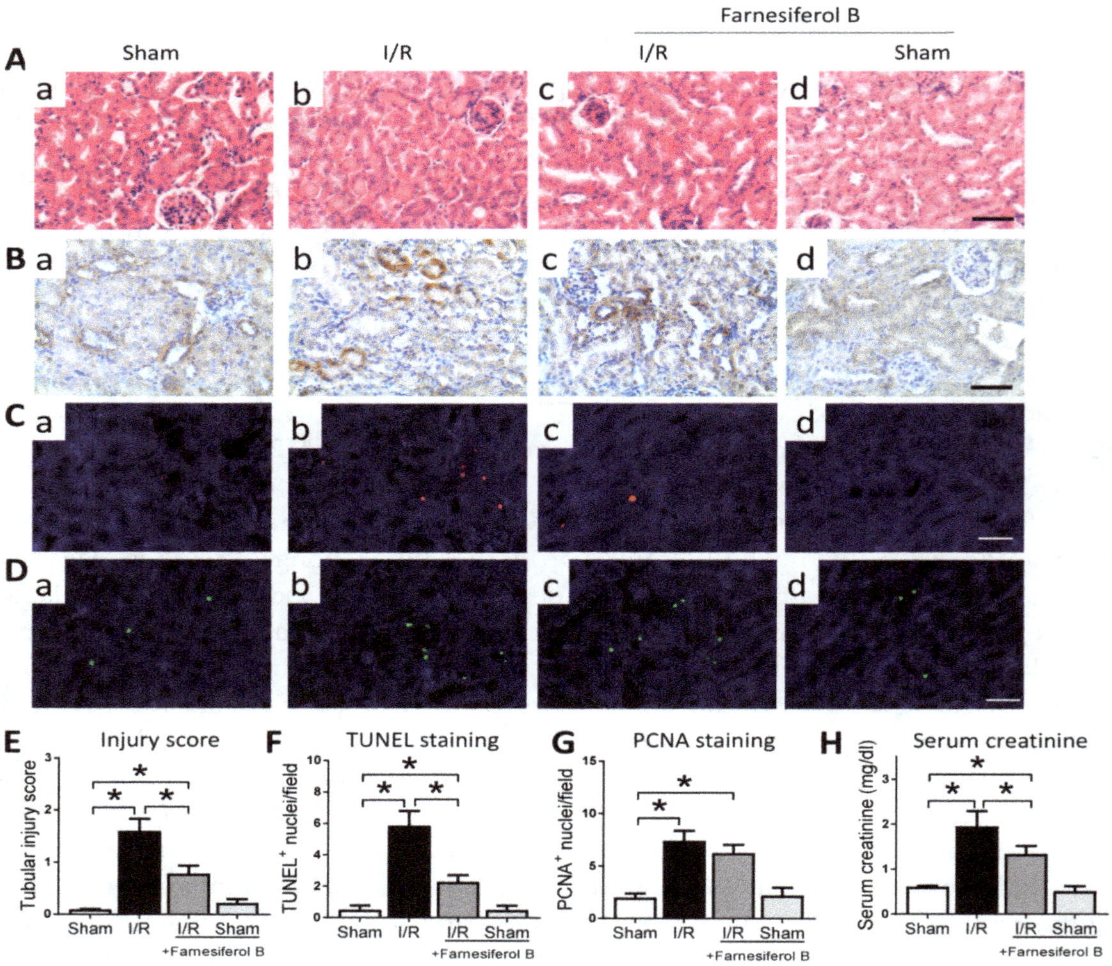

Figure 1. Farnesiferol B protects kidney from I/R-induced kidney damage. Representative images showing (**A**) Haemotoxylin and Eosin (HE) staining and (**B**) Kim1, (**C**) TUNEL, (**D**) PCNA immunostaining on renal sections from (**a**) sham, (**b**) I/R, (**c**) I/R + Farnesiferol B and (**d**) sham + Farnesiferol B groups (scale bar 50 μm). Quantitative analysis of (**E**) tubular injury scores, (**F**) TUNEL staining, (**G**) PCNA staining, and (**H**) serum creatinine from different groups. $n = 6$ mice/group. Data are means ± SD, one-way ANOVA with Bonferroni's test. * $p < 0.05$.

2.2. Farnesiferol B Reduces Oxidative Stress and Lipid Oxidative Signaling Pathways in I/R Kidney

I/R is often associated with oxidative stress, with existing evidence suggesting that oxidative stress is a paramount contributor in causing kidney damage [25]. Therefore, the effect of Farnesiferol B on oxidative stress in the kidney after I/R was evaluated. Immunohistochemical staining for NGAL neutrophil gelatinase-associated lipocalin (NGAL), an oxidative stress risk factor, showed that I/R may induced significant increases of oxidative stress in I/R kidneys (Figure 2A(b),B). The level of NGAL was reduced in mice treated with Farnesiferol B (Figure 2A(c),B). The potential mechanisms involved in the inhibitory effects of Farnesiferol B on I/R-induced oxidative stress were investigated. The I/R greatly increased the oxidative stress production and impaired antioxidant capacity in the injured kidney (Figure 2C–E). Farnesiferol B administration significantly diminished oxidative stress in the urine of injured group, namely H_2O_2 (hydrogen peroxide). Treatment with Farnesiferol B significantly increased the expression of Nrf2 and its downstream HO-1 (Figure 2D,E).

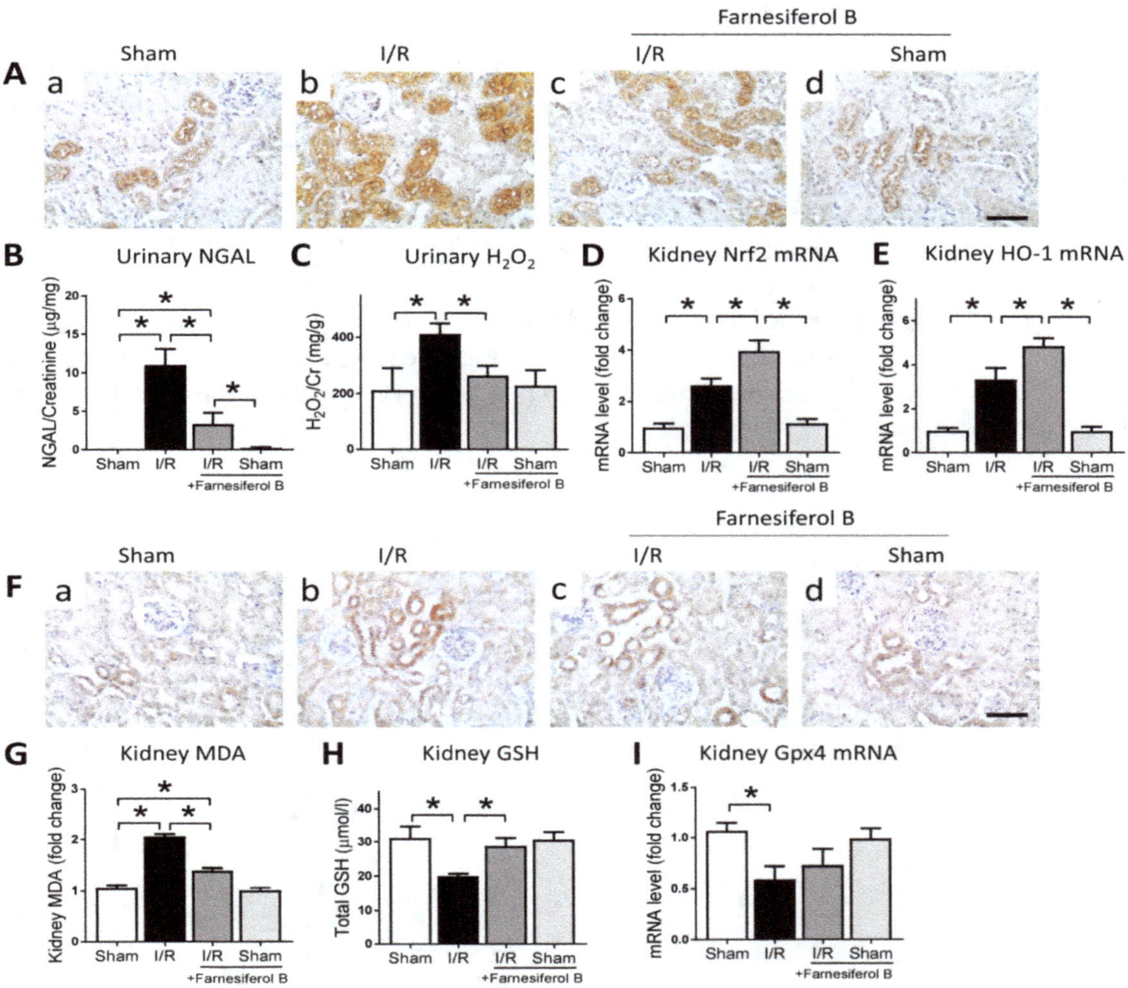

Figure 2. Farnesiferol B reduces oxidative stress in ischemia/reperfusion (I/R) kidney. (**A**) Representative images of immunostaining for NGAL on renal sections from (**a**) sham, (**b**) I/R, (**c**) I/R + Farnesiferol B and (**d**) sham + Farnesiferol B groups (scale bar 50 μm). (**B**) urinary neutrophil gelatinase-associated lipocalin (NGAL), (**C**) urinary H_2O_2, and kidney mRNA levels of (**D**) Nrf2 and (**E**) HO-1 were analyzed. $n = 6$ mice/group. Data are means ± SD, one-way ANOVA with Bonferroni's test. * $p < 0.05$. (**F**) Representative images of immunostaining for 4-HNE on renal sections from (**a**) sham, (**b**) I/R, (**c**) I/R + Farnesiferol B and (**d**) sham + Farnesiferol B groups (scale bar 50 μm). (**G**) kidney malondialdehyde (MDA), (**H**) kidney GSH, and kidney mRNA levels of (**I**) Gpx4 were analyzed. $n = 6$ mice/group. Data are means ± SD, one-way ANOVA with Bonferroni's test. * $p < 0.05$.

Reactive oxygen species accumulation can lead to lipid peroxidation and ferroptosis, a kind of regulated cell death [26]. The lipid peroxidation marker, 4-HNE (4-hydroxynonenal) and MDA (malondialdehyde), and markers related to ferroptosis were examined. The results show that 4-HNE and MDA levels were induced and GSH (glutathione) levels were reduced in the injured kidney (Figure 2F–H). Farnesiferol B administration reduced kidney lipid peroxidation and induced GSH level in the renal tissue homogenate. Furthermore, mRNA expression of Gpx4, the key ferroptosis regulator, was examined (Figure 2I). Gpx4 mRNA level was significantly down-regulated after I/R injury, whereas the expression seemed to be increased by Farnesiferol B treatment (not significantly). Taken together, the results indicated that anti-lipid peroxidation effects seen in Farnesiferol B treatment group could be an indirect result of its regulation on antioxidant pathways.

2.3. Farnesiferol B Protectes Kidney from I/R-Induced Inflammation and Inhibits NF-κB Signaling Pathway

The other oxidative stress-producer is the inflammatory cell such as monocytes and macrophages, which infiltrate into tissue, especially during acute inflammation [27]. Next, we analyzed the degree of kidney inflammation. I/R increased the positive stainings of macrophages and neutrophils in the kidney (Figure 3A–D). I/R also induced levels of TNFα and MCP-1 in mouse serum and kidney, as well as the proinflammatory mediator LTB_4 in the kidney (Figure 3E–I). The number of macrophages and neutrophils, as well as the serum and kidney levels of TNFα, MCP-1, and LTB4 were significantly reduced by Farnesiferol B treatment (Figure 3E–I). Inflammation-related genes expressed in the kidney were also measured. Quantitative analysis showed that I/R stimulated the expression of kidney TNFα, IL-6, and Icam mRNA levels, while levels of these mRNA decreased under treatment with Farnesiferol B (Figure 3J–L). The evidence presented here suggests a positive role of Farnesiferol B in attenuating renal inflammation.

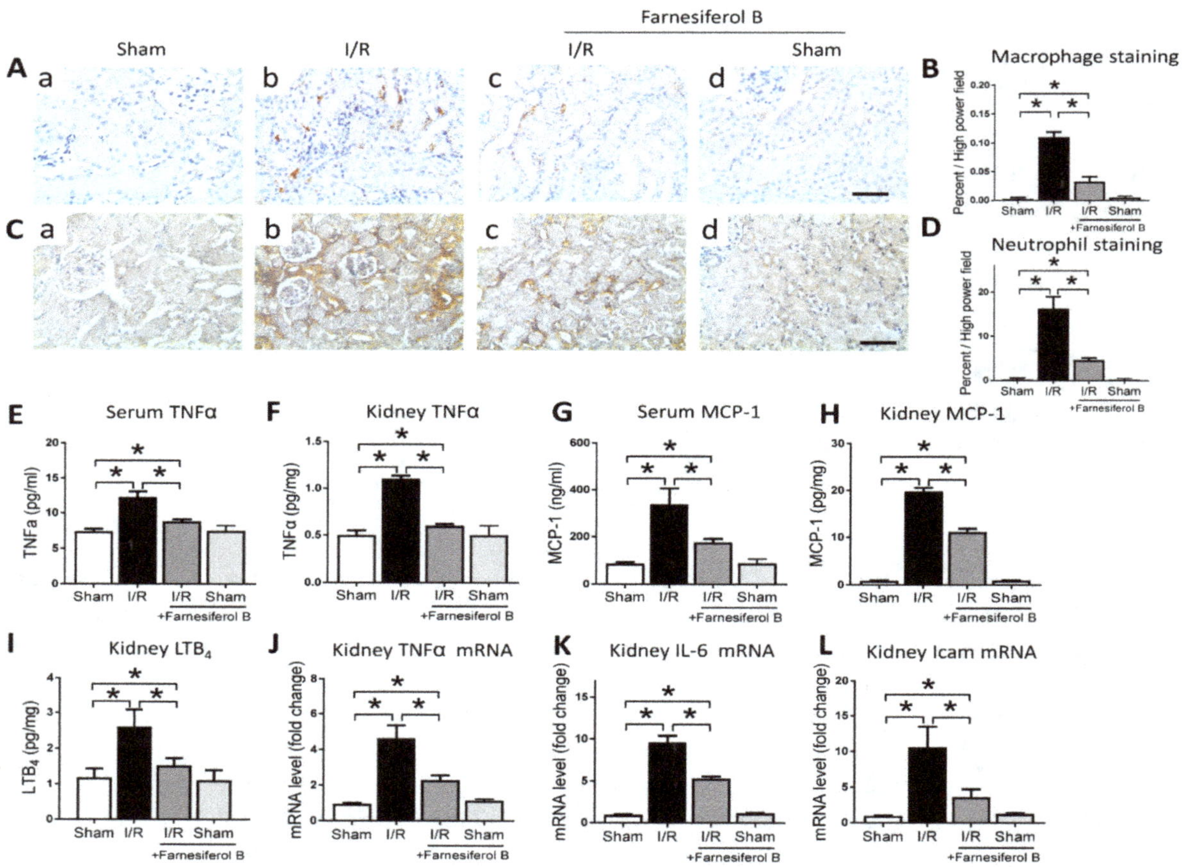

Figure 3. Farnesiferol B protects kidney from I/R-induced inflammation. (**A**) Representative images and (**B**) the quantitative analysis of positive immunostaining for macrophages on renal sections from (**a**) sham, (**b**) I/R, (**c**) I/R + Farnesiferol B, and (**d**) sham + Farnesiferol B groups (scale bar 50 μm). (**C**) Representative images and (**D**) the quantitative analysis of positive immunostaining for neutrophils on renal sections from (**a**) sham, (**b**) I/R, (**c**) I/R + Farnesiferol B, and (**d**) sham + Farnesiferol B groups (scale bar 50 μm). Levels of (**E**) serum TNFα, (**F**) kidney TNFα, (**G**) serum MCP-1, (**H**) kidney MCP-1, (**I**) kidney LTB_4, (**J**) kidney TNFα mRNA, (**K**) kidney IL-6 mRNA, and (**L**) kidney Icam mRNA from different treatment groups. $n = 6$ mice/group. Data are means ± SD, one-way ANOVA with Bonferroni's test. * $p < 0.05$.

NF-κB signaling pathway is one of the key inflammatory pathways during AKI. To examine the inhibitory effects of Farnesiferol B on I/R-induced inflammation, p65 levels from different treatment groups were evaluated. I/R induced increased tubulointerstitial staining of p65 in the kidney sections (Figure 4A(b)) and p65 translocation in the nuclei (Figure 4B). The I/R+Farnesiferol B group showed reduced levels of p65 immunostaining in kidney sections as well as nuclei translocation, indicating that part of anti-inflammatory effect is reacted on inflammatory cells.

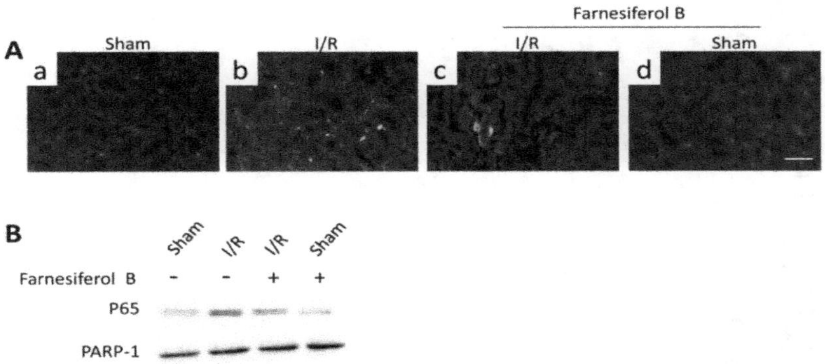

Figure 4. Farnesiferol B inhibits NF-κB signaling pathway in I/R kidney. (**A**) Representative images showing immunostaining of p65 on renal sections from (**a**) sham, (**b**) I/R, (**c**) I/R + Farnesiferol B and (**d**) sham + Farnesiferol B groups (scale bar 50 μm). (**B**) Representative immunoblotting image of nuclear protein for NF-κB p65 expression in kidney tissue. PARP-1 protein is used as the loading control.

2.4. Farnesiferol B Inhibits the Activity of Inflammatory Cells by Activating TGR5

To examine the direct effect of Farnesiferol B on macrophages, we conducted in vitro experiments using the J774 cell line. J774 macrophages were treated with LPS and/or Farnesiferol B and migration ability in a transwell system was monitored as a proxy for infiltration capability. Representative images show that migration induced by LPS was abolished by co-incubation with Farnesiferol B (Figure 5A). LPS-induced migration was associated with higher mRNA expression levels of TNFα, Ccl2, Ccl3 in macrophages, compared with that from the untreated cells. Treatment with Farnesiferol B lowered mRNA expression of these inflammatory cytokines significantly (Figure 5B–D).

Farnesiferol B was previously reported to be a TGR5 agonist, which can inhibit macrophage infiltration through inhibiting NF-κB activation [28]. Based on this, we speculated that the anti-inflammatory effect of Farnesiferol B may be related to its ability to activate TGR5. Therefore, we evaluated the regulatory effect of Farnesiferol B on LPS-induced NF-κB activation in J774 macrophages. Immunoblotting of nuclear protein for NF-κB p65 indicated an LPS-induced nuclear translocation in J774 macrophages (Figure 5E). Similar to INT777, a known TGR5 agonist, Farnesiferol B also significantly reduced p65 translocation in a dose-dependent way (Figure 5E). PARP-1 was stably expressed between groups as a nucleoprotein control (Figure 5E). An NF-κB binding assay also revealed that LPS-induced NF-κB binding activity was blocked by Farnesiferol B or INT777 co-incubation (Figure 5F), which was consistent with previous publications [29].

In order to further verify the target of Farnesiferol B in macrophages, RAW264.7 cells, which do not express TGR5 [30], were exposed to LPS with and without Farnesiferol B. As shown in Figure 6, Farnesiferol B could not inhibit LPS-induced cell migration, suggesting that Farnesiferol B suppresses LPS-mediated macrophage migration by activating TGR5. Benzoxathiole derivative (BOT), an NF-κB inhibitor, was used as a positive control to block LPS-induced migration (Figure 6c). Taken together, Farnesiferol B inhibits the LPS-induced NF-κB pathway by activating TGR5.

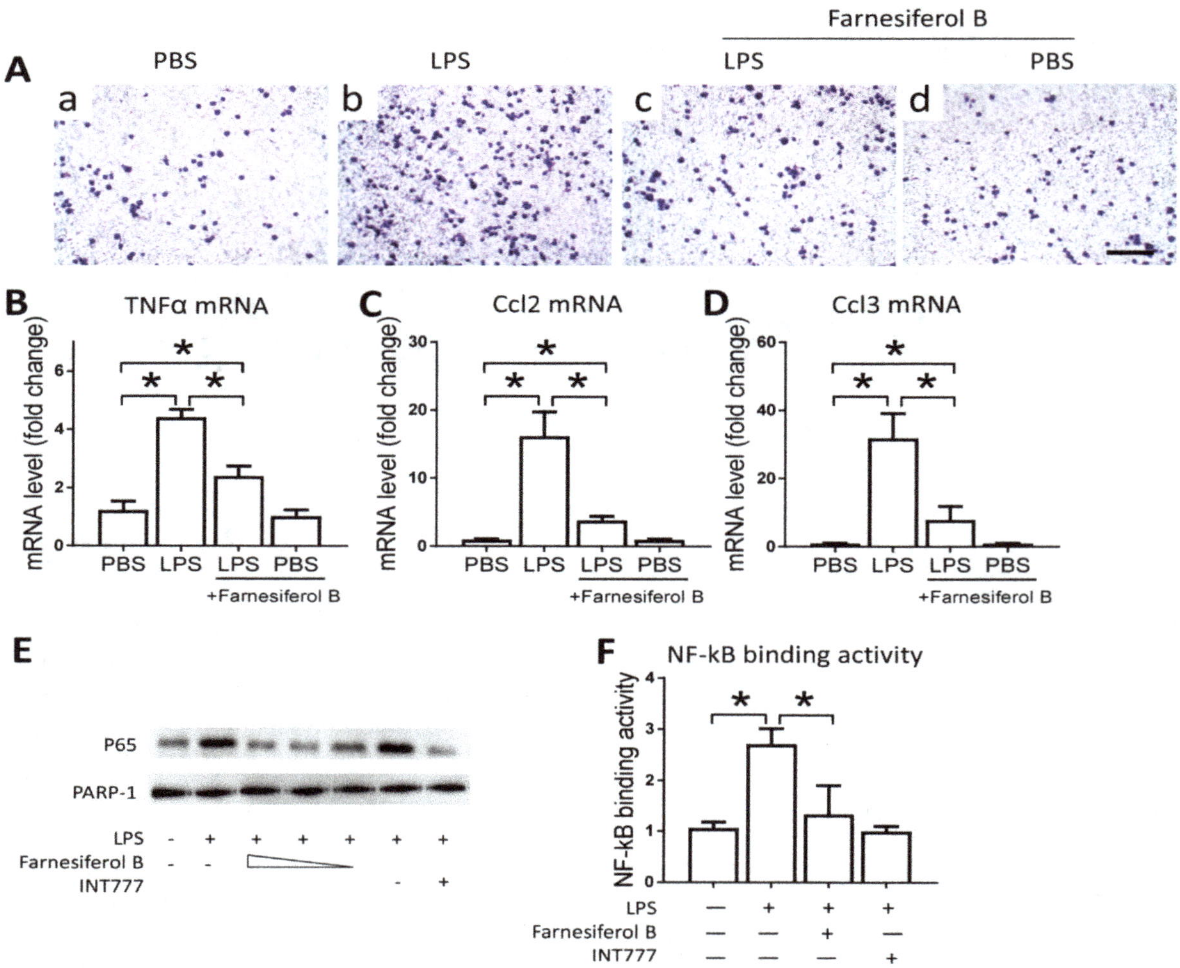

Figure 5. Farnesiferol B inhibits the activity of inflammatory cells by activating TGR5. (**A**) Representative images of J774 cells seeded in 3-μm pore polycarbonate membrane and stained with crystal violet for migration analysis (scale bar 100 μm) after treatment with (a) PBS, (b) LPS, (c) LPS+Farnesiferol B, or (d) PBS+Farnesiferol B. Level of mRNA for (**B**) TNFα, (**C**) Ccl2 and (**D**) Ccl3 with different treatments. (**E**) Representative immunoblotting image of nuclear protein for NF-κB p65 expression. J774 cells were treated with 100 ng/mL LPS with or without co-incubation with Farnesiferol B at 5 μM, 10 μM and 20 μM, or INT777 for 2 h. (**F**) NF-κB DNA binding activity. Data are means ± SD of at least three independent experiments, one-way ANOVA with Bonferroni's test. * $p < 0.05$.

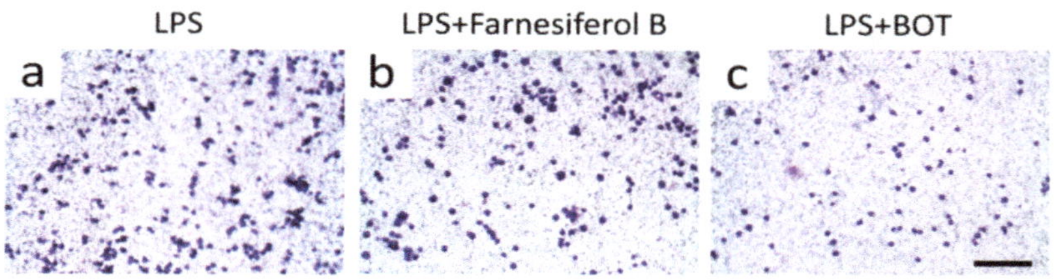

Figure 6. Farnesiferol does not inhibit migration of inflammatory cells not expressing TGR5. Representative images of RAW 264.7 macrophages seeded in 3-μm pore polycarbonate membrane with different treatment for 2 h, and stained with crystal violet for migration assay (scale bar 100 μm). Cells were treated with (**a**) 100 ng/mL LPS, (**b**) LPS with 20 μM Farnesiferol co-incubation, and (**c**) LPS with a NF-κB inhibitor, benzoxathiole derivative (BOT).

3. Discussion

In the current study, our results point out that Farnesiferol B treatment play a beneficial role in renal I/R injury. Compared with I/R treated mice, Farnesiferol B-treated mice showed lower score of renal injury, while significantly decreased levels of histological tubular injury, oxidative stress, and inflammation (Figure 7). In line with and based on our experiments in mice, the in vitro analysis show that Farnesiferol B reduces LPS-induced macrophage migration. Moreover, Farnesiferol B can inhibit NF-κB nuclear translocation through activating TGR5 in macrophages. Thus, Farnesiferol B might represent a novel natural compound against I/R-induced kidney damage.

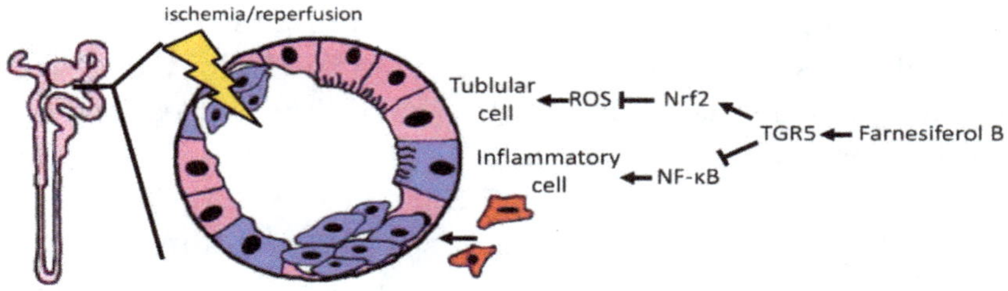

Figure 7. Model of the Farnesiferol B-mediated protection against ischemia/reperfusion-induced AKI. I/R induces ROS generation that causes tubular cell damage (shown in purple-blue). In parallel, inflammatory cell infiltration (shown in red) also promotes oxidative stress and post-hypoxic kidney damage after I/R. Farnesiferol B-mediated TGR5 activation induces the antioxidant Nrf2 pathway and inhibits the proinflammatory NF-κB signaling pathway, which in turn protects the kidney from tubular damage and inflammation.

Ischaemia-reperfusion (I/R) injury is the main cause of AKI under common clinical conditions [31,32]. Nowadays, the pathogenesis of AKI is characterized by renal tubular damage, inflammation, and vascular dysfunction [33,34]. In vivo experiment, we examined the kidney of AKI mice and found that Farnesiferol B effectively reduced the regulated cell death and oxidative stress. Although it was hard to identify the exact type of cell death, both results of TUNEL assay and ferroptosis marker Gxp4 showed that Farnesiferol B have protective effects on tubular cell damage during AKI. NGAL is an early biomarker of AKI which is produced in the distal nephron and its synthesis is upregulated in response to kidney injury [35]. Recent evidence demonstrates that high NGAL level is a risk factor for oxidative stress in patients [36]. In our case, I/R increased highly expression of NGAL in mice. Furthermore, Farnesiferol B reduced the NGAL level both in kidney and in urine, as well as the other oxidative stress marker MDA. Furthermore, with treatment of Farnesiferol B, GSH levels was increased and Nrf2 and HO-1 expression were restored in the I/R injured kidney, while at the same time, reduced oxidative stress (H_2O_2) and lipid peroxidation (4-HNE and MDA). These data indicated that antioxidant related pathways may be regulated by Farnesiferol B-TGR5 signaling pathway. Nrf2 and its target gene, HO-1, has generally been considered to be an adaptive cellular response to oxidative stress [26]. Recently, Nrf2/HO-1 has also been shown to be protective in AKI and diabetic nephropathy [37–39]. It has been reported that treatment with either FXR/TGR5 dual agonist INT-767 or TGR5 specific agonist INT-777 could prevent diabetic nephropathy through inducing Nrf2-mediated antioxidant generation, and reducing renal expression of oxidative stress [23,40]. We have seen similar effects in the I/R-induced mouse AKI model with treatment with FXR/TGR5 dual agonist [25]. In the study, treatment with 6alpha-ethyl-chenodeoxycholic acid (6-ECDCA), a potent dual FXR/TGR5 agonist [41], significantly improved Nrf2-mediated antioxidant capacity. Silencing of Nrf2 blocked the antioxidant effect of 6-ECDCA in proximal tubule cells exposed to hypoxia. Based on these findings, TGR5 could be a potent target to induce antioxidant pathways. However, to identify the renal signaling pathways regulated by FXR and TGR5 respectively and specify the regulatory effects of TGR5 on antioxidant pathways need to be further studied.

Renal inflammation after I/R is directly related to monocyte infiltration and macrophage activation [25,42]. TGR5, also called GPBAR1 or GPR131, is a bile acid–responsive G protein-coupled receptor, which plays a crucial role in protection against diet-induced diabetes through different cellular mechanisms [43]. The role of TGF5 activation in modulating inflammatory pathways was confirmed in experiments on mice and immune cells [21,28]. Recent evidence suggests that activation of TGR5 regulates inflammatory cell signaling pathways such as NF-κB, AKT and extracellular signal-regulated kinase (ERK) [44,45]. Macrophages play a pivotal role in kidney injury, inflammation, and fibrosis [46]. In the present study, we can clearly notice that, after I/R, the mice shown an increased inflammation level on renal tissue (e.g., the infiltration of macrophages and neutrophils in Figure 3 and high expression of p65 in Figure 5), as well as high level of proinflammatory factors (TNFα, MCP-1, IL-6) both in serum and kidney tissue. While the treatment with Farnesiferol B demonstrated a critical anti-inflammatory effects by reducing those inflammatory factors or NF-κB activation. However, NF-κB signaling can be activated in all cell types during AKI, thereby immunostaining or immunoblotting providing only limited information about cell-specific NF-κB functions in the kidney during AKI [47]. Therefore, we employed the in vitro experiments. Our results shown that Farnesiferol B effectively inhibited the expression of inflammatory cytokines, such as MCP-1, LTB4, and TNFα. Farnesiferol B inhibited LPS-induced NF-κB activation and decreased p65 translocation in J774 macrophages, possessing similar effects as other TGR5 agonists [40]. Moreover, the anti-inflammatory effect of Farnesiferol B was blocked in RAW264.7 cells, which do not express TGR5 [21,30]. Taken together, these results indicate that Farnesiferol B inhibits LPS-induced NF-κB activation through activating TGR5, which is consistent with previous predictive results [17].

Ferula species from the family Apiaceae are rich sources of biologically active natural products including sesquiterpene coumarins (SCs) and sesquiterpenes [48]. Some studies have shown that SCs are able to enhance the cytotoxicity of anticancer compounds [49]. Recently Kasaian et al. showed enhancement of doxorubicin cytotoxicity in MCF-7/Adr cells (doxorubicin resistant derivatives of MCF-7 cells overexpressing P-gp) when combined with non-toxic concentrations of farnesiferols, proving the significant activity of Farnesiferol B on multi-drug resistant cells [50]. Previous studies show that sesquiterpene coumarins and their derivative from *Ferula fukanensis* reduces IL-6 and TNFα, while inducing nitric oxide synthase in RAW264.7 cells, possessing inhibitory effects on LPS and IFN-γ induced pro-inflammatory cytokine release and nitric oxide production [51,52]. A recent study also showed the anti-inflammatory effect of *Ferula szowitsiana* in vitro, which indicates that Farnesiferol B might inhibit neuroinflammation via reducing the generation of inflammatory cytokines [53]. In this study, we show the active effect of Farnesiferol B on TGR5, which suppresses the NF-κB p65 binding activity and inhibits macrophage migration.

4. Materials and Methods

4.1. Animals Study Approval and Tissue Samples

All animal experiments conformed to both Swiss and Chinese animal protection laws and were approved (May, 2015) by the Scientific Animal Study Committee of Shandong University, Jinan, China (study number 2015064).

Six-week-old female C57/BJ mice were randomly assigned to I/R or sham procedures. They were divided into four groups with six animals each: sham, I/R, I/R + Farnesiferol B and sham + Farnesiferol B. AKI was induced by unilateral nephrectomy and contralateral ischemia and reperfusion, as previously described [25]. For Farnesiferol B treatment, mice were injected intraperitoneally (i.p.) with Farnesiferol B (10 mg/kg, Golexir Pars Co., Mashhad, Iran) 2 h before the procedure. All mice were killed under anesthesia 24 h after surgery. Kidneys were harvested for further analysis.

4.2. Measurements in Serum, Urine, and Kidney Samples

Urinary H_2O_2 and NGAL levels were measured in the resulting urine samples with the Amplex Red H_2O_2 assay kit (A12214, Invitrogen, Carlsbad, CA, USA) and Mouse Lipocalin-2/NGAL ELISA Kit (ab119601, Abcam, Cambridge, UK). Serum creatinine, MCP-1, TNFα, and LTB4 levels were measured with a creatinine assay kit (ab65340, Abcam, Cambridge, UK), Mouse MCP1 ELISA Kit (ab100721, Abcam), Mouse TNF alpha ELISA Kit (ab46105, Abcam), and LTB4 Parameter Assay Kit (KGE006B; R&D Systems, Minneapolis, MN, USA), respectively. Kidney malondialdehyde (MDA) levels were measured by a Lipid Peroxidation (MDA) Assay Kit (ab118970, Abcam).

4.3. Renal Pathological Assessments and Immunostaining

Tissue sections were stained with hematoxylin and eosin (HE) using standard protocols. TUNEL staining was performed with an ApopTag kit (Millipore, Billerica, MA, USA) based on the manufacturer's instructions. The antibodies for immunohistochemistry used in this study were those against Kim-1 (ab78494, Abcam), 4-hydroxynonenal (4-HNE, ab46545, Abcam), neutrophil gelatinase-associated lipocalin (NGAL, ab63929, Abcam), Ly-6B (NBP2-13077), NFκB p65 (sc-372, Santa Cruz, CA, USA), and MAC387 (ab22506, Abcam). Sections were treated with the Envision+ DAB kit (Dako, Basel, Switzerland) according to the manufacturer's instructions.

4.4. Cell Culture and Migration Assay

J774 cells were grown in Dulbecco's modified Eagle's medium and RAW264.7 macrophages were maintained in RPMI 1640 medium. Both cell culture media were supplemented with 10% FCS, 100 U/mL penicillin, and 100 mg/mL streptomycin. Cells were cultured at 37 °C in a humidified atmosphere with 5% CO_2.

For LPS treatment, J774 or RAW cells were treated with 100 ng/mL LPS with or without co-incubation of 20 μM Farnesiferol B for 2 h. Afterwards, RNA and protein were extracted for further analysis. For the migration assay, cells were seeded in 3-μm pore polycarbonate membrane inserts (Costar Corning, Darmstadt, Germany) on 12-well plates and treated with 100 ng/mL LPS (L3254, Sigma, St. Louis, MO, USA) or 20 μM Farnesiferol for 2 h at 37 °C. The inserts were washed, fixed, and stained with crystal violet for analysis.

4.5. NF-κB DNA Binding Assay

The assay was performed with a NF-κB p65 Transcription Factor Assay kit (ab133112, Abcam). Briefly, nuclear extracts from cells were incubated with a double stranded DNA sequence containing the NF-κB response element overnight. After washing, an NF-κB antibody was added and incubated for 1 h. Then an HRP-conjugated secondary antibody was added for 1 h and washed twice. After incubation with developing solution for 30 min, stop solution was added and the results were analyzed with a microplate reader (Glomax, Promega, Madison, WI, USA).

4.6. Isolation of RNA from Kidney Tissue and Quantitative Real-Time Polymerase Chain Reaction (qRT-PCR)

Total RNA was prepared using Trizol (Invitrogen, Carlsbad, CA, USA). The mRNA was quantified based on absorbance at 260 nm. After DNAse (Promega) treatment, 2 μg total RNA was reverse transcribed using oligo-dT priming and Superscript II (Invitrogen). First-strand complementary DNA was used as the template for real-time polymerase chain reaction analysis with TaqMan master mix and primers (Life Technologies, Carlsbad, CA, USA). Primers used were TNFα (No. Mm00443258-m1), Icam1 (No. Mm00516023_m1), IL-6 (No. Mm00446190_m1), Ccl2 (No. Mm00441242_m1), Ccl3 (No. Mm00441259_g1), Gpx4 (No. Mm00515041_m1), Nrf2 (No. Mm00477784_m1), HO-1 (No. Mm00516005_m1). Transcript levels, determined in two independent complementary DNA preparations, were calculated and expressed relative to levels of RNA for the housekeeping gene beta-actin (No. Mm00607939-s1) or GAPDH (No. Mm99999915-g1).

4.7. Western Blotting

Protein lysates (20 μg protein) from cells nuclear were separated by SDS-PAGE and blotted on polyvinylidene difluoride membranes (Millipore, Burlingtob, MA, USA). The membranes were incubated overnight at 4 °C with the respective primary antibodies and secondary antibodies accordingly. Staining was then developed using the ECL Plus detection system (Amersham Biosciences, Little Chalfont, UK). The antibodies used were anti-p65 (sc-372, Santa Cruz, Recife, Pernambuco) and PARP-1 (AV33754, Sigma-Aldrich).

4.8. Statistics

Data are expressed as means ± SD. For data relating to baseline characteristics and histological analysis, groups were compared by one-way ANOVA followed by Bonferroni's test. Statistical analyses were performed using GraphPad software (GraphPad Software Inc., San Diego, CA, USA).

5. Conclusions

In vivo, the present study clearly demonstrates that Farnesiferol B protects kidney from I/R-induced damage by reducing oxidative stress and inflammation. In vitro, Farnesiferol B ameliorates macrophage migration by activating TGR5.

Author Contributions: All authors (L.Z., X.F., T.G., T.W., Z.W., G.A.K.-U. and Z.G.) were responsible for: acquisition of data, or analysis and interpretation of data, final approval of the version to be published. Additionally, L.Z., X.F., T.W. and Z.G. were responsible for substantial contributions to conception and design and drafting the manuscript. Especially, L.Z., T.G., and Z.G. were responsible for revising the manuscript critically for important intellectual content.

Acknowledgments: We thank Sophia Samodelov for proofreading of the manuscript.

Abbreviations

4-HNE	4-hydroxynonenal
AKI	Acute kidney injury
ERK	Extracellular signal-regulated kinase
GPBAR1	G protein–coupled bile acid receptor 1
H_2O_2	Hydrogen peroxide
Icam	Intercellular adhesion molecule
IL-6	Interleukin-6
i.p.	Intraperitoneally
I/R	Ischemia/reperfusion
IRI	Ischemia/reperfusion injury
Kim1	Kidney injury molecule-1
MDA	Malondialdehyde
NF-κB	Nuclear factor-kappa B
NGAL	Neutrophil gelatinase-associated lipocalin
RIR	Renal ischemia reperfusion
ROS	Reactive oxygen species
TNFα	Tumor necrosis factor alpha

References

1. Bonventre, J.V. Pathophysiology of AKI: Injury and normal and abnormal repair. *Contrib. Nephrol.* **2010**, *165*, 9–17. [PubMed]
2. Saat, T.C.; van den Akker, E.K.; JN, I.J.; Dor, F.J.; de Bruin, R.W. Improving the outcome of kidney transplantation by ameliorating renal ischemia reperfusion injury: Lost in translation? *J. Transl. Med.* **2016**, *14*, 20. [CrossRef] [PubMed]
3. Smith, S.F.; Hosgood, S.A.; Nicholson, M.L. Ischemia-reperfusion injury in renal transplantation: 3 key signaling pathways in tubular epithelial cells. *Kidney Int.* **2019**, *95*, 50–56. [CrossRef] [PubMed]
4. Yang, B.; Lan, S.; Dieude, M.; Sabo-Vatasescu, J.P.; Karakeussian-Rimbaud, A.; Turgeon, J.; Qi, S.; Gunaratnam, L.; Patey, N.; Hebert, M.J. Caspase-3 Is a Pivotal Regulator of Microvascular Rarefaction and Renal Fibrosis after Ischemia-Reperfusion Injury. *J. Am. Soc. Nephrol.* **2018**, *29*, 1900–1916. [CrossRef]

5. Minutoli, L.; Puzzolo, D.; Rinaldi, M.; Irrera, N.; Marini, H.; Arcoraci, V.; Bitto, A.; Crea, G.; Pisani, A.; Squadrito, F.; et al. ROS-Mediated NLRP3 Inflammasome Activation in Brain, Heart, Kidney, and Testis Ischemia/Reperfusion Injury. *Oxid Med. Cell Longev.* **2016**, *2016*, 2183026. [CrossRef]
6. Raup-Konsavage, W.M.; Wang, Y.; Wang, W.W.; Feliers, D.; Ruan, H.; Reeves, W.B. Neutrophil peptidyl arginine deiminase-4 has a pivotal role in ischemia/reperfusion-induced acute kidney injury. *Kidney Int.* **2018**, *93*, 365–374. [CrossRef]
7. Masola, V.; Zaza, G.; Bellin, G.; Dall'Olmo, L.; Granata, S.; Vischini, G.; Secchi, M.F.; Lupo, A.; Gambaro, G.; Onisto, M. Heparanase regulates the M1 polarization of renal macrophages and their crosstalk with renal epithelial tubular cells after ischemia/reperfusion injury. *FASEB J.* **2018**, *32*, 742–756. [CrossRef]
8. Bonventre, J.V.; Weinberg, J.M. Recent advances in the pathophysiology of ischemic acute renal failure. *J. Am. Soc. Nephrol.* **2003**, *14*, 2199–2210. [CrossRef]
9. Ratliff, B.B.; Abdulmahdi, W.; Pawar, R.; Wolin, M.S. Oxidant Mechanisms in Renal Injury and Disease. *Antioxid. Redox Signal.* **2016**, *25*, 119–146. [CrossRef]
10. Mittal, M.; Siddiqui, M.R.; Tran, K.; Reddy, S.P.; Malik, A.B. Reactive oxygen species in inflammation and tissue injury. *Antioxid. Redox Signal.* **2014**, *20*, 1126–1167. [CrossRef]
11. Paller, M.S. Effect of neutrophil depletion on ischemic renal injury in the rat. *J. Lab. Clin. Med.* **1989**, *113*, 379–386. [PubMed]
12. Lever, J.M.; Boddu, R.; George, J.F.; Agarwal, A. Heme Oxygenase-1 in Kidney Health and Disease. *Antioxid. Redox Signal.* **2016**, *25*, 165–183. [CrossRef] [PubMed]
13. Li, C.; Jackson, R.M. Reactive species mechanisms of cellular hypoxia-reoxygenation injury. *Am. J. Physiol. Cell Physiol.* **2002**, *282*, C227–C241. [CrossRef] [PubMed]
14. Abd El-Razek, M.H.; Ohta, S.; Ahmed, A.A.; Hirata, T. Sesquiterpene coumarins from the roots of Ferula assa-foetida. *Phytochemistry* **2001**, *58*, 1289–1295. [CrossRef]
15. Ahmed, A.A.; Hegazy, M.E.; Zellagui, A.; Rhouati, S.; Mohamed, T.A.; Sayed, A.A.; Abdella, M.A.; Ohta, S.; Hirata, T. Ferulsinaic acid, a sesquiterpene coumarin with a rare carbon skeleton from Ferula species. *Phytochemistry* **2007**, *68*, 680–686. [CrossRef]
16. Dastan, D.; Salehi, P.; Reza Gohari, A.; Zimmermann, S.; Kaiser, M.; Hamburger, M.; Reza Khavasi, H.; Ebrahimi, S.N. Disesquiterpene and sesquiterpene coumarins from Ferula pseudalliacea, and determination of their absolute configurations. *Phytochemistry* **2012**, *78*, 170–178. [CrossRef]
17. Kirchweger, B.; Kratz, J.M.; Ladurner, A.; Grienke, U.; Langer, T.; Dirsch, V.M.; Rollinger, J.M. In Silico Workflow for the Discovery of Natural Products Activating the G Protein-Coupled Bile Acid Receptor 1. *Front. Chem.* **2018**, *6*, 242. [CrossRef]
18. Porez, G.; Prawitt, J.; Gross, B.; Staels, B. Bile acid receptors as targets for the treatment of dyslipidemia and cardiovascular disease. *J. Lipid Res.* **2012**, *53*, 1723–1737. [CrossRef]
19. Pols, T.W.; Noriega, L.G.; Nomura, M.; Auwerx, J.; Schoonjans, K. The bile acid membrane receptor TGR5 as an emerging target in metabolism and inflammation. *J. Hepatol.* **2011**, *54*, 1263–1272. [CrossRef]
20. Keitel, V.; Reinehr, R.; Gatsios, P.; Rupprecht, C.; Gorg, B.; Selbach, O.; Haussinger, D.; Kubitz, R. The G-protein coupled bile salt receptor TGR5 is expressed in liver sinusoidal endothelial cells. *Hepatology* **2007**, *45*, 695–704. [CrossRef]
21. Kawamata, Y.; Fujii, R.; Hosoya, M.; Harada, M.; Yoshida, H.; Miwa, M.; Fukusumi, S.; Habata, Y.; Itoh, T.; Shintani, Y.; et al. A G protein-coupled receptor responsive to bile acids. *J. Biol. Chem.* **2003**, *278*, 9435–9440. [CrossRef] [PubMed]
22. Keitel, V.; Donner, M.; Winandy, S.; Kubitz, R.; Haussinger, D. Expression and function of the bile acid receptor TGR5 in Kupffer cells. *Biochem. Biophys. Res. Commun.* **2008**, *372*, 78–84. [CrossRef] [PubMed]
23. Wang, X.X.; Edelstein, M.H.; Gafter, U.; Qiu, L.; Luo, Y.; Dobrinskikh, E.; Lucia, S.; Adorini, L.; D'Agati, V.D.; Levi, J.; et al. G Protein-Coupled Bile Acid Receptor TGR5 Activation Inhibits Kidney Disease in Obesity and Diabetes. *J. Am. Soc. Nephrol.* **2016**, *27*, 1362–1378. [CrossRef] [PubMed]
24. Su, J.; Zhang, Q.; Qi, H.; Wu, L.; Li, Y.; Yu, D.; Huang, W.; Chen, W.D.; Wang, Y.D. The G-protein-coupled bile acid receptor Gpbar1 (TGR5) protects against renal inflammation and renal cancer cell proliferation and migration through antagonizing NF-kappaB and STAT3 signaling pathways. *Oncotarget* **2017**, *8*, 54378–54387. [CrossRef]
25. Gai, Z.; Chu, L.; Xu, Z.; Song, X.; Sun, D.; Kullak-Ublick, G.A. Farnesoid X receptor activation protects the kidney from ischemia-reperfusion damage. *Sci. Rep.* **2017**, *7*, 9815. [CrossRef]
26. Dixon, S.J.; Stockwell, B.R. The role of iron and reactive oxygen species in cell death. *Nat. Chem. Biol.* **2014**, *10*, 9–17. [CrossRef]

27. Scindia, Y.; Dey, P.; Thirunagari, A.; Liping, H.; Rosin, D.L.; Floris, M.; Okusa, M.D.; Swaminathan, S. Hepcidin Mitigates Renal Ischemia-Reperfusion Injury by Modulating Systemic Iron Homeostasis. *J. Am. Soc. Nephrol.* **2015**, *26*, 2800–2814. [CrossRef]
28. Perino, A.; Pols, T.W.; Nomura, M.; Stein, S.; Pellicciari, R.; Schoonjans, K. TGR5 reduces macrophage migration through mTOR-induced C/EBPbeta differential translation. *J. Clin. Investig.* **2014**, *124*, 5424–5436. [CrossRef]
29. Pols, T.W.; Nomura, M.; Harach, T.; Lo Sasso, G.; Oosterveer, M.H.; Thomas, C.; Rizzo, G.; Gioiello, A.; Adorini, L.; Pellicciari, R.; et al. TGR5 activation inhibits atherosclerosis by reducing macrophage inflammation and lipid loading. *Cell Metab.* **2011**, *14*, 747–757. [CrossRef]
30. Miyazaki-Anzai, S.; Masuda, M.; Levi, M.; Keenan, A.L.; Miyazaki, M. Dual activation of the bile acid nuclear receptor FXR and G-protein-coupled receptor TGR5 protects mice against atherosclerosis. *PLoS ONE* **2014**, *9*, e108270. [CrossRef]
31. Verma, S.K.; Molitoris, B.A. Renal endothelial injury and microvascular dysfunction in acute kidney injury. *Semin. Nephrol.* **2015**, *35*, 96–107. [CrossRef] [PubMed]
32. Liano, F.; Pascual, J. Epidemiology of acute renal failure: A prospective, multicenter, community-based study. Madrid Acute Renal Failure Study Group. *Kidney Int.* **1996**, *50*, 811–818. [CrossRef] [PubMed]
33. Martin-Sanchez, D.; Fontecha-Barriuso, M.; Carrasco, S.; Sanchez-Nino, M.D.; Massenhausen, A.V.; Linkermann, A.; Cannata-Ortiz, P.; Ruiz-Ortega, M.; Egido, J.; Ortiz, A.; et al. TWEAK and RIPK1 mediate a second wave of cell death during AKI. *Proc. Natl. Acad. Sci. USA* **2018**, *115*, 4182–4187. [CrossRef]
34. Linkermann, A.; Stockwell, B.R.; Krautwald, S.; Anders, H.J. Regulated cell death and inflammation: An auto-amplification loop causes organ failure. *Nat. Rev. Immunol.* **2014**, *14*, 759–767. [CrossRef]
35. Devarajan, P. Neutrophil gelatinase-associated lipocalin (NGAL): A new marker of kidney disease. *Scand. J. Clin. Lab. Invest.* **2008**, *68* (Suppl. 241), 89–94. [CrossRef]
36. Nevo, A.; Armaly, Z.; Abd El Kadir, A.; Douvdevani, A.; Tovbin, D. Elevated Neutrophil Gelatinase Lipocalin Levels Are Associated with Increased Oxidative Stress in Hemodialysis Patients. *J. Clin. Med. Res.* **2018**, *10*, 461–465. [CrossRef]
37. Ibrahim, Z.S.; Alkafafy, M.E.; Ahmed, M.M.; Soliman, M.M. Renoprotective effect of curcumin against the combined oxidative stress of diabetes and nicotine in rats. *Mol. Med. Rep.* **2016**, *13*, 3017–3026. [CrossRef]
38. Sun, Q.; Meng, Q.T.; Jiang, Y.; Liu, H.M.; Lei, S.Q.; Su, W.T.; Duan, W.N.; Wu, Y.; Xia, Z.Y.; Xia, Z.Y. Protective effect of ginsenoside Rb1 against intestinal ischemia-reperfusion induced acute renal injury in mice. *PLoS ONE* **2013**, *8*, e80859. [CrossRef]
39. Shalaby, R.H.; Rashed, L.A.; Ismaail, A.E.; Madkour, N.K.; Elwakeel, S.H. Hematopoietic stem cells derived from human umbilical cord ameliorate cisplatin-induced acute renal failure in rats. *Am. J. Stem. Cells* **2014**, *3*, 83–96.
40. Wang, X.X.; Wang, D.; Luo, Y.; Myakala, K.; Dobrinskikh, E.; Rosenberg, A.Z.; Levi, J.; Kopp, J.B.; Field, A.; Hill, A.; et al. FXR/TGR5 Dual Agonist Prevents Progression of Nephropathy in Diabetes and Obesity. *J. Am. Soc. Nephrol.* **2018**, *29*, 118–137. [CrossRef]
41. Gioiello, A.; Rosatelli, E.; Nuti, R.; Macchiarulo, A.; Pellicciari, R. Patented TGR5 modulators: A review (2006–present). *Expert Opin. Pat.* **2012**, *22*, 1399–1414. [CrossRef] [PubMed]
42. Zhang, R.; He, G.; Wang, Y.; Wang, J.; Chen, W.; Xu, Y. The effect of different treatments of lymph after intestinal ischemia-reperfusion in rats on macrophages in vitro. *PLoS ONE* **2019**, *14*, e0211195. [CrossRef] [PubMed]
43. Harach, T.; Pols, T.W.; Nomura, M.; Maida, A.; Watanabe, M.; Auwerx, J.; Schoonjans, K. TGR5 potentiates GLP-1 secretion in response to anionic exchange resins. *Sci. Rep.* **2012**, *2*, 430. [CrossRef] [PubMed]
44. Kida, T.; Tsubosaka, Y.; Hori, M.; Ozaki, H.; Murata, T. Bile acid receptor TGR5 agonism induces NO production and reduces monocyte adhesion in vascular endothelial cells. *Arter. Thromb. Vasc. Biol.* **2013**, *33*, 1663–1669. [CrossRef] [PubMed]
45. Masyuk, A.I.; Huang, B.Q.; Radtke, B.N.; Gajdos, G.B.; Splinter, P.L.; Masyuk, T.V.; Gradilone, S.A.; LaRusso, N.F. Ciliary subcellular localization of TGR5 determines the cholangiocyte functional response to bile acid signaling. *Am. J. Physiol. Gastrointest. Liver Physiol.* **2013**, *304*, G1013–G1024. [CrossRef]
46. Cao, Q.; Harris, D.C.; Wang, Y. Macrophages in kidney injury, inflammation, and fibrosis. *Physiology* **2015**, *30*, 183–194. [CrossRef]
47. Marko, L.; Vigolo, E.; Hinze, C.; Park, J.K.; Roel, G.; Balogh, A.; Choi, M.; Wubken, A.; Cording, J.; Blasig, I.E.; et al. Tubular Epithelial NF-kappaB Activity Regulates Ischemic AKI. *J. Am. Soc. Nephrol.* **2016**

27, 2658–2669. [CrossRef]

48. Sattar, Z.; Iranshahi, M. Phytochemistry and pharmacology of Ferula persica Boiss.: A review. *Iran. J. Basic Med. Sci.* **2017**, *20*, 1–8.
49. Behnam Rassouli, F.; Matin, M.M.; Iranshahi, M.; Bahrami, A.R.; Neshati, V.; Mollazadeh, S.; Neshati, Z. Mogoltacin enhances vincristine cytotoxicity in human transitional cell carcinoma (TCC) cell line. *Phytomedicine* **2009**, *16*, 181–187. [CrossRef]
50. Kasaian, J.; Mosaffa, F.; Behravan, J.; Masullo, M.; Piacente, S.; Ghandadi, M.; Iranshahi, M. Reversal of P-glycoprotein-mediated multidrug resistance in MCF-7/Adr cancer cells by sesquiterpene coumarins. *Fitoterapia* **2015**, *103*, 149–154. [CrossRef]
51. Motai, T.; Daikonya, A.; Kitanaka, S. Sesquiterpene coumarins from Ferula fukanensis and their pro-inflammatory cytokine gene expression inhibitory effects. *Chem. Pharm. Bull.* **2013**, *61*, 618–623. [CrossRef] [PubMed]
52. Motai, T.; Kitanaka, S. Sesquiterpene coumarins from Ferula fukanensis and nitric oxide production inhibitory effects. *Chem. Pharm. Bull.* **2004**, *52*, 1215–1518. [CrossRef] [PubMed]
53. Xing, Y.; Li, N.; Zhou, D.; Chen, G.; Jiao, K.; Wang, W.; Si, Y.; Hou, Y. Sesquiterpene Coumarins from Ferula sinkiangensis Act as Neuroinflammation Inhibitors. *Planta Med.* **2017**, *83*, 135–142. [CrossRef]

Permissions

All chapters in this book were first published by MDPI; hereby published with permission under the Creative Commons Attribution License or equivalent. Every chapter published in this book has been scrutinized by our experts. Their significance has been extensively debated. The topics covered herein carry significant findings which will fuel the growth of the discipline. They may even be implemented as practical applications or may be referred to as a beginning point for another development.

The contributors of this book come from diverse backgrounds, making this book a truly international effort. This book will bring forth new frontiers with its revolutionizing research information and detailed analysis of the nascent developments around the world.

We would like to thank all the contributing authors for lending their expertise to make the book truly unique. They have played a crucial role in the development of this book. Without their invaluable contributions this book wouldn't have been possible. They have made vital efforts to compile up to date information on the varied aspects of this subject to make this book a valuable addition to the collection of many professionals and students.

This book was conceptualized with the vision of imparting up-to-date information and advanced data in this field. To ensure the same, a matchless editorial board was set up. Every individual on the board went through rigorous rounds of assessment to prove their worth. After which they invested a large part of their time researching and compiling the most relevant data for our readers.

The editorial board has been involved in producing this book since its inception. They have spent rigorous hours researching and exploring the diverse topics which have resulted in the successful publishing of this book. They have passed on their knowledge of decades through this book. To expedite this challenging task, the publisher supported the team at every step. A small team of assistant editors was also appointed to further simplify the editing procedure and attain best results for the readers.

Apart from the editorial board, the designing team has also invested a significant amount of their time in understanding the subject and creating the most relevant covers. They scrutinized every image to scout for the most suitable representation of the subject and create an appropriate cover for the book.

The publishing team has been an ardent support to the editorial, designing and production team. Their endless efforts to recruit the best for this project, has resulted in the accomplishment of this book. They are a veteran in the field of academics and their pool of knowledge is as vast as their experience in printing. Their expertise and guidance has proved useful at every step. Their uncompromising quality standards have made this book an exceptional effort. Their encouragement from time to time has been an inspiration for everyone.

The publisher and the editorial board hope that this book will prove to be a valuable piece of knowledge for researchers, students, practitioners and scholars across the globe.

List of Contributors

Jong Han Lee
College of Pharmacy, Gachon University, Incheon 21936, Korea
Lee Gil Ya Cancer and Diabetes Institute, Gachon University, Incheon 21999, Korea

Donghee Kim
Lee Gil Ya Cancer and Diabetes Institute, Gachon University, Incheon 21999, Korea

Yoon Sin Oh
Department of Food and Nutrition, Eulji University, Seongnam 13135, Korea

Hee-Sook Jun
College of Pharmacy, Gachon University, Incheon 21936, Korea
Lee Gil Ya Cancer and Diabetes Institute, Gachon University, Incheon 21999, Korea
Gachon University Gil Medical Center, Gachon Medical and Convergence Institute, Incheon 21565, Korea

Patrick C. Baer, Benjamin Koch, Janina Freitag and Helmut Geiger
Division of Nephrology, Department of Internal Medicine III, University Hospital, Goethe-University, 60596 Frankfurt/M., Germany

Ralf Schubert
Division of Allergology, Pneumology and Cystic Fibrosis, Department for Children and Adolescents, University Hospital, Goethe-University, 60596 Frankfurt/M., Germany

Chia-Jung Chang and Akiyoshi Taniguchi
Cellular Functional Nanobiomaterials Group, Research Center for Functional Materials, National Institute for Materials Science, 1-1 Namiki, Tsukuba, Ibaraki 305-0044, Japan
Graduate School of Advanced Science and Engineering,Waseda University, 3-4-1 Okubo, Shinjuku-ku, Tokyo 169-8555, Japan

Pi-Chao Wang
Graduate School of Life and Environmental Sciences, University of Tsukuba, 1-1-1 Tennoudai, Tsukuba, Ibaraki 305-8572, Japan

Tzou-Chi Huang
Department of Biological Science and Technology, National Pingtung University of Science and Technology, Neipu, Pingtung 912-01, Taiwan

Michael Ignarski and Rashidul Islam
Department II of Internal Medicine and Center for Molecular Medicine, University of Cologne, Faculty of Medicine and University Hospital Cologne, 50931 Cologne, Germany
Cologne Excellence Cluster on Cellular Stress Responses in Aging-Associated Diseases, University of Cologne, Faculty of Medicine and University Hospital Cologne, 50931 Cologne, Germany

Roman-Ulrich Müller
Department II of Internal Medicine and Center for Molecular Medicine, University of Cologne, Faculty of Medicine and University Hospital Cologne, 50931 Cologne, Germany
Cologne Excellence Cluster on Cellular Stress Responses in Aging-Associated Diseases, University of Cologne, Faculty of Medicine and University Hospital Cologne, 50931 Cologne, Germany
Systems Biology of Ageing Cologne, University of Cologne, 50931 Cologne, Germany

Keiichiro Matoba, Yusuke Takeda, Yosuke Nagai and Rimei Nishimura
Division of Diabetes, Metabolism, and Endocrinology, Department of Internal Medicine, The Jikei University School of Medicine, Tokyo 105-8461, Japan

Daiji Kawanami
Department of Endocrinology and Diabetes Mellitus, Fukuoka University School of Medicine, Fukuoka 814-0180, Japan

Kazunori Utsunomiya
Center for Preventive Medicine, The Jikei University School of Medicine, Tokyo 105-8461, Japan

Minnie M. Sarwal and Joshua Y. C. Yang Department of Surgery, University of California San Francisco, San Francisco, CA 94143, USA
KIT Bio, 665 3rd St, Suite 280, San Francisco, CA 94107, USA

Reuben D. Sarwal
Department of Surgery, University of California San Francisco, San Francisco, CA 94143, USA

Fernando C. Fervenza
Division of Nephrology and Hypertension, Mayo Clinic, Rochester, MN 55905, USA

Richard A. Lafayette
Division of Nephrology and Hypertension, Stanford University, Stanford, CA 94305, USA

Yu Mizuno, Takeshi Yamamotoya, Yusuke Nakatsu, Koji Ueda, Tomoichiro Asano and Masa-Ki Inoue
Department of Medical Science, Graduate School of Medicine, University of Hiroshima, 1-2-3 Kasumi, Minami-ku, Hiroshima City, Hiroshima 734-8551, Japan

Yasuka Matsunaga
Department of Medical Science, Graduate School of Medicine, University of Hiroshima, 1-2-3 Kasumi, Minami-ku, Hiroshima City, Hiroshima 734-8551, Japan
Center for Translational Research in Infection & Inflammation, School of Medicine, Tulane University, 6823 St. Charles Avenue, New Orleans, LA 70118, USA

Hideyuki Sakoda
Division of Neurology, Respirology, Endocrinology, and Metabolism, Department of Internal Medicine, Faculty of Medicine, University of Miyazaki, 5200 Kihara, Kiyotake, Miyazaki 889-1692, Japan

Midori Fujishiro
Division of Diabetes and Metabolic Diseases, Nihon University School of Medicine, Itabashi, Tokyo 173-8610, Japan

Hiraku Ono
Department of Clinical Cell Biology, Graduate School of Medicine, Chiba University, 1-8-1 Inohana, Chuo-ku, Chiba City, Chiba 260-8670, Japan

Takako Kikuchi
Division of Diabetes and Metabolism, The Institute for Adult Diseases, Asahi Life Foundation, 2-2-6, Nihonbashi Bakurocho, Chuo-ku, Tokyo 103-0002, Japan

Masahiro Takahashi and Akifumi Kushiyama
Department of Pharmacotherapy, Meiji Pharmaceutical University, 2-522-1 Noshio, Kiyose City, Tokyo 204-8588, Japan

Kenichi Morii, Kensuke Sasaki and Takao Masaki
Department of Nephrology, Hiroshima University Hospital, 1-2-3 Kasumi, Minami-ku, Hiroshima City, Hiroshima 734-8551, Japan

Po-KuanWu
School of Medicine, College of Medicine, Taipei Medical University, Taipei 11042, Taiwan

Shu-Ching Yeh
Division of Nephrology, Department of Internal Medicine, Taipei Medical University Hospital, Taipei 11042, Taiwan

Shan-Jen Li
Department of Emergency Medicine, Taipei Medical University Hospital, Taipei 11042, Taiwan

Yi-No Kang
Evidence-Based Medicine Center,Wan Fang Hospital, Taipei Medical University, Taipei 11696, Taiwan

Christelle Cauffiez
EA 4483-IMPECS-IMPact of Environmental ChemicalS on Human Health, Univ. Lille, 59045 Lille CEDEX, France

Cynthia Van der Hauwaert
EA 4483-IMPECS-IMPact of Environmental ChemicalS on Human Health, Univ. Lille, 59045 Lille CEDEX, France
Département de la Recherche en Santé, CHU Lille, 59037 Lille, France

François Glowacki
EA 4483-IMPECS-IMPact of Environmental ChemicalS on Human Health, Univ. Lille, 59045 Lille CEDEX, France
Service de Néphrologie, CHU Lille, 59037 Lille, France

Nicolas Pottier
EA 4483-IMPECS-IMPact of Environmental ChemicalS on Human Health, Univ. Lille, 59045 Lille CEDEX, France
Service de Toxicologie et Génopathies, CHU Lille, 59037 Lille, France

Giovanna Priante, Lisa Gianesello, Monica Ceol, Dorella Del Prete and Franca Anglani
Kidney Histomorphology and Molecular Biology Laboratory, Clinical Nephrology, Department of Medicine - DIMED, University of Padua, via Giustiniani 2, 35128 Padova, Italy

Lena Schiffer
Nephrology, Hannover Medical School, 30625 Hannover, Germany
Pediatric Nephrology, Hannover Medical School, 30625 Hannover, Germany

Flavia Wiehler, Wilfried Gwinner, Robert Greite, Kirill Kreimann, Anja Thorenz, Beina Teng, Song Rong, Sibylle von Vietinghoff, Hermann Haller and Faikah Gueler
Nephrology, Hannover Medical School, 30625 Hannover, Germany

Lars Pape and Christian Lerch
Pediatric Nephrology, Hannover Medical School, 30625 Hannover, Germany

Jan Hinrich Bräsen
Pathology, Hannover Medical School, 30625 Hannover, Germany

Katja Derlin
Radiology, Hannover Medical School, 30625 Hannover, Germany

Michael Mengel
Laboratory Medicine & Pathology, University of Alberta, Edmonton, AB T6G 2R3, Canada

Mario Schiffer
Nephrology, Hannover Medical School, 30625 Hannover, Germany
Nephrology and Hypertension, University Hospital Erlangen, 91054 Erlangen, Gerrmany

Alexander Mocker, Carlos Menendez-Castro, JoachimWoelfle, Andrea Hartner and Fabian B. Fahlbusch
Department of Pediatrics and Adolescent Medicine, University Hospital of Erlangen, 91054 Erlangen, Germany

Karl F. Hilgers, Nada Cordasic and Rainer Wachtveitl
Department of Nephrology and Hypertension, University Hospital of Erlangen, 91054 Erlangen, Germany

Nadezda V. Andrianova
Faculty of Bioengineering and Bioinformatics, Lomonosov Moscow State University, 119992 Moscow, Russia
A.N. Belozersky Institute of Physico-Chemical Biology, Lomonosov Moscow State University, 119992 Moscow, Russia

Marina I. Buyan
Faculty of Bioengineering and Bioinformatics, Lomonosov Moscow State University, 119992 Moscow, Russia

Ljubava D. Zorova, Irina B. Pevzner, Vasily A. Popkov, Valentina A. Babenko, Denis N. Silachev and Dmitry B. Zorov
A.N. Belozersky Institute of Physico-Chemical Biology, Lomonosov Moscow State University, 119992 Moscow, Russia
V.I. Kulakov National Medical Research Center of Obstetrics, Gynecology and Perinatology, 117997 Moscow, Russia

Egor Y. Plotnikov
A.N. Belozersky Institute of Physico-Chemical Biology, Lomonosov Moscow State University, 119992 Moscow, Russia
V.I. Kulakov National Medical Research Center of Obstetrics, Gynecology and Perinatology, 117997 Moscow, Russia
Sechenov First Moscow State Medical University, Institute of Molecular Medicine, 119991 Moscow, Russia

Wen-Shin Chang, Chia-Wen Tsai and Te-Chun Shen
Terry Fox Cancer Research Laboratory, Translational Medicine Research Center, China Medical University Hospital, Taichung 40447, Taiwan

Wei-Lan Yeh
Institute of New Drug Development, China Medical University, Taichung 40402, Taiwan

Chien-Chih Yu and Hui-Yi Lin
School of Pharmacy, China Medical University, Taichung 40402, Taiwan

Hsi-ChinWu
Terry Fox Cancer Research Laboratory, Translational Medicine Research Center, China Medical University Hospital, Taichung 40447, Taiwan
School of Medicine, China Medical University, Taichung 40402, Taiwan

Da-Tian Bau
Terry Fox Cancer Research Laboratory, Translational Medicine Research Center, China Medical University Hospital, Taichung 40447, Taiwan
Graduate Institute of Biomedical Sciences, China Medical University, Taichung 40402, Taiwan
Department of Bioinformatics and Medical Engineering, Asia University, Taichung 41354, Taiwan

Lu Zhang and Zhibo Gai
College of Traditional Chinese Medicine; Shandong Co-Innovation Center of TCM Formula; Institute for Literature and Culture of Chinese Medicine; Key Laboratory of Traditional Chinese Medicine for Classical Theory, Ministry of Education, Shandong University of Traditional Chinese Medicine, Jinan 250355, China
Department of Clinical Pharmacology and Toxicology, University Hospital Zurich, University of Zurich, 8006 Zurich, Switzerland

Xianjun Fu, Ting Gui, Tianqi Wang and Zhenguo Wang
College of Traditional Chinese Medicine; Shandong Co-Innovation Center of TCM Formula; Institute for Literature and Culture of Chinese Medicine; Key Laboratory of Traditional Chinese Medicine for Classical Theory, Ministry of Education, Shandong University of Traditional Chinese Medicine, Jinan 250355, China

Gerd A. Kullak-Ublick
Department of Clinical Pharmacology and Toxicology, University Hospital Zurich, University of Zurich, 8006 Zurich, Switzerland
Mechanistic Safety, CMO & Patient Safety, Global Drug Development, Novartis Pharma, 4056 Basel, Switzerland

Index

L

M

N

O

P

R

S

T

X

www.ingramcontent.com/pod-product-compliance
Lightning Source LLC
LaVergne TN
LVHW081036210926
848485LV00004B/1033